W9-AVF-257

Breed Predispositions to Disease in Dogs and Cats

Breed Predispositions to Disease in Dogs and Cats

Alex Gough
MA VetMB CertSAM MRCVS
&
Alison Thomas
BVSc CertSAM MRCVS

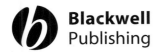

© 2004 by Blackwell Publishing Ltd

Editorial offices:
Blackwell Publishing Ltd, 9600 Garsington Road, Oxford OX4 2DQ, UK
Tel: +44 (0) 1865 776868
Blackwell Publishing Professional, 2121 State Avenue, Ames, Iowa, 50014-8300, USA
Tel: +1 515 292 0140
Blackwell Publishing Asia Pty Ltd, 550 Swanston Street, Carlton, Victoria 3053, Australia
Tel: +61 (0)3 8359 1011

The right of the Author to be identified as the Author of this Work has been asserted in accordance with the UK Copyright, Designs, and Patents Act 1988.

All rights reserved. No part of this publication may be reproduced, stored in a retrieval system, or transmitted, in any form or by any means, electronic, mechanical, photocopying, recording or otherwise, except as permitted by the UK Copyright, Designs, and Patents Act 1988, without the prior permission of the publisher.

First published 2004 by Blackwell Publishing Ltd

7   2008

ISBN: 978-1-4051-0748-8

Library of Congress Cataloging-in-Publication Data
Gough, Alex.
   Breed predispositions to disease in dogs and cats / by Alex Gough & Alison Thomas.
      p. cm.
   ISBN 1-4051-0748-0 (pbk. : alk. paper)
   1. Dogs—Diseases. 2. Cats—Diseases.   I. Thomas, Alison, 1964–   II. Title.

   SF991 .G67 2004
   636.7'0896—dc22

                                                                         2003022236

A catalogue record for this title is available from the British Library

Set in 9/11pt Ehrhardt
by Graphicraft Limited, Hong Kong
Printed and bound by Sheridan Books, Inc.
United States of America

The publisher's policy is to use permanent paper from mills that operate a sustainable forestry policy, and which has been manufactured from pulp processed using acid-free and elementary chlorine-free practices. Furthermore, the publisher ensures that the text paper and cover board used have met acceptable environmental accreditation standards.

For further information on
Blackwell Publishing, visit our website:
www.blackwellpublishing.com

Contents

Contents

Acknowledgements

The authors wish to thank the following people for their helpful comments in the writing of this book: Mark Bossley BVM&S CertVOphthal MRCVS, Malcolm Cobb MA VetMB PhD DVC MRCVS, Clive Elwood MA VetMB MSc DipACVIM DipECVIM PhD CertSAC MRCVS, Heidi Featherstone BVetMed, DVOphthal MRCVS, Nick Jeffery BVSc PhD CertSAO DSAS DECVS DECVN FRCVS and Retha Queenan BVSc CertVOphthal MRCVS. Any errors remain the responsibility of the authors themselves.

Introduction

It is well known that most breeds of dogs and cats have diseases and disorders to which they are particularly prone. Breed predispositions are often listed under specific disease conditions in the published literature and textbooks. However, it is hard to find a source of information that lists these conditions by breed.

This book aims to correct this deficiency. It is intended to be of use to prospective or current pet owners and breeders who wish to be fully informed of the diseases to which their chosen or favourite breeds may be prone. Its main utility, though, will be to veterinary surgeons, and it is at this group of people that the book is aimed. Much of the language used is of necessity technical, and non-veterinary readers wishing to use this book are urged to contact their vets if they have any queries regarding the information. Breeders wishing to institute programmes to select against inherited diseases should also speak to their vet or a suitably qualified professional.

For veterinary surgeons, this book should be useful in several ways. Most importantly, it should assist in producing and prioritising a list of differential diagnoses after a history has been taken and physical examination made, and allow the selection of the most appropriate tests to achieve a diagnosis. It will also be important in advising clients wishing to buy new pets, and owners of existing pets can be warned of preventative measures to reduce the risk of diseases, or to monitor closely for the onset of clinical signs to allow early treatment to be instituted.

For the purposes of this book, a breed predisposition has been defined as an increased risk for a condition in a breed. This does not mean that breed predispositions are necessarily inherited diseases (although many are). For example, the uses to which a breed is put can influence the conditions to which it is prone. A Foxhound may be prediposed to fox bites, but this doesn't mean that it inherits them!

The data in this book have been categorised by body systems affected as far as possible, although some diseases span more than one category. The category 'physiological conditions' is intended to describe those abnormalities specific to a breed which are non-pathological, or are accepted as part of a breed standard.

Caution should be exercised when using the information in this book. Many diseases which do not have breed predispositions are not in the text, and will also need to be included in differential diagnosis lists. Also, some predispositions are weak, with only a slightly increased risk in the breed. Where there are data on the relative risk (the ratio of the risk of the disease occurring in the breed to the risk of the disease occurring in the general population), these have been included. However, the existence of a breed predisposition should not lead the clinician to exclude other disease possibilities, nor should the absence of a predisposition in a breed be taken to mean that the breed cannot contract the disease.

It may be noted that some breeds are absent from this book – this is because the authors have not found any data on any predispositions in these breeds.

Some rare diseases, which have only been reported in one or a limited number of individuals, have been included. These cases do not represent a true breed predisposition, however were considered relevant breed-related information. Where an entry is based on a single report, this is indicated in the text.

The evidence for the data in this book is taken from published literature and the major veterinary textbooks. There are many anecdotal reports of breed predispositions, but, unless the authors have found published evidence of these, they have been omitted.

A final limitation of the data presented in this book is that of geographical variation. Some populations may exhibit predispositions to diseases that others do not. Where possible this has been indicated in the text.

Basic Genetics

All mammalian life is based on the genetic code stored within the nucleus of a cell. This genetic code is stored in a long molecule called *deoxyribonucleic acid* (DNA). DNA is composed of four units called bases, and these bases attract each other, *guanine* to *cytosine* and *adenine* to *thymine*. When attached together, they form the famous *double helix*. The order in which these bases (or base pairs, since they always match together) occur along the molecule provides the code for the synthesis of proteins. Proteins are then responsible for most of the functions of the body, from the structure of tissues, to the biological catalysts called enzymes, to the hormones which regulate the body's metabolic processes.

A length of DNA which codes for a particular protein is called a *gene*. Long strings of genes, interspersed with areas of DNA which do not code for proteins, make up *chromosomes*. Each nucleus of a mammalian cell contains a set number of chromosomes, except the sex cells (*gametes*) – sperm and ova. For dogs this number is 78 and for cats it is 38.

When a somatic (body) cell divides, the chromosomes shorten and thicken within the nucleus, so they become visible under a microscope. They then replicate, and one copy of each chromosome separates into a new nucleus before the cell splits. This process is called *mitosis*. However, in the production of the gametes (the process of *meiosis*), the chromosomes line themselves up in the middle of the cell with a companion. This companion is always the same, and two chromosomes that associate together are called *homologous pairs*. These homologous pairs separate, so the gametes have half the number of chromosomes as normal cells. This means that when a sperm and ova combine at fertilisation, the newly-formed cell (the *zygote*) has the correct number of chromosomes.

Homologous pairs code for related genes, but are not identical. The two genes, one on each chromosome, interact in different ways. Sometimes one gene is *dominant* to the other, the less dominant gene being termed *recessive*, and the expression of the gene, i.e. the protein that is produced, will be determined by the dominant gene. In other cases both genes will play a role in the production of the protein, a situation called *co-dominance*.

The exception to the homologous pairs are two chromosomes called the sex chromosomes (all the other chromosomes are called the *autosomes*). These chromosomes determine the sex of an animal. A female's cells are composed of two X chromosomes, a male's of an X and a Y. At meiosis, the ova inherit a single X chromosome from the mother, whereas the sperm inherit either an X or a Y from the father. This has significance for the inheritance of conditions carried on the X chromosome, and means that some inherited diseases can be more prevalent in one sex than another.

Although any one animal will carry only up to two versions of a gene, many more can exist within a population because of mutation and natural selection. These different versions of the gene are called *alleles*.

In conditions and characteristics that are inherited in a simple way, i.e. the conditions are autosomal dominant or recessive, then a system of genetics devised by the monk Mendel (hence Mendelian genetics) can be used to predict the likely offspring of two parents, if the parents' genetic make-up is known. For example, the gene that codes for Labrador coat colours is dominant for black and recessive for brown. If a Labrador has two alleles for black colour (call the allele B) it is described as being BB and hence the coat will be black. If it has one allele for black and one for brown (call the allele b), it will be described as Bb but the coat colour will still be black since this colour is dominant. However, if the dog possesses two alleles for brown (bb), it will be brown. The genetic make-up is called the *genotype*, whereas the physical expression of the genes is called the *phenotype*.

The situation is slightly more complex when looking at matings, and a matrix can be used to aid prediction of offspring types. Take the example of a BB black male crossed with a bb brown female. The BB male will produce sperm each carrying a single B gene, and the female will produce ova each carrying a single b gene. These are then recombined at random to produce offspring. The matrix would therefore look like this:

		Male	
		B	B
Female	b	Bb	Bb
	b	Bb	Bb

This means that all the offspring would be Bb. They all carry the b gene for brown coat, but because this gene is recessive, the coat colour is black. An animal with two alleles the same (e.g. BB) is called a *homozygote* while an animal with two different alleles (e.g. Bb) is called a *heterozygote*. If a black Bb female was then crossed with a black Bb male a different pattern would emerge:

		Male	
		B	b
Female	B	BB	Bb
	b	Bb	bb

On average three of the offspring would be black, one a homozygote BB and two heterozygotes Bb. One would be a homozygote for brown coat colour, and, since this gene is not now being suppressed by the dominant gene, the brown coat colour phenotype is expressed.

In fact, since the fertilisation process is random, a litter of 4 pups may not be born in the exact 1:2:1 ratio, but if this was repeated enough times the proportions of pups of the various colours would be close to this.

Generally, the alleles separate randomly from each other, so just because one condition is expressed in an offspring, it doesn't mean that another shown by its parent will be. However, some alleles that are closely positioned on a chromosome have a tendency to be passed on together. Thus two traits controlled by different genes may often be found together in the same individual, and the presence of one of these traits may act as a marker for the other. This process is known as linkage.

When one allele is not dominant over another co-dominance exists. For example, certain flowers that have alleles for red flowers (R) and white flowers (W) will be coloured red if homozygous for red (RR), white if homozygous for white (WW) but pink if heterozygous (RW).

Some genes, even if dominant, do not always produce a physical effect in the host. For example, the condition polycystic kidney disease in cats is inherited as an autosomal dominant trait, but not all cats with the genes have cysts in the kidneys. This situation is called *incomplete penetrance*. Penetrance is the proportion of individuals with a particular genotype that demonstrate the characteristics normally expected with that genotype.

Some characteristics are carried on the X chromosome, and this can lead to the phenomenon of sex-linkage. For example, there is a condition called X-linked muscular dystrophy, to which Golden Retrievers are predisposed. The allele for muscular dystrophy (call it M) is carried on the X chromosome, as is the allele for a normal dog not suffering from the condition (call it N). M is recessive to N. Therefore, a female carrying a single affected X chromosome (genetic make up $X^M X^N$) would not show the effects of the disease. If this female was mated with a normal male, ($X^N Y$) then the matrix for their offspring would be as follows:

		Male	
		X^N	Y
Female	X^M	$X^M X^N$	$X^M Y$
	X^N	$X^N X^N$	$X^N Y$

All of the females born to this cross will be clinically unaffected by the disease but 50% of the females will be carriers of the disease. These will not show the disease since they have a normal gene on the other X chromosome which suppresses the abnormal, recessive gene. However, the males only possess a single X chromosome, so the 50% of males born $X^M Y$ will show the disease (since they do not possess another X chromosome with a normal gene). The 50% of males born $X^N Y$ will not show the disease and will not carry it.

Because of this process, sex-linked diseases usually affect only males, and males cannot normally be asymptomatic carriers. Females are often carriers but the only way they can express the disease is if their mother was a carrier and their father was affected. This situation is rare in nature, especially for uncommon genes, but can occur in domestic animals due to inbreeding.

Some disease inheritances are more complex still, because more than one gene may determine the expression of a disease, or the interaction of genes and environment can determine the outcome in an individual. An example of this is hip dysplasia in dogs. More than one gene is considered to be responsible, but the dog's nutrition, exercise and other factors can also influence the severity of the disease.

Finally, some diseases are not inherited through the DNA of the nucleus at all, but through the DNA present within the *mitochondria* (which are intracellular organelles responsible for energy production). Mitochondria are entirely inherited from the mother, hence characteristics and diseases caused by mitochondrial DNA can only be passed down from the mother. Although conditions caused by mitochondrial DNA are rare, some canine myopathies are thought to be inherited this way.

In summary, an autosomal dominant trait is transmitted from generation to generation without skipping. Each affected offspring has at least one affected parent, unless the disorder has arisen because of mutation. If the disorder is lethal, then it will be very rare. An autosomal recessive disorder may skip generations. If the two parents are affected then all the offspring are affected. With an X-linked dominant condition, affected males mated to normal females transmit the gene to their daughters, who are all affected, but not their sons. Affected females then pass the condition on to approximately half of their sons and half of their daughters. In the population as a whole, the incidence in females tends to be twice that of males. With an X-linked recessive disorder, the condition may skip generations. The incidence is more common in males. Affected males do not transmit the disease when mated to a normal female, but all female offspring will be carriers. Females showing the disease who are mated with normal males will pass the condition on to all their sons, and all their daughters will be carriers.

Clinical genetics

Genetic diseases are probably more frequently encountered in domestic animals than in most wild populations. The process of domestication involves selecting animals for their most desirable traits from a human point of view. Initially, these traits would have been practical: speed in a horse, fertility and milk production in a cow, herding instincts in a sheepdog and so on. Over time, when animals came to be kept for their companionship and aesthetic appeal, the pressures of selection altered to produce breeds that were poorly adapted to survive in the wild, but fitted in well to the human environment, for example achondroplasia in many dog breeds. As breeding practices were refined and the science of genetics was discovered, inbreeding was used to create breeds that bred true with respect to certain desired characteristics.

Unfortunately, inbreeding reduces the genetic variation within a breed, and tends to accentuate the presence of recessive genes which are often deleterious. Population bottlenecks occur due to overuse of a desirable individual such as a show champion (particularly males which are capable of producing many more offspring than a female). Most of the recognised genetic diseases of the dog are inherited as an autosomal recessive. This may be because of inbreeding, but is also due to the difficulty in identifying and eliminating recessive traits in breeding programmes. The often repeated saying that crossbreed dogs are healthier than pedigrees may have some basis in truth because outbreeding tends to mask the effect of many recessive genes. However, crossbreed dogs can still be predisposed to the diseases of their parent breeds.

It should be noted that inbreeding of itself does not cause genetic disease, and some degree of inbreeding is necessary for the concentration of desirable genes. In fact, some inbred strains of mice and rats are entirely homozygous and yet are healthy. Inbreeding promotes homozygosity, and thus deleterious recessive genes are exposed. However, by exposing these genes it is possible to eliminate them by further selective breeding.

Data are currently sparse regarding the prevalance of disease caused by new mutations, but studies of some diseases suggest this is very rare. In those limited cases studied, the mutation seems to be uniform within a breed. This suggests that a 'founder effect' applies, i.e. a single initial mutation was propagated throughout the breed. In some cases, closely related breeds may have the same mutation causing a disease, for example phosphofructokinase deficiency in English Springers and American Cocker Spaniels, suggesting that a common ancestor was responsible for the original mutation. Some diseases, however, have more than one mutation in the same gene (*allelic heterogeneity*).

When determining whether or not a disease is hereditary, certain typical characteristics increase suspicion of a genetic predisposition. Often the first thing to suggest that a disease is inherited is that the disorder occurs with a higher frequency in a group of related animals than in the general population. This can help distinguish an inherited disease from a breed predisposition. For example, Saint Bernards are predisposed to osteosarcomas, but it was possible this was merely a reflection of their large size: the faster growth rate leading to more mistakes being made in DNA replication, leading to the cancer. However, analysis of pedigrees shows that there is a familial clustering pattern to cases of the disease, which suggests a specific gene or group of genes being responsible. Second, a hereditary defect often involves the same anatomic site in a group of related animals. This is often seen in congenital heart disease in dogs. Third, the disease is often seen to increase in frequency with inbreeding. Fourth, hereditary diseases often have an early onset, and those that do not often have a consistent age of onset.

Genetic diseases usually affect a few individuals within a litter, as opposed to intoxications and infectious diseases which frequently affect them all. Some genetic diseases will cause abortion or resorption, and these are often never diagnosed. Similarly, some genetic disorders will cause a failure to thrive, the 'fading kitten (or puppy) syndrome', and again it can be hard to determine the cause in these cases.

There is an extremely wide range of hereditary diseases, from the relatively benign to the invariably fatal. Diagnosis of a hereditary disease is usually based on history, clinical signs, history of disease in related individuals, test matings and specific tests for diseases.

Test matings are often suggested in order to identify autosomal recessives but it does have problems. With late-onset defects, the results of the mating will be known too late to be useful in selecting which individuals to use for breeding. Test matings can be more useful for early-onset diseases, but the ethics of keeping a known affected animal purely for test purposes, and what to do with affected offspring, can be problematic. Furthermore, the results of test matings may be unreliable. For example, a mating of a suspected carrier (N?) to a known carrier (Nn) which produced six normal puppies would only give an 82.2% certainty that the N? was not a carrier (NN). However, a single abnormal pup would confirm carrier status.

The results of random matings, if performed often enough and with respect to a sufficiently prevalent gene, can provide useful information without the need to maintain a carrier or affected animal, and with less likelihood of breeding unwanted affected individuals. It would require central banks of information and more openness from breeders and breed organisations for this approach to work, however.

Specific tests for diseases include ultrasonography and histopathology for polycystic kidney disease, or von Willebrand factor assay for von Willebrand's disease. Some laboratories will test samples using enzyme and immunological assays to detect disorders, and the results may indicate whether an individual is a homozygote or heterozygote. An example of this is testing for haemophilia B. A defect in an affected protein's size, function or amount allows the identification of carriers of a disease in some cases, although there may be an overlap with normal values. Also, compensatory rises in other proteins, such as a related isoenzyme to pyruvate kinase in pyruvate kinase deficiency, may reduce the accuracy of this sort of test.

In some of the inherited diseases, the molecular defects which cause them have been identified. Those identified on the X chromosome include haemophilia B, severe combined X-linked immunodeficiency and hereditary nephropathy. Those autosomal recessive traits for which the mutation has been identified include copper toxicosis in Bedlington Terriers, progressive retinal atrophy in Irish Setters, von Willebrand's disease in Scottish Terriers and pyruvate kinase deficiency in Basenjis.

Specific DNA tests currently available to identify genetic diseases include linkage-based tests, which look for a marker gene which is physically in close proximity to the gene of interest. An example of a currently-available test using this method is for copper toxicosis in Bedlington Terriers. Mutation-based tests look for a specific mutation causing a disease, but these tests must be used with caution, since there may be more than one type of mutation responsible for a disease, particularly between breeds.

DNA testing shows great promise for the identification and elimination of genetic diseases in dogs and cats. The inherited disorders can be identified before an animal is bred, and affected animals can either be removed from the breeding pool, or, in the case of recessive traits, bred only to normal individuals, in order to preserve desirable characterisics. This allows the genetic diversity of breeds to be retained while inherited disorders are eliminated.

The limitations of DNA testing, such as limited availablity of tests, and utility largely to single gene disorders, mean that there is still a vital role for screening programmes to eliminate inherited disorders. Screening programmes currently in operation in the UK include the British Veterinary Association/Kennel Club programmes for hip and elbow dysplasia and eye diseases, and the Feline Advisory Bureau scheme for polycystic kidney disease in cats. (See under Ocular conditions in Part 3 for an explanation of the BVA/KC/ISDS Eye Schemes.)

PART I
DOGS

AFFENPINSCHER

Ocular conditions
Cataract
- Inheritance suspected

AFGHAN HOUND

Cardiovascular conditions
Dilated cardiomyopathy
- Prevalence of 1.7% in this breed compared to 0.16% in mixed breeds and 0.65% in pure breeds
- Increased prevalence with age
- Approximately twice as common in males as females
- Thought to be familial or genetic

Dermatological conditions
Generalised demodicosis
- Afghans are in the ten breeds at highest statistical risk of this disease in the Cornell, USA population

Testosterone-responsive dermatosis of male animals
- Rare
- Unknown cause
- Seen in castrated males

Nasal depigmentation
- Also known as Dudley nose
- Cause unknown

Skin tumours
- See under Neoplastic conditions

Endocrine diseases
Central diabetes insipidus (CDI)
- One report of CDI, in two sibling Afghan pups under 4 months of age, with a suggested hereditary basis

Hypothyroidism
- Reported in some texts to be at increased risk
- Often middle-aged (2–6 years)

Neoplastic conditions
Tricholemmoma
- Rare
- Affects middle-aged to older dogs

11

Neurological conditions
Afghan myelopathy (causing pelvic limb ataxia)
- Autosomal recessive inheritance suggested
- Age of clinical onset: 6–9 months
- Seen occasionally

Ocular conditions
Medial canthal pocket syndrome
- Breed predisposition due to head shape

Corneal dystrophy
- Breed predisposition
- Stromal lipid dystrophy

Cataract
- Simple autosomal recessive inheritance has been suggested
- Localisation: initially equatorial, later anterior and posterior cortical
- Age of onset: 4–24 months. Rapid progression possible, leading to visual impairment

Generalised progressive retinal atrophy (GPRA)
- Mode of inheritance unknown, but presumed to be recessive
- Clinically evident at 3 years of age

Respiratory conditions
Largyngeal paralysis
- Idiopathic

Chylothorax
- Usually idiopathic

Lung-lobe torsion
- Rare
- May be associated with chylothorax in this breed

AIREDALE TERRIER

Cardiovascular conditions
Dilated cardiomyopathy
- Increased prevalence with age
- Approximately twice as common in males as females
- Thought to be familial or genetic

Dermatological conditions
Generalised demodicosis
- Airedales are in the ten breeds at highest statistical risk of this disease in the Cornell, USA population

Canine follicular dysplasia
- A marked predilection in this breed implies a genetic basis for this group of diseases
- Hair loss begins at 2–4 years of age and occurs mainly on the flank

Seasonal flank alopecia
- Tends to occur in spring or autumn

Scrotal vascular naevus
- More common in older dogs

Grass awn migration
- Common in the summer months

Skin tumours
- See under Neoplastic conditions

Endocrine conditions
Hypothyroidism
- Reported to be at increased risk in some texts
- Often middle-aged (2–6 years)

Gastrointestinal conditions
Pancreatic carcinoma
- Possible breed predisposition
- Seen in older dogs (mean age 10 years)
- Females may be predisposed

Haematological conditions
Von Willebrand's disease
- This breed is susceptible to type I disease
- Possibly inherited as an autosomal recessive trait
- This breed appears not to show clinical signs of disease, even when von Willebrand's factor is low

Musculoskeletal conditions
Spondylosis deformans
- Usually clinically insignificant

Umbilical hernia

Neoplastic conditions
Cutaneous melanoma
- Breed predisposition
- Average age 8–9 years

Cutaneous haemangioma
- Possible breed predisposition
- Average age was 8.7 years in one study

Nasal cavity tumours
- Reported to be at increased risk for nasal carcinoma
- Usually older dogs
- Dogs in urban areas may be at increased risk

Lymphosarcoma (malignant lymphoma)
- Higher incidence noted in this breed
- Most cases are seen in middle-aged dogs (mean 6–7 years)

Pancreatic carcinoma
- See under Gastrointestinal conditions

Neurological conditions
Cerebellar malformation
- Congenital
- Uncommon
- Age of clinical onset: < 3 months

Cerebellar degeneration
- Reported in this breed
- Age of clinical onset: < 3 years

Ocular conditions
Entropion (lower lids)
- Breed predisposition; polygenic inheritance likely
- Usually seen in the first year

Distichiasis
- Breed predisposition

Chronic superficial keratitis (pannus)
- Breed predisposition
- Age of onset: 1–2 years

Corneal dystrophy
- Sex-linked inheritance has been suggested
- Lipid dystrophy affecting the corneal stroma
- Age of onset: 4–12 months; progressive

Generalised progressive retinal atrophy (GPRA)
- Mode of inheritance unknown but presumed to be recessive
- Age of clinical onset: 3 years

Reproductive conditions
XXX syndrome
- Congenital abnormality of chromosomal sex which has been reported in this breed

Vaginal hyperplasia
- Possible breed predisposition

ALASKAN MALAMUTE

Dermatological conditions
Generalised demodicosis
- Malamutes are in the ten breeds at highest statistical risk of this disease in the Cornell, USA population

Follicular dysplasia
- May affect multiple dogs in a litter
- Clipped areas tend not to regrow

Zinc-responsive dermatosis
- Syndrome I affects Malamutes
- Skin lesions develop despite adequate levels of zinc in the diet
- Malamutes have a genetic defect causing zinc malabsorption

Skin tumours
- See under Neoplastic conditions

Endocrine diseases
Hypothyroidism
- Reported in some text to be at increased risk
- Often middle-aged (2–6 years)

Diabetes mellitus
- Possible breed predisposition
- Usual age range 4–14 years, peak incidence 7–9 years
- Old entire females are predisposed

Haematological conditions
Hereditary stomatocytosis
- Causes minimal anaemia

DOGS

Haemophilia B
- Factor IX deficiency
- Also known as Christmas disease
- Inherited as a sex-linked trait
- Less common than haemophilia A

Musculoskeletal conditions
Alaskan Malamute chondrodysplasia
- Causes disproportionate dwarfism
- Haemolytic anaemia usually present
- May be zinc responsive
- Autosomal recessive inheritance with complete penetrance and variable expression

Cartilaginous exostosis

Neoplastic conditions
Sebaceous gland tumours
- Possible breed predisposition to sebaceous epithelioma
- Seen in older dogs (average age 10 years)

Anal sac adenocarcinoma
- Breed predisposition suggested in one survey of 232 cases
- Average age was 10.5 years
- Some surveys suggest a predisposition for females

Neurological conditions
Narcolepsy-cataplexy
- Reported in this breed
- Age of clinical onset: <1 year

Ocular conditions
Refractory corneal ulceration
- Breed predisposition
- Age of onset: 7–9 years

Corneal dystrophy
- Breed predisposition
- Lipid dystrophy
- Age of onset: 2 years

Glaucoma
- Breed predisposition
- Age of onset: 6 years

Cataract
- Inheritance suspected
- Localisation: posterior subcapsular

- Age of onset: 1 year; slowly progressive; complete blindness is rare
- Schedule 3 of the BVA/KC/ISDS Eye Scheme

Hemeralopia (day blindness)
- Autosomal recessive inheritance
- Age of onset: 8 weeks

Generalised progressive retinal atrophy (GPRA)
- Mode of inheritance unknown but presumed to be recessive
- Clinically evident at 4 years of age

Renal and urinary conditions
Familial renal disease (renal dysplasia)
- Reported in 3 sibling pups
- Presented at 4–11 months with renal failure

AMERICAN STAFFORDSHIRE TERRIER

Dermatological conditions
Truncal solar dermatitis
- A combination of factors are required to cause this condition
- Flank and abdomen most severely affected

Skin tumours
- See under Neoplastic conditions

Musculoskeletal conditions
Cranial cruciate ligament rupture
- Common cause of hind-limb lameness
- Neutered individuals may be predisposed
- Young animals may be predisposed in this breed

Neoplastic conditions
Actinic keratosis (solar keratosis)
- Reported to be at increased risk
- Seen more commonly in pale-skinned animals with the opportunity for long periods of intense sun exposure

Cutaneous haemangioma
- Possible breed predisposition
- Average age was 8.7 years in one study

Canine cutaneous histiocytoma
- Possible breed predisposition
- More common in young dogs, 1–2 years of age

Mast cell tumours
- Occur at an average of 8 years of age, and are rarely reported in puppies

Ocular conditions
Cataract
- Inheritance suspected

Generalised progressive retinal atrophy (GPRA)
- Mode of inheritance unknown but presumed to be recessive
- Clinically evident at 1.5 years of age

Persistent hyperplastic primary vitreous (PHPV)
- Congenital defect, inheritance suspected

AMERICAN WATER SPANIEL

Dermatological conditions
Pattern baldness
- Hair loss occurs at about 6 months of age
- Ventral neck, thighs and tail are affected

Adult-onset growth-hormone-responsive dermatosis
- See under Endocrine conditions

Endocrine conditions
Adult-onset growth-hormone-responsive dermatosis
- Breed predisposition
- Males may be predisposed
- Clinical signs seen at 1–5 years

Ocular conditions
Cataract
- Inheritance suspected
- Localisation: anterior sutures
- Age of onset: <1 year

Focal retinal dysplasia (retinal folds)
- Reported in the USA as a minor, non-progressive condition

AUSTRALIAN CATTLE DOG

Ocular conditions
Cataract
- Inheritance suspected

Lens luxation
- Reported in middle-aged dogs in Australia

Generalised progressive retinal atrophy (GPRA)
- Autosomal recessive inheritance has been suggested
- Clinically evident at 2–4 years of age (with a second group seen at 6 years)
- High incidence reported in USA and Australia
- Schedule 1 BVA/KC/ISDS Eye Scheme

Neurological conditions
Congenital deafness
- Signs seen from birth

Renal and urinary conditions
Cystine urolithiasis
- Cystinuria results from an inherited defect in renal tubular transport of cystine and predisposes to cystine urolithiasis
- Higher incidence reported in this breed in some USA surveys
- Average age at diagnosis is 1–8 years
- Males seem predisposed

AUSTRALIAN KELPIE

Ocular conditions
Generalised progressive retinal atrophy (GPRA)
- Mode of inheritance unknown but presumed to be recessive
- Ophthalmoscopic signs visible at 1.5 years, progresses to blindness by 4 years

Neurological conditions
Cerebellar degeneration
- Autosomal recessive inheritance suggested
- Uncommon
- Signs seen at 6–12 weeks

DOGS

AUSTRALIAN SHEPHERD DOG

Cardiovascular conditions
Patent ductus arteriosus
- Common congenital abnormality
- Relative risk 2.0
- Females predisposed
- Mode of inheritance polygenic

Dermatological conditions
Mucocutaneous hypopigmentation
- Nasal form is a common problem in Australian Shepherd Dogs
- May have concurrent seasonal nasal hypopigmentation

Nasal solar dermatitis
- Develops in dogs that are amelanotic

Drug reactions
Ivermectin and milbemycin
- High doses can cause tremors, ataxia, coma and death

Infectious diseases
Coccidiomycosis
- Increased incidence in this breed, possibly due to an increased likelihood of exposure
- Mainly seen in young male dogs
- Geographic distribution: California, Arizona, Texas, New Mexico, Nevada, Utah, Mexico and parts of Central and South America. Not reported in the UK

Musculoskeletal conditions
Polydactyly/syndactyly
- Inherited, possibly as an X-linked gene

Neurological conditions
Congenital deafness
- Signs seen from birth

Ocular conditions
Cataract
- Inheritance suspected
- Schedule 3 of the BVA/KC/ISDS Eye Scheme

Collie eye anomaly (choroidal hypoplasia and sometimes optic nerve colobomas)
- Congenital condition; inheritance suspected
- A low incidence has been reported in this breed

Colobomas
- Congenital, mode of inheritance unknown; not known if related to the same conditions found associated with microphthalmia
- May affect iris, choroid or optic disc
- Schedule 3 of the BVA/KC/ISDS Eye Scheme

Multiple ocular defects
- Autosomal recessive inheritance with incomplete penetrance has been suggested
- Seen in homozygous merles (the result of merle to merle breeding) with predominantly white coats
- Defects may include microphthalmia, microcornea, cataract, persistent pupillary membranes, equatorial staphylomas, colobomas and retinal dysplasia

Renal and urinary conditions
Cystine urolithiasis
- Cystinuria results from an inherited defect in renal tubular transport of cystine and predisposes to cystine urolithiasis
- Higher incidence reported in this breed in some American surveys
- Average age at diagnosis is 1–8 years
- Males seem predisposed

BASENJI

Gastrointestinal conditions
Hypertrophic gastritis
- Possible breed predisposition
- Generally affects older dogs
- Males may be predisposed

Lymphangiectasia (protein-losing enteropathy)
- Breed predisposition

Immunoproliferative enteropathy (of Basenjis)
- Specific disease of Basenjis
- Usually presents before 3 years

Haematological conditions
Pyruvate kinase deficiency
- Affected dogs have abnormal red blood cells with a lifespan of about 20 days
- DNA test available in this breed

Musculoskeletal conditions
Pyruvate kinase deficiency
- Inherited
- Causes intramedullary osteosclerosis

Inguinal hernia

Umbilical hernia

Ocular conditions
Persistent pupillary membranes
- Inherited, mode unclear
- Widespread defect in this breed (40–90% prevalence reported in the USA, similar prevalence in UK and Australia)
- Severity and effect on vision varies
- Schedule 1 of the BVA/KC/ISDS Eye Scheme

Cataract
- Inheritance suspected

Optic nerve coloboma
- Congenital defect, possibly inherited in this breed

Physiological conditions
Pelger-Huet anomaly
- Decreased segmentation of granulocyte nuclei are seen
- Does not appear to be clinically significant

Renal and urinary conditions
Fanconi syndrome
- Familial, with 10–30% Basenjis in the USA affected
- Most dogs present at 1–5 years with polyuria/polydipsia. Cases may progress to acute renal failure or pyelonephritis

Cystine urolithiasis
- Cystinuria results from an inherited defect in renal tubular transport of cystine and predisposes to cystine urolithiasis

- Higher incidence reported in this breed in some American surveys
- Average age at diagnosis is 1–8 years
- Males seem predisposed

Reproductive conditions
Variation in the interoestrus interval
- This breed normally cycles only once per year

BASSET HOUND

Cardiovascular conditions
Ventricular septal defect
- Marked risk in this breed (relative risk >5)
- No sex predilection
- Not known to be inherited in this breed

Pulmonic stenosis
- Third most frequent cause of canine congenital heart disease
- May be polygenic mode of inheritance

Dermatological conditions
Pododermatitis
- Can affect any age or sex
- Males predisposed
- Front feet more commonly affected

Malassezia dermatitis (see figure 1)
- Affects adults of any age or sex
- May be seasonal

Primary seborrhoea
- Probably inherited as an autosomal recessive trait
- Signs first appear at an early age and get worse

Congenital hypotrichosis
- Symmetrical hair loss
- Usually hair loss is apparent at birth and gets worse over the following few weeks

Black hair follicular dysplasia
- Rare
- Early onset
- Familial

DOGS

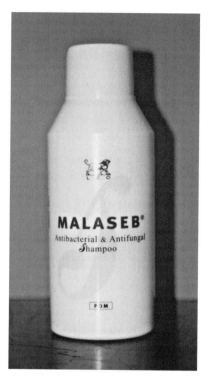

Figure 1
Shampoos containing miconazole are useful for the treatment of *Malassezia*.

Intertrigo
- Body-fold intertrigo occurs in Bassets occasionally
- Obesity predisposes

Skin tumours
- See under Neoplastic conditions

Gastrointestinal conditions
Tuberculosis
- Possible breed predisposition to gastrointestinal infection with the avian form of tuberculosis

Haematological/immunological conditions
Severe combined immunodeficiency
- Inherited as an X-linked recessive trait
- Thymic hypoplasia and lymphopaenia seen

Basset hound thrombopathia
- Inherited as an autosomal recessive trait
- Aetiology unknown
- May be a variant of Glanzmann's thrombasthenia

Tuberculosis
- See under Infectious conditions and Gastrointestinal conditions

Infectious conditions
Mycobacterium avium
- Rare condition
- Possible breed predisposition

Infectious skin diseases
- See under Dermatological conditions

Musculoskeletal conditions
Temporomandibular dysplasia/luxation
- Congenital dysplasia may predispose to luxation

Ununited anconeal process
- A true fracture of the process occurs in this breed

Inguinal hernia

Neoplastic conditions
Mast cell tumours
- Possible breed predisposition
- May be seen at any age (from 4 months onwards), but usually seen in older animals

Trichoepithelioma
- Possible breed predisposition
- Average age is 9 years
- This breed may be predisposed to multiple trichoepitheliomas

Pilomatrixoma
- Possible breed predisposition
- Average age is 6 years

Actinic keratosis (solar keratosis)
- Reported to be at increased risk
- Seen more commonly in pale-skinned animals with the opportunity for long periods of intense sun exposure

Cutaneous haemangioma
- Possible breed predisposition
- Average age was 8.7 years in one study

Non-epitheliotropic lymphoma
- Affects older dogs

Nasal cavity tumours
- Reported to be at increased risk for nasal carcinoma
- Usually older dogs
- Dogs in urban areas may be at increased risk

Lymphosarcoma (malignant lymphoma) (see plate 1)
- Higher incidence noted in this breed
- Most cases are seen in middle-aged dogs (mean 6–7 years)

Neurological conditions
Intervertebral disc disease
- Breed predisposition
- Common
- Adults affected

Discospondylitis
- Breed predisposition possibly due to concurrent immunodeficiency
- Young/middle-aged dogs affected
- Males may be predisposed

Lysosomal storage disease – neuronal glycoproteinosis (Lafora's disease)
- Inheritance suspected
- Rare
- Signs seen at 5 months–9 years

Cervical vertebral malformation (wobbler syndrome)
- Breed predisposition
- Seen occasionally in this breed

Ocular conditions
Entropion (may be associated with 'diamond eye')
- Breed predisposition; polygenic inheritance likely

Ectropion (may be associated with 'diamond eye')
- Breed predisposition; polygenic inheritance likely

Combined entropion–ectropion ('diamond eye')
- Breed predisposition; genetic basis incompletely understood

Eversion of the cartilage of the nictitating membrane
- Breed predisposition
- Usually occurs in young dogs

Primary glaucoma/goniodysgenesis
- Inheritance suspected
- Age of onset: 5–7 years
- Schedule 1 of the BVA/KC/ISDS Eye Scheme

Cataract
- Inheritance suspected

Generalised progressive retinal atrophy (GPRA)
- Mode of inheritance unknown, but presumed to be recessive
- Age of clinical onset: 3 years, with a second type occurring at 6–8 years

Physiological conditions
Chondrodystrophy/hypochondroplasia
- Accepted as breed standard
- Short, bowed legs but normal skulls seen

Renal and urinary conditions
Cystine urolithiasis
- Cystinuria results from an inherited defect in renal tubular transport of cystine and predisposes to cystine urolithiasis
- Higher incidence reported in this breed in some American surveys
- Average age at diagnosis is 1–8 years
- Males seem predisposed

BEAGLE

Cardiovascular conditions
Pulmonic stenosis
- Third most frequent cause of canine congenital heart disease
- Polygenic mode of inheritance shown in this breed

DOGS

Coronary artery vasculitis
- Asymptomatic
- Unknown aetiology
- Recognised in 34% of young Beagles

Canine juvenile polyarteritis syndrome
- Causes a pain syndrome
- Reported in USA, France and UK

Dermatological conditions
Congenital hypotrichosis
- Symmetrical hair loss
- Usually hair loss is apparent at birth and gets worse over the following few weeks

Black hair follicular dysplasia
- Rare
- Early onset
- Familial

Ehler-Danlos syndrome
- Also known as cutaneous asthenia
- Inherited
- Various modes of inheritance

Familial vasculopathy
- Necrotising vasculitis of small- and medium-sized arteries
- Early onset of signs

Canine truncal solar dermatitis
- Photosensitisation implicated
- Worse in sunny climates

Zinc-responsive dermatosis
- In Beagles, occurs in puppies fed zinc-deficient diets

Skin tumours
- See Neoplastic conditions

Endocrine conditions
Lymphocytic thyroiditis (causing hypothyroidism)
- Demonstrated to be inherited polygenically in laboratory Beagles

Thyroid neoplasia (may be associated with hyper- or hypothyroidism, but most are euthyroid)
- Possible breed predisposition
- Average age 10 years

Hyperadrenocorticism: pituitary-dependent (PDH)
- Possible breed predisposition
- Middle–aged/older; median age 10 years
- 55–60% female

Diabetes mellitus
- Reported in some texts to be at increased risk
- Usual age range: 4–14 years; peak incidence: 7–9 years
- Old entire females are predisposed

Gastrointestinal conditions
Chronic hepatitis
- Increased incidence noted in this breed

Haematological/immunological conditions
Severe combined immunodeficiency
- Inherited as an X-linked recessive trait
- Thymic hypoplasia and lymphopaenia seen

Selective IgA deficiency
- Leads to chronic respiratory conditions and dermatitis
- May be associated with autoimmunity

Pyruvate kinase deficiency
- Affected dogs have abnormal red blood cells with a lifespan of about 20 days

Non-spherocytic haemolytic anaemia
- Due to a defect in the ATPase calcium pump system in this breed

Factor VII deficiency
- Seen in families of laboratory dogs
- Inherited as an autosomal dominant trait
- Heterozygotes are asymptomatic

Primary idiopathic hyperlipidaemia
- Familial

Infectious conditions
Coccidiomycosis
- Increased incidence in this breed possibly due to an increased likelihood of exposure
- Mainly seen in young male dogs
- Geographic distribution: California, Arizona, Texas, New Mexico, Nevada, Utah, Mexico and parts of Central and South America. Not reported in the UK

DOGS

Musculoskeletal conditions
Polyarthritis/meningitis
- Idiopathic
- Affects dogs from 6–9 months old

Multiple epiphyseal dysplasia
- Inherited as an autosomal recessive trait

Brachyury
- Inherited as an autosomal dominant trait

Neoplastic conditions
Mast cell tumours
- Possible breed predisposition
- May be seen at any age (from 4 months onwards), but usually seen in older animals

Actinic keratosis (solar keratosis)
- Reported to be at increased risk
- Seen more commonly in pale-skinned animals with the opportunity for long periods of intense sun exposure

Sebaceous gland tumours
- Possible breed predisposition to nodular sebaceous hyperplasia
- Seen in older dogs (average age 10 years)

Haemangiopericytoma
- Occur at a mean age of 7–10 years

Perianal (hepatoid) gland adenomas
- Breed predisposition suggested in one survey of 2700 cases
- Average age was 10.5 years
- Entire males were predisposed

Cutaneous haemangioma
- Possible breed predisposition
- Average age was 8.7 years in one study

Thyroid neoplasia
- See under Endocrine conditions

Pituitary tumour resulting in hyperadrenocorticism
- See under Endocrine conditions

Lymphosarcoma (malignant lymphoma)
- Higher incidence noted in this breed
- Most cases are seen in middle-aged dogs (mean 6–7 years)

Neurological conditions
Congenital vestibular disease
- Signs seen <3 months
- May be seen with congenital deafness

Congenital deafness
- Signs seen from birth

Intervertebral disc disease
- Breed predisposition
- Relatively common condition
- Adults affected

Lysosomal storage disease – GM$_1$ gangliosidosis
- Autosomal recessive inheritance
- Rare
- Signs seen at 3–6 months

Lysosomal storage disease – neuronal glycoproteinosis (Lafora's disease)
- Inheritance suspected
- Rare
- Signs seen at 5–12 months

Cerebellar degeneration
- Reported in Japan
- Signs seen at 3 weeks

True epilepsy
- Inherited
- Age of onset: 6–36 months
- Reported to affect males more than females

Narcolepsy-cataplexy
- Reported in this breed
- Age of onset: <1 year

Lissencephaly
- Rare disease reported in this breed
- Age of onset: <1 year

Hound ataxia
- Reported in the UK
- Age of onset: 2–7 years

Meningitis and polyarteritis
- Reported in this breed
- Age of onset: <1 year

Spina bifida
- Congenital

Ocular conditions

Prolapse of the gland of the nictitating membrane ('cherry eye')
- Breed predisposition; possibly inherited
- Usually presents in the first year of life

Corneal dystrophy
- Inheritance suspected
- Stromal lipid dystrophy
- Reports suggest occurs in approximately 17% of Beagles aged 8–15 years
- Rarely affects vision

Glaucoma
- Autosomal recessive inheritance suggested
- Primary open–angle glaucoma seems to occur in this breed
- Clinical signs seen at 2–5 years

Lens luxation
- Breed predisposition
- Often seen in the later stages of glaucoma, but some texts suggest it also occurs as a primary condition

Cataract
- Inheritance suspected
- Congenital anterior-capsular cataracts; unilateral; rarely affect vision
- Posterior cortical cataracts affect mature dogs, are usually bilateral and may cause intraocular inflammation and visual deficiencies

Multifocal retinal dysplasia
- Congenital condition, inheritance as an autosomal recessive trait suspected
- Schedule 3 of the BVA/KC/ISDS Eye Scheme

Tapetal degeneration
- Autosomal recessive inheritance suspected
- Associated with lightly-pigmented iridal tissues
- Minor condition with no effect on vision

Generalised progressive retinal atrophy (GPRA)
- Mode of inheritance unknown but presumed to be recessive
- Age of clinical onset: 3–5 years

Micropapilla
- Congenital condition, not known if inherited
- Seen occasionally in this breed

Optic nerve hypoplasia
- Congenital condition, not known if inherited
- Seen occasionally in this breed

Congenital cataract with microphthalmia
- Dominant inheritance suspected

Microphthalmia-microphakia-persistent pupillary membrane (PPM) syndrome
- Dominant inheritance suspected
- Heterozygotes have PPM and congenital cataract/microphakic lens
- Homozygotes are microphthalmic, have multiple ocular defects and are blind

Multiple ocular defects of the posterior segment
- Mode of inheritance unknown but autosomal recessive inheritance suspected
- Defects include retention of the hyaloid system, excessive myelination of the optic disc and neovascularisation of the retina, with a tendency for intraocular haemorrhage

Physiological conditions

Hypochondroplasia
- Accepted as breed standard
- Short, bowed legs but normal skulls seen

Renal and urinary conditions

Renal (glomerular) amyloidosis
- Has been reported in families of older Beagles
- Dogs presented with proteinuria and renal failure

Unilateral renal agenesis
- Uncommon condition
- High prevalence reported in some families of Beagles

Reproductive conditions

XX sex reversal
- Congenital condition reported in this breed

BEARDED COLLIE

Dermatological conditions
Pemphigus foliaceous
- Probably the most common immune-mediated skin disorder in cats and dogs, but still uncommon
- Incidence of 0.04% in hospitalised dogs
- No age or sex predisposition

Black hair follicular dysplasia
- Rare
- Early onset
- Familial

Musculoskeletal conditions
Congenital elbow luxation
- Type II luxation in this breed (proximal radius displaced caudolaterally)
- Usually 4–5 months old at presentation

Ocular conditions
Corneal dystrophy
- Breed predisposition
- Lipid dystrophy
- Age of onset: >1 year

Cataract
- Inheritance suspected
- Localisation: anterior subcapsular
- Age of onset: 2–5 years

Generalised progressive retinal atrophy (GPRA)
- Mode of inheritance unknown, but presumed to be recessive
- Age of onset: 1 year

BEAUCERON

Dermatological conditions
Atopy
- Age of onset 6 months to 7 years
- Females possibly predisposed

Junctional epidermolysis bullosa
- Genital and mucocutaneous lesions at 6 weeks of age
- Probably autosomal recessive inheritance

Dystrophic epidermolysis bullosa
- Lesions at mucocutaneous junctions, pressure points and claws

BEDLINGTON TERRIER

Dermatological conditions
Melanotrichia
- Often following healing of deep inflammation

Gastrointestinal conditions
Copper storage hepatopathy
- Chronic hepatitis resulting from a primary defect in copper excretion and abnormal copper retention in the hepatocytes. This defect is inherited as an autosomal recessive trait
- Clinical onset seen in young to middle-aged dogs
- High prevalence worldwide

Musculoskeletal conditions
Osteogenesis imperfecta
- Rare
- Group of inherited diseases

Ocular conditions
Entropion (usually lateral lower lids)
- Breed predisposition; polygenic inheritance likely

Distichiasis
- Possible breed predisposition

Lacrimal punctal aplasia
- Congenital condition

Cataract
- Inheritance suspected
- Localisation: posterior subcapsular
- Age of onset: 3–24 months

Total retinal dysplasia with retinal detachment and absence of the secondary vitreous
- Autosomal recessive inheritance
- Schedule 1 of the BVA/KC/ISDS Eye Scheme

Generalised progressive retinal atrophy (GPRA)
- Mode of inheritance unknown, but presumed to be recessive
- Clinically evident at 1–2 years of age

DOGS

BELGIAN SHEPHERD DOG

Dermatological conditions
Congenital hypotrichosis
- Present at birth or develops in the first month of life
- Predisposition for males suggests sex linkage

Gastrointestinal conditions
Gastric carcinoma
- See under Neoplastic conditions

Musculoskeletal conditions
Gracilis and semitendinosus myopathy
- Occasionally reported in this breed

Neoplastic conditions
Gastric carcinoma
- Breed predisposition
- Male dogs more commonly affected
- Mean age of occurrence: 8–10 years

Ocular conditions
Plasma cell infiltration of the nictitating membrane (plasmoma)
- Possible breed predisposition
- May be associated with pannus

Chronic superficial keratitis (pannus)
- Breed predisposition
- Age of onset: 2–5 years

Cataract
- Inheritance suspected
- Localisation: posterior polar
- Schedule 1 of the BVA/KC/ISDS Eye Scheme

Generalised progressive retinal atrophy (GPRA)
- Mode of inheritance unknown, but presumed to be recessive

Retinopathy
- Autosomal recessive inheritance suspected
- Photoreceptor dysplasia
- Complete blindness may be present from 8 weeks

Micropapilla
- Congenital condition

BELGIAN TERVUREN

Dermatological conditions
Atopy
- Age of onset 6 months to 7 years
- Females possibly predisposed

Granulomatous sebaceous adenitis
- Affects young to middle-aged dogs

Hypopigmentary disorders
- Various causes
- Suspected to be hereditary in this breed

Primary lymphoedema
- No sex predisposition
- Appears within first 12 weeks of life

Vitiligo
- Presumed to be hereditary
- Antimelanocyte antibodies found in all 17 affected Belgian Tervurens tested and none of the 11 normal Belgian Tervurens tested

Neurological conditions
True epilepsy
- Inherited
- Age of onset: 6 months to 3 years

Ocular conditions
Chronic superficial keratitis (pannus)
- Possible breed predisposition
- Age of onset: 2–5 years

Cataract
- Inheritance suspected
- Posterior subcapsular cataracts may be seen at 2 years and progress slowly along the suture lines
- Anterior subcapsular cataracts have been seen in 3-year-old dogs

Generalised progressive retinal atrophy (GPRA)
- Mode of inheritance unknown, but presumed to be recessive

Micropapilla
- Congenital condition

Physiological conditions
Leucopaenia
- Six out of 9 healthy Belgian Tervurens sampled had white blood cell counts $2.4-5.4 \times 10^9/l$

BERNESE MOUNTAIN DOG

Dermatological conditions
Colour dilution alopecia
- Probably much less common in this breed than in Dobermanns

Seasonal nasal hypopigmentation
- Also known as snow nose
- Usually occurs in winter

Skin tumours
- See under Neoplastic conditions

Musculoskeletal conditions
Elbow dysplasia
- Also known as osteochondrosis
- Genetically determined in this breed
- Medial coronoid process disease is common in this breed

Polyarthritis/meningitis
- Idiopathic
- This breed is predisposed to a more severe form of the disease

Shoulder osteochondrosis
- Male:female ratio 2.24:1
- 50% bilateral
- Age of onset usually 4–7 months, but can be older

Lateral torsion and tarsal valgus deformity
- Unknown aetiology
- Cosmetic fault only

Hip dysplasia
- A large 1989 study showed a prevalence of 25.3% in this breed

Neoplastic conditions
Cutaneous haemangiosarcoma
- Possible breed predisposition
- Average age 9–10 years

Malignant histiocytosis
- Rare condition
- Breed predisposition; possibly inherited polygenically
- Affects older dogs (7–8 years)
- More common in males

Systemic histiocytosis
- Rare condition
- Has only been reported in this breed, possibly inherited polygenically
- Affects younger dogs (3–4 years)

Neurological conditions
Hypomyelination of the central nervous system
- Inheritance suspected
- Signs seen at 2–8 weeks

Meningitis and polyarteritis
- Has been reported
- Age of clinical onset: <1 year

Ocular conditions
Entropion
- Breed predisposition, polygenic inheritance likely

Systemic histiocytosis (ocular signs may include uveitis, chemosis and scleritis)
- See under Neoplastic conditions

Cataract
- Inheritance suspected
- Localisation: posterior subcapsular cortex
- Age of onset: 1 year; may progress and affect vision

Generalised progressive retinal atrophy (GPRA)
- Mode of inheritance unknown, but presumed to be recessive
- Age of clinical onset: 1 year of age

DOGS

Renal and urinary conditions
Familial renal disease (membranoproliferative glomerulonephritis)
- Autosomal recessive inheritance suggested
- This condition was reported in a group of 20 Bernese Mountain Dogs. Affected dogs presented at 2–5 years with renal failure and marked proteinuria
- Most of the dogs had a high titre to *Borrelia burgdorferi* suggesting that it may have had a role in the development of the condition

Respiratory conditions
Malignant histiocytosis
- See under Neoplastic conditions

BICHON FRISE

Cardiovascular conditions
Patent ductus arteriosus
- Common congenital abnormality
- Relative risk 5.5
- Females predisposed
- Mode of inheritance is polygenic

Dermatological conditions
Congenital hypotrichosis
- Present at birth or develops in the first month of life
- Predisposition for males suggests sex linkage

Skin tumours
- See under Neoplastic conditions

Haematological/immunological conditions
Haemophilia B
- Factor IX deficiency
- Also known as Christmas disease
- Inherited as a sex-linked trait
- Less common than haemophilia A

Neoplastic conditions
Basal cell tumour
- Possible breed predisposition

Neurological conditions
Shaker dog disease
- Has been reported
- Age of onset: 9 months to 2 years

Atlantoaxial subluxation
- Congenital
- Age of onset: <1 year

Ocular conditions
Entropion (usually medial lower lids)
- Breed predisposition; polygenic inheritance likely

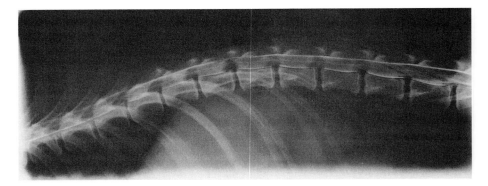

Figure 2a
Although not listed as a predisposed breed, the Bichon Frise may be commonly affected by intervertebral disc disease. This myelogram of an eleven-year-old neutered male Bichon Frise shows loss of the dorsal column of contrast at T12–T13 consistent with disc herniation at this site (lateral view).

DOGS

DOGS

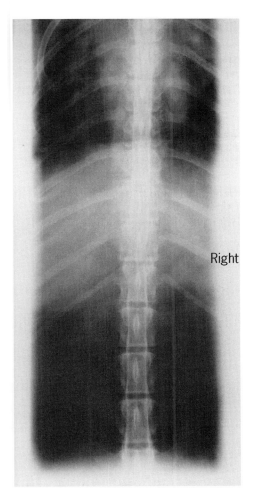

Right

Figure 2b
Dorsoventral view showing extradural
compression on the right side at the level
of T12–T13.

Congenital, sub-epithelial, geographic corneal
dystrophy
- Congenital condition; predisposed breed
- Occurs in young puppies (<10 weeks); transient condition

Corneal dystrophy
- Inheritance suspected
- Paracentral, lipid dystrophy
- Age of onset: 2 years

Cataract (see pate 2)
- Inheritance suspected
- Localisation: posterior subcapsular
- Age of onset: 6 months to 3 years
- Rate of advancement varies
- Schedule 3 of the BVA/KC/ISDS Eye
  Scheme

Renal and urinary conditions
Cystine urolithiasis
- Cystinuria results from an inherited defect in
  renal tubular transport of cystine and predis-
  poses to cystine urolithiasis
- Higher incidence reported in this breed in
  some American surveys
- Average age at diagnosis is 1–8 years
- Males seem predisposed

Calcium oxalate urolithiasis
- Higher incidence has been noted in this
  breed in some surveys
- Average age at diagnosis is 5–12 years
- Males may be predisposed

Struvite (magnesium ammonium phosphate)
urolithiasis
- Higher incidence has been noted in this breed
- Average age at diagnosis is 2–8 years
- Females seem to be predisposed

Calcium phosphate urolithiasis
(hydroxyapatite and carbonate apatite)
- Higher incidence has been noted in this
  breed in some surveys
- Average age at diagnosis is 7–11 years

Calcium phosphate urolithiasis
(brushite)
- Higher incidence has been noted in this
  breed in some surveys
- Average age at diagnosis is 7–11 years
- Males may be predisposed

Respiratory conditions
Primary ciliary dyskinesia
- Inherited defect
- Usually signs seen within first few weeks of
  life

BLOODHOUND

Cardiovascular conditions
Aortic stenosis
- Common congenital disease
- Relative risk >5.0
- No sex predilection
- Inheritance possibly autosomal dominant with modifying genes, or polygenic

Gastrointestinal conditions
Gastric dilatation/volvulus
- Possible breed predisposition

Neoplastic conditions
Cutaneous haemangioma
- Possible breed predisposition
- Average age was 8.7 years in one study

Ocular conditions
Entropion (usually upper eyelids, may be associated with macropalpebral fissure)
- Breed predisposition; polygenic inheritance likely

Ectropion (may be associated with macropalpebral fissure)
- Breed predisposition; polygenic inheritance likely

Macropalpebral fissure resulting in combined entropion–ectropion ('diamond eye')
- Breed predisposition; genetic basis incompletely understood

Keratoconjunctivitis sicca
- Breed predisposition

Eversion of the cartilage of the nictitating membrane
- Breed predisposition; inheritance suspected
- Usually occurs in young dogs

Prolapse of the gland of the nictitating membrane ('cherry eye')
- Breed predisposition
- Usually presents before 2 years of age

Multiple ocular defects
- Congenital defects
- Schedule 3 of the BVA/KC/ISDS Eye Scheme

BORDER COLLIE

Haematological/immunological conditions
Canine cyclic neutropaenia
- Inherited as autosomal recessive
- Associated with grey Collies

Musculoskeletal conditions
Shoulder osteochondrosis
- Male:female ratio 2.24:1
- 50% bilateral
- Age of onset usually 4–7 months but can be older

Carpal soft-tissue injury
- Especially seen in working dogs

Neurological conditions
Congenital deafness
- Signs seen from birth

Cerebellar degeneration
- Familial
- Uncommon
- Signs seen at 6–8 weeks

Lysosomal storage disease – ceroid lipofuscinosis
- Autosomal recessive inheritance
- Rare
- Signs seen at 1–2 years

Ocular conditions
Nodular episclerokeratitis
- Breed predisposition
- Usually presents at 2–5 years

Chronic superficial keratitis (pannus)
- Breed predisposition

Primary lens luxation
- Simple autosomal recessive inheritance suggested
- Age of onset: 3–5 years
- Often followed by glaucoma
- Schedule 1 of the BVA/KC/ISDS Eye Scheme

Cataract
- Inheritance suspected
- Localisation: anterior subcapsular
- Age of onset: 4–6 years
- Schedule 3 of the BVA/KC/ISDS Eye Scheme

Collie eye anomaly
- Congenital disorder, inheritance suspected
- Low incidence in this breed
- Schedule 1 of the BVA/KC/ISDS Eye Scheme

Generalised progressive retinal atrophy (GPRA)
- Mode of inheritance unknown but presumed to be recessive
- Clinically evident at 2 years of age

Central progressive retinal atrophy (CPRA) or retinal pigment epithelial dystrophy (RPED)
- Mode of inheritance unknown
- Age of clinical onset: 1–2 years
- More prevalent in the UK than in the USA. Becoming less prevalent following the introduction of control schemes
- Schedule 1 of the BVA/KC/ISDS Eye Scheme

Multiple ocular defects
- Congenital condition, seen in homozygous merles (the result of merle to merle breeding) with predominantly white coats
- Defects may include microphthalmia, microcornea, cataract, equatorial staphylomas and coloboma

Neuronal ceroid lipofuscinosis
- Autosomal recessive inheritance suspected

BORDER TERRIER

Ocular conditions
Cataract
- Inheritance suspected
- Localisation: posterior subcapsular
- Age of onset: 3–5 years; slowly progressive
- Schedule 3 of the BVA/KC/ISDS Eye Scheme

BORZOI

Dermatological conditions
Primary lymphoedema
- No apparent sex predisposition
- Usually occurs within first 12 weeks of life

Endocrine conditions
Lymphocytic thyroiditis (causing hypothyroidism)
- Reported to be inherited in one family of Borzois

Gastrointestinal conditions
Gastric dilatation/volvulus
- Possible breed predisposition

Neurological conditions
Cervical vertebral malformation (wobbler syndrome)
- Seen occasionally in this breed
- Age of clinical onset: 5–8 years

Ocular conditions
Plasma cell infiltration of the nictitating membrane (plasmoma)
- Breed predisposition

Cataract
- Inheritance suspected
- Localisation: posterior cortex
- Age of onset: 1–4 years; slowly progressive
- Nuclear cataracts may be seen in older Borzois

Retinopathy of Borzois
- Inheritance suspected
- Unilateral or bilateral progressive retinal degeneration causing visual defects; blindness uncommon
- Seen most commonly in young dogs (1–2 years of age)
- Males may be affected twice as frequently as females

Multiple ocular defects
- Congenital condition; inheritance suspected
- Defects may include microphthalmia, cataract, multifocal retinal dysplasia and persistent pupillary membranes

DOGS

Respiratory conditions
Aspergillosis
- Uncommon fungal infection

BOSTON TERRIER

Dermatological conditions
Generalised demodicosis
- Boston Terriers are in the ten breeds at highest statistical risk of this disease in the Cornell, USA population

Atopy
- Females probably predisposed
- Age of onset from 6 months to 7 years
- May or may not be seasonal

Canine pinnal alopecia
- Onset usually >1 year of age

Pattern baldness
- Usually affects females in this breed
- Gradual hair loss from 6 months of age
- Affects mainly the ventrum and caudomedial thighs

Colour-dilution alopecia
- Coat-colour genes play an important role in pathogenesis
- Incidence much lower in this breed than in Dobermanns

Intertrigo
- Tail-fold intertrigo results from corkscrew tails

Calcinosis circumscripta
- Uncommon condition
- No sex predisposition
- In this breed lesions usually occur on the cheek

Retrognathia
- Possibly inherited as an autosomal recessive trait

Skin tumours
- See under Neoplastic conditions

Endocrine conditions
Hyperadrenocorticism: pituitary-dependent (PDH)
- Possible breed predisposition
- Middle-aged/older
- 55–60% female

Gastrointestinal conditions
Vascular ring anomaly
- Breed predisposition; inheritance suspected
- Clinical presentation at time of weaning

Pyloric stenosis (antral pyloric hypertrophy syndrome)
- Congenital hypertrophy of pyloric muscle, resulting in gastric-outflow obstruction and vomiting
- Clinical presentation shortly after weaning or within first 6–12 months

Musculoskeletal conditions
Craniomandibular osteopathy
- Aetiology unknown in this breed
- Usually affects dogs aged 3–8 months

Congenital elbow luxation
- Uncommon, accounts for 15% of non-traumatic elbow lameness
- Severe disability in this breed (type I)
- Present at birth or in the first 3 months of life

Perineal hernia
- Intact males predisposed

Hemivertebrae
- Mode of inheritance not known

Sacrocaudal dysgenesis
- Congenital
- See also under Neurological conditions

Neoplastic conditions
Mast cell tumours
- Possible breed predisposition
- May be seen at any age (from 4 months onwards), but usually seen in older animals

Melanoma
- Breed predisposition
- Average age 8–9 years

Canine cutaneous histiocytoma
- Possible breed predisposition
- More common in young dogs 1–2 years of age

Fibroma
- Females predisposed
- Affects older animals

Chemodectoma
- Higher incidence noted in this breed
- Older dogs usually affected (10–15 years)
- Males may be predisposed to aortic-body tumours

Primary brain tumour
- See under Neurological conditions

Pituitary tumour resulting in hyperadrenocorticism
- See under Endocrine diseases

Neurological conditions
Congenital deafness
- Signs seen from birth

Hydrocephalus
- Congenital
- Relatively common
- Onset of signs: <3 months

Cerebellar malformation
- Congenital
- Uncommon
- Onset of clinical signs: 3–4 weeks

Hemivertebrae
- Congenital
- Occasionally seen

Primary brain tumour
- Higher incidence noted in this breed
- Older dogs affected (mean 9–10 years)

Sacrocaudal dysgenesis
- Congenital
- Occasionally reported

Arachnoid cysts
- Rare condition reported in this breed
- Age of clinical onset: <1 year

Ocular conditions
Caruncular trichiasis
- Breed predisposition

Keratoconjunctivitis sicca
- Breed predisposition

Prolapse of the gland of the nictitating membrane
- Breed predisposition; possibly inherited
- Usually presents before 2 years of age

Pigmentary keratitis
- Breed predisposition

Refractory corneal ulceration
- Breed predisposition
- Age of onset: 6–8 years

Corneal dystrophy
- Breed predisposition
- Endothelial dystrophy with progressive corneal oedema
- Age of onset: 5–9 years

Iris cysts (see plate 3)
- Breed predisposition; inheritance suspected
- Age of onset: approximately 9 years

Cataract
- Simple autosomal recessive inheritance
- Localisation: posterior suture lines and nucleus
- Age of onset: 8–10 weeks; progression occurs affecting vision
- Late-onset cataracts may occur in the anterior and posterior cortices, but the mode of inheritance is unknown
- Schedule 1 of the BVA/KC/ISDS Eye Scheme

Vitreal syneresis
- Breed predisposition
- Occurs in older dogs
- Vitreal degeneration results in strands of vitreous extending into the anterior chamber predisposing to glaucoma and cataracts

Physiological conditions
Achondroplasia
- Genetic dwarfism
- Skull and limbs affected
- Accepted as a breed standard

DOGS

Renal and urinary conditions
Urethral prolapse
- Possible breed predisposition
- Generally seen in male dogs at 4 months to 5 years of age

Hypospadias
- Congenital defect with a high incidence in this breed suggesting a possible genetic basis

Reproductive conditions
Dystocia
- Breed predisposition due to combination of narrow pelvis and large head/wide shoulders

Hypospadias
- See under Renal and urinary conditions

Urethral prolapse
- See under Renal and urinary conditions

Respiratory conditions
Brachycephalic upper airway syndrome
- Complex of anatomical deformities
- Common in this breed
- Likely a consequence of selective breeding for certain facial characteristics

Hypoplastic trachea
- This breed accounts for 15% of cases

BOUVIER DES FLANDRES

Dermatological conditions
Seasonal flank alopecia
- May occur in autumn or spring

Skin tumours
- See under Neoplastic conditions

Gastrointestinal conditions
Oesophageal/pharyngeal muscle degeneration and dysphagia
- Breed predisposition

Musculoskeletal conditions
Muscular dystrophy
- Primary myopathy affecting the muscles of swallowing
- Limb muscles not affected

Degenerative polymyopathy
- Reported in four related Bouviers
- Causes generalised weakness and megaoesophagus

Hip dysplasia
- This breed has the fourteenth worst breed mean score in the BVA/KC Hip Dysplasia Scheme as of October 2001
- Breed mean score 18

Neoplastic conditions
Squamous cell carcinoma of the digit
- Occurs at an average of 9 years of age

Ocular conditions
Entropion (usually lateral canthal area of both upper and lower lids)
- Breed predisposition; polygenic inheritance likely
- Usually occurs in the first year of life

Primary glaucoma (see figure 3)
- Breed predisposition (especially in the Netherlands)
- An association with goniodysgenesis has been suggested in this breed

Cataract
- Inheritance suspected

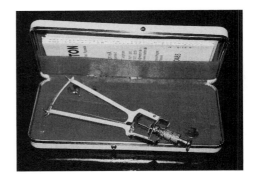

Figure 3
A Schiotz tonometer is an inexpensive tool for estimating intra-ocular pressure in suspected cases of glaucoma.

Respiratory conditions
Laryngeal paralysis
• Neurogenic and hereditary in this breed

BOXER

Cardiovascular conditions
Atrial septal defect
• Uncommon disease
• Congenital
• Not yet proven to be inherited
• Relative risk 25.0

Aortic stenosis
• Common congenital disease
• Relative risk 9.3
• Males strongly predisposed in this breed
• Particular prevalence in this breed in Scotland
• Inheritance possibly autosomal dominant with modifying genes, or polygenic

Dilated cardiomyopathy (see figures 4a and 4b)
• Prevalence of 3.4% in this breed compared to 0.16% in mixed breeds and 0.65% in pure breeds

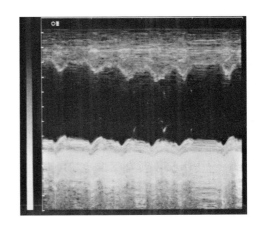

Figure 4b
M-mode echocardiogram (left ventricular short axis) of a twelve-year-old Boxer with dilated cardiomyopathy (5.0 MHz).

• Increased prevalence with age
• Approximately twice as common in males as females
• Thought to be familial or genetic

Sick sinus syndrome
• Middle-aged to old dogs
• Relative risk 2.6 in this breed
• No sex predisposition in this breed

Pericardial effusion
• Relative risk only 1.5
• Usually affects middle–aged dogs

Boxer cardiomyopathy

Dermatological conditions
Muzzle folliculitis/furunculosis
• Also known as canine acne
• Local trauma, hormones and genetics may play a role in pathogenesis

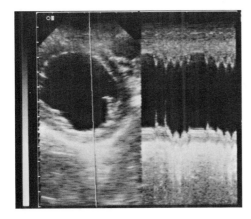

Figure 4a
B-mode and M-mode echocardiogram (left ventricular short axis) of a twelve-year-old Boxer with dilated cardiomyopathy (5.0 MHz).

Pododermatitis
• Males predisposed
• Front feet more commonly affected

Coccidiomycosis (disseminated)
- See under Infectious conditions

Atopy
- Females probably predisposed
- Age of onset from 6 months to 7 years
- May or may not be seasonal
- Relative risk 5.8

Food hypersensitivity
- No sex predisposition, but many cases occur in young dogs
- Some studies have not shown a breed predisposition
- One study shows relative risk 4.3

Oestrogen-responsive dermatosis
- Usually occurs in the young adult

Canine follicular dysplasia
- Presumed genetic basis
- Alopecia starts at 2–4 years of age and is restricted to the flank in this breed

Demodicosis
- Possible breed predisposition

Seasonal flank alopecia
- May occur in autumn or spring

Ehler-Danlos syndrome
- Also known as cutaneous asthenia
- A group of inherited diseases with various modes of inheritance

Truncal solar dermatitis
- Affects white boxers
- Incidence of disease increases in sunny climates

Callus dermatitis/pyoderma
- Sternal calluses often become infected

Idiopathic sterile granuloma and pyogranuloma
- Uncommon
- No age or sex predisposition

Follicular cyst
- No age or sex predisposition

Dermoid cyst
- Rare
- Solitary or multiple
- Occur on the dorsal midline

Calcinosis circumscripta
- Most common in younger dogs
- Lesions at the base of the pinna are most common in this breed

Skin tumours
- See under Neoplastic conditions

Drug reactions
Acepromazine and other phenothiazines (see figure 5)
- This breed is very sensitive even to small doses of ACP

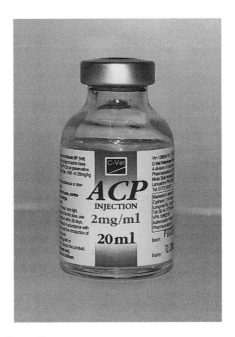

Figure 5
Boxers are sensitive to even small doses of Acepromazine (ACP).

DOGS

Endocrine conditions

Hypothyroidism
- Reported in some texts to be at increased risk
- Often middle-aged (2–6 years)
- One report of congenital secondary hypothyroidism due to TSH deficiency

Thyroid neoplasia (may be associated with hyper- or hypothyroidism, but most are euthyroid)
- Possible breed predisposition
- Average age 10 years

Hyperadrenocorticism: pituitary-dependent (PDH)
- Possible breed predisposition
- Middle-aged/older
- 55–60% female

Insulinoma
- Higher incidence seen in this breed
- Middle aged/older dogs affected

Phaeochromocytoma
- Uncommon
- An increased incidence has been suggested in two studies
- Older dogs affected

Gastrointestinal conditions

Gingival and oropharyngeal neoplasia
- Possible breed predisposition

Pyloric stenosis (antral pyloric hypertrophy syndrome)
- Congenital hypertrophy of pyloric muscle, resulting in gastric outflow obstruction and vomiting
- Clinical presentation shortly after weaning or within first 6–12 months

Histiocytic colitis
- Breed predisposition
- Most common in young dogs

Chronic idiopathic (lymphocytic-plasmacytic) colitis
- Breed predisposition
- Most common in young to middle-aged dogs

Infectious conditions

Coccidiomycosis
- Increased incidence in this breed, possibly due to increased likelihood of exposure
- Seen mainly in young, male dogs
- Geographic distribution: California, Arizona, Texas, New Mexico, Nevada, Utah, Mexico, and parts of Central and South America. Not reported in the UK

Infectious skin disease
- See under Dermatological conditions

Musculoskeletal conditions

Temporomandibular dysplasia/luxation
- Congenital dysplasia may predispose to luxation

Polyarthritis/meningitis
- Idiopathic
- Affects dogs from 6 months onwards

Congenital elbow luxation
- Type II luxation occurs in this breed (proximal radius displaced caudolaterally)
- Usually 4–5 months old at presentation

Spondylosis deformans
- Usually clinically insignificant

Neoplastic conditions

Mast cell tumours
- Possible breed predisposition
- May be seen at any age (from 4 months onwards), but usually seen in older animals

Melanoma
- Breed predisposition
- Average age 8–9 years

Cutaneous haemangioma
- Possible breed predisposition
- Average age was 8.7 years in one study

Cutaneous haemangiosarcoma
- Possible breed predisposition
- Average age 9–10 years

Canine cutaneous histiocytoma
- Higher incidence seen in this breed
- More common in young dogs of 1–2 years of age

Squamous cell carcinoma of the skin
- Occurs at an average of 9 years of age

Fibroma
- Females predisposed
- Affects older animals

Non-epitheliotropic lymphoma
- Affects older dogs

Haemangiopericytoma
- Occurs at a mean age of 7–10 years

Chemodectoma
- Higher incidence noted in this breed
- Older dogs usually affected (10–15 years)
- Males may be predisposed to aortic-body tumours

Thyroid neoplasia
- See under Endocrine conditions

Phaeochromocytoma
- See under Endocrine conditions

Insulinoma
- See under Endocrine conditions

Pituitary tumour resulting in hyperadrenocorticism
- See under Endocrine conditions

Gingival and oropharyngeal neoplasia
- Possible breed predisposition

Osteosarcoma of the skull
- Higher incidence noted in this breed

Chondrosarcoma of the rib
- Higher incidence noted in this breed

Primary brain tumour
- See under Neurological conditions

Lymphosarcoma (malignant lymphoma)
- Higher incidence noted in this breed
- Most cases are seen in middle-aged dogs (mean 6–7 years)

Canine anterior uveal melanoma
- Breed predisposition

Fibromatous/ossifying epulis
- Breed predisposition to the development of multiple tumours
- Seen in middle-aged/older dogs

Testicular neoplasia
- Believed to be a breed at increased risk

Neurological conditions
Congenital deafness
- Signs seen from birth

Primary brain tumour
- Higher incidence noted in this breed
- Older dogs affected (mean 9–10 years)

Sensory neuropathy of Boxers (progressive axonopathy)
- Autosomal recessive inheritance
- Rare
- Age of clinical onset: 2 months

Meningitis and polyarteritis
- Reported in this breed
- Age of onset: <1 year

Ocular conditions
Entropion
- Breed predisposition; polygenic inheritance likely
- Usually presents in the first year of life

Ectropion
- Breed predisposition; polygenic inheritance likely

Prolapse of the gland of the nictitating membrane ('cherry eye')
- Breed predisposition; possibly inherited
- Usually presents before 2 years of age

Distichiasis
- Breed predisposition

Refractory corneal ulceration
- Breed predisposition
- Age of onset: 4–8 years

Corneal endothelial dystrophy
- Breed predisposition
- Endothelial dystrophy with progressive corneal oedema

Canine anterior uveal melanoma
- Breed predisposition

Physiological conditions
Vertebral heart score
- The healthy dog has a higher mean score than most other breeds

Renal and urinary conditions
Urethral sphincter mechanism incompetence (causing urinary incontinence)
- Possible breed predisposition in female dogs

Reproductive conditions
Vaginal hyperplasia
- Breed predisposition

Cryptorchidism
- Developmental defect believed to be inherited as a sex-limited, autosomal recessive trait
- Believed to be a breed at increased risk of the condition

Testicular neoplasia
- Believed to be a breed at increased risk

BOYKIN SPANIEL

Cardiovascular conditions
Pulmonic stenosis
- Third most frequent cause of canine congenital heart disease
- May be a polygenic mode of inheritance

Musculoskeletal conditions
Incomplete ossification of the humeral condyle
- Cause unknown
- Polygenic recessive mode of inheritance
- Mean age of presentation is 6 years

BRIARD

Musculoskeletal conditions
Hip dysplasia
- This breed has the eighth worst breed mean score in the BVA/KC Hip Dysplasia Scheme as of October 2001
- Breed mean score 20
- Breed mean score is currently improving

Ocular conditions
Central progressive retinal atrophy (CPRA) or retinal pigment epithelial dystrophy (RPED)
- Breed predisposition; autosomal recessive inheritance has been sugggested
- Age of onset varies
- Previously prevalent in the UK, now uncommon
- Schedule 1 of the BVA/KC/ISDS Eye Scheme

Hereditary retinal dystrophy of Briards (congenital stationary night blindness)
- Autosomal recessive inheritance supected
- Congenital night blindness with variable effects on day vision
- Slowly progressive
- Possibly involves a defect in retinal polyunsaturated fatty acid metabolism

BRITTANY SPANIEL

Dermatological conditions
Histoplasmosis
- See under Infectious conditions

Grass awn migration
- Common in the summer months

Discoid lupus erythematosus
- Uncommon
- No age or sex predisposition recognised

Skin tumours
- See under Neoplastic conditions

Haematological conditions
Deficiency of third component of complement
- Discovered in a colony of Brittany Spaniels with inherited spinal muscular atrophy

DOGS

- Inherited as an autosomal recessive
- Inherited separately from the spinal atrophy gene

Infectious conditions
Histoplasmosis
- Uncommon
- Mainly restricted to central United States
- Usually affects dogs less than 4 years old

Musculoskeletal conditions
Hip dysplasia
- This breed has the fifteenth worst breed mean score in the BVA/KC Hip Dysplasia Scheme as of October 2001
- Breed mean score 18

Incomplete ossification of the humeral condyle
- Cause unknown
- Polygenic recessive mode of inheritance
- Mean age of presentation is 6 years

Spinal muscular atrophy
- See under Neurological conditions

Neoplastic conditions
Liposarcoma
- Average age of onset: 10 years
- Males may be predisposed

Neurological conditions
Cerebellar degeneration (late-onset)
- Uncommon
- Signs seen at 7–13 years

Spinal muscular atrophy
- Autosomal dominant inheritance suggested
- Rare
- Age of clinical onset: <1 year

Ocular conditions
Lens luxation
- Possible breed predisposition

Generalised progressive retinal atrophy (GPRA)
- Mode of inheritance unknown but presumed to be recessive

Vitreal syneresis
- Possible breed predisposition
- Occurs in older dogs
- Vitreal degeneration results in strands of vitreous extending into the anterior chamber predisposing to glaucoma and cataracts

Renal and urinary conditions
Familial renal disease (membranoproliferative glomerulonephritis)
- Reported in this breed
- Autosomal recessive inheritance suggested
- Affected dogs present at 4–9 years

BULLDOG (ENGLISH)

Cardiovascular conditions
Ventricular septal defect
- Marked risk in this breed (relative risk 5.0)
- No sex predilection
- Not known to be inherited in this breed

Tetralogy of Fallot
- Uncommon
- Congenital

Aortic stenosis
- Common congenital disease
- Relative risk >5.0
- No sex predilection
- Inheritance possibly autosomal dominant with modifying genes, or polygenic

Pulmonic stenosis
- Third most frequent cause of canine congenital heart disease
- May be polygenic mode of inheritance
- Relative risk 12.9
- May be associated anomalous coronary artery development in this breed

Dermatological conditions
Muzzle folliculitis and furunculosis
- Possible genetic susceptibility

Pododermatitis
- Males predisposed
- Front feet more commonly affected

Generalised demodicosis
- Bulldogs are in the ten breeds at highest statistical risk of this disease in the Cornell, USA, population

Hyperoestrogenism
- Rare
- Affects older, intact females

Canine follicular dysplasia
- A marked predilection in this breed implies a genetic basis for this group of diseases

Seasonal flank alopecia
- Tends to occur in spring or autumn

Primary lymphoedema
- No apparent sex predisposition
- Only seen in certain populations

Intertrigo
- May occur due to intentional breeding for excessive skin folding

Skin tumours
- See under Neoplastic conditions

Endocrine diseases
Hypothyroidism
- Reported in some texts to be at increased risk
- Often middle-aged (2–6 years)

Gastrointestinal conditions
Cleft palate
- Congenital disorder with inheritance suspected in this breed

Musculoskeletal conditions
Ununited anconeal process
- A true fracture of the process occurs in this breed

Congenital elbow luxation
- Type II luxation occurs in this breed (proximal radius displaced caudolaterally)
- Usually 4–5 months old at presentation

Hemivertebrae
- Mode of inheritance not known

Sacrocaudal dysgenesis
- Congenital
- See also under Neurological conditions

Brachyury

Hip dysplasia
- Although not ranked in the top 20 in the BVA/KC Hip Dysplasia Scheme, due to small numbers sampled, the breed mean score was 41

Neoplastic conditions
Mast cell tumours
- Possible breed predisposition
- May be seen at any age (from 4 months onwards), but usually seen in older animals

Primary brain tumour
- See under Neurological conditions

Lymphosarcoma (malignant lymphoma)
- Higher incidence noted in this breed
- Most cases are seen in middle-aged dogs (mean 6–7 years)

Neurological conditions
Congenital deafness
- Signs seen from birth

Hydrocephalus
- Congenital
- Relatively common
- Onset of clinical signs: <3 months

Hemivertebrae
- Congenital
- Occasionally seen

Spina bifida (and myelodysplasia)
- Congenital

Sacrocaudal dysgenesis
- Congenital
- Occasionally reported

Stenosis of the vertebral canal
- Congenital

Primary brain tumour
- Higher incidence noted in this breed
- Older dogs affected (mean 9–10 years)

DOGS

DOGS

Ocular conditions

Entropion (usually lower lid)
- Breed predisposition; polygenic inheritance likely

Macropalpebral fissure resulting in combined entropion–ectropion ('diamond eye')
- Breed predisposition; genetic basis incompletely understood

Distichiasis
- Breed predisposition

Trichiasis
- Breed predisposition; inheritance suspected

Keratoconjunctivitis sicca
- Breed predisposition
- Age of onset: 4–7 years

Prolapse of the gland of the nictitating membrane (see plate 4)
- Breed predisposition; possibly inherited
- Usually presents before 2 years of age

Refractory corneal ulceration
- Breed predisposition
- Usually middle-aged

Multifocal retinal dysplasia
- Simple autosomal recessive inheritance suspected

Physiological conditions

Achondroplasia
- Genetic dwarfism
- Skull and limbs affected
- Accepted as a breed standard

Renal and urinary conditions

Ectopic ureters
- Congenital anomaly; higher incidence reported in this breed
- Usually presents <1 year of age
- More commonly diagnosed in females

Urethrorectal fistula
- Possible breed predisposition
- Males more commonly affected than females

Urethral prolapse
- Possible breed predisposition
- Generally seen in male dogs at 4 months to 5 years of age

Sacrocaudal dysgenesis (causing urinary incontinence)
- Congenital
- Occasionally reported

Cystine urolithiasis
- Cystinuria results from an inherited defect in renal tubular transport of cystine and predisposes to cystine urolithiasis
- Higher incidence reported in this breed in some American surveys
- Average age at diagnosis is 1–8 years
- Males seem predisposed

Urate urolithiasis
- Higher incidence noted in this breed; familial predisposition suspected
- Average age at diagnosis is 3–6 years
- Males seem to be predisposed

Reproductive conditions

Dystocia
- Breed predisposition due to combination of narrow pelvis and large head/wide shoulders

Vaginal hyperplasia
- Possible breed predisposition

Cryptorchidism
- Developmental defect believed to be inherited as a sex-limited, autosomal recessive trait
- Believed to be a breed at increased risk of the condition

Urethral prolapse
- See under Renal and urinary conditions

Respiratory conditions

Hypoplastic trachea
- This breed accounts for 55% of cases

Brachycephalic upper airway syndrome
- Complex of anatomical deformities
- Common in this breed

- Likely to be a consequence of selective breeding for certain facial characteristics
- May be associated with non-cardiogenic pulmonary oedema in this breed
- Aerophagia associated with this condition may lead to excessive flatulence

BULL MASTIFF

Cardiovascular conditions
Pulmonic stenosis
- Third most frequent cause of canine congenital heart disease
- May be polygenic mode of inheritance

Dermatological conditions
Muzzle folliculitis and furunculosis
- Possible genetic susceptibility

Pododermatitis
- Males predisposed
- Front feet more commonly affected

Gastrointestinal conditions
Gastric dilatation-volvulus
- Possible breed predisposition

Musculoskeletal conditions
Congenital elbow luxation
- Type II luxation occurs in this breed (proximal radius displaced caudolaterally)
- Usually 4–5 months old at presentation

Hip dysplasia
- This breed has the fourth worst breed mean score in the BVA/KC Hip Dysplasia Scheme as of October 2001
- Breed mean score 28

Cranial cruciate ligament rupture
- Common cause of hind-limb lameness

Neoplastic conditions
Lymphosarcoma (malignant lymphoma)
- Familial incidence reported in this breed

Neurological conditions
Cerebellar degeneration
- Autosomal recessive inheritance suggested
- Uncommon

- Signs seen at 4–9 weeks
- May be seen with hydrocephalus

Ocular conditions
Entropion (may be associated with macropalpebral fissure)
- Breed predisposition; polygenic inheritance likely

Ectropion (may be associated with macropalpebral fissure)
- Breed predisposition; polygenic inheritance likely

Macropalpebral fissure resulting in combined entropion–ectropion ('diamond eye')
- Breed predisposition; genetic basis incompletely understood

Distichiasis
- Breed predisposition

Persistent pupillary membranes (PPM)
- Inheritance suspected
- Schedule 3 of the BVA/KC/ISDS Eye Scheme

Glaucoma
- Possible breed predisposition

Multifocal retinal dysplasia
- Breed predisposition; autosomal recessive inheritance suspected

Renal and urinary conditions
Cystine urolithiasis
- Cystinuria results from an inherited defect in renal tubular transport of cystine and predisposes to cystine urolithiasis
- Higher incidence reported in this breed in some American surveys
- Average age at diagnosis is 1–8 years
- Males seem predisposed

Reproductive conditions
Vaginal hyperplasia
- Breed predisposition

DOGS

BULL TERRIER

Cardiovascular conditions
Mitral dysplasia
- Congenital
- Genetic basis suspected

Aortic stenosis
- Common congenital disease
- Inheritance possibly autosomal dominant with modifying genes, or polygenic

Dermatological conditions
Nasal folliculitis and furunculosis
- Uncommon
- Unknown cause

Pododermatitis
- Males predisposed
- Front feet more commonly affected

Demodicosis
- Possible breed predisposition

Ichthyosis
- Rare; congenital

Acrodermatitis
- Inherited as an autosomal recessive trait

Waardenburg-Klein syndrome
- Inherited as an autosomal dominant trait with incomplete penetrance

Truncal solar dermatitis
- Affects white Bull Terriers
- More common in sunny climates

Zinc responsive dermatosis
- In Bull Terriers, occurs in puppies fed zinc-deficient diets

Skin tumours
- See under Neoplastic conditions

Haematological/immunological conditions
Acrodermatitis
- Inherited
- T-lymphocytes are depleted

Musculoskeletal conditions
Osteochondrodysplasia
- Does not cause dwarfing in this breed
- Familial but inheritance not known

Congenital elbow luxation
- Type II luxation occurs in this breed (proximal radius displaced caudolaterally)
- Usually 4–5 months old at presentation

Avulsion of tibial tuberosity
- A growth-plate avulsion fracture

Hock osteochondritis dissecans
- Affects dogs 4–6 months of age
- Reasonably common cause of lameness

Neoplastic conditions
Actinic keratosis (solar keratosis)
- Reported to be at increased risk
- Seen more commonly in pale-skinned animals with the opportunity for long periods of intense sun exposure

Mast cell tumours
- Possible breed predisposition
- May be seen at any age (from 4 months onwards), but usually seen in older animals

Neurological conditions
Congenital deafness
- Autosomal recessive inheritance suggested
- Signs seen from birth

Cerebellar malformation
- Congenital
- Uncommon
- Age of clinical onset: <3 months

Ocular conditions
Micropalpebral fissure
- Breed predisposition

Entropion (usually lateral lower lids, may be associated with micropalpebral fissure)
- Breed predisposition; polygenic inheritance likely

Ectropion (mild, usually disappears with maturity)
- Breed predisposition; polygenic inheritance likely

Prolapse of the gland of the nictitating membrane
- Breed predisposition
- Usually presents before 2 years of age

Renal and urinary conditions
Polycystic kidney disease
- Autosomal dominant inheritance suggested
- Polycystic kidney disease is associated with nodular thickenings of the mitral and aortic valves. Cases present, with haematuria and recurrent urinary tract infections more commonly than with uraemia, at 6–15 months of age. Some cases present with cardiac disease. Hepatic cysts have not been seen in these cases

Familial renal disease
- Autosomal dominant inheritance
- The condition is believed to be a glomerular basement-membrane disorder
- Proteinuria may be an early indicator with cases progressing to renal failure at 1–8 years of age

CAIRN TERRIER

Dermatological conditions
Atopy
- Common
- May be more prevalent in females

Endocrine conditions
Diabetes mellitus
- Possible breed predisposition
- Usual age range: 4–14 years; peak incidence: 7–9 years
- Old, entire females are predisposed

Gastrointestinal conditions
Congenital bronchoesophageal fistula
- Possible breed predisposition

Congenital portosystemic shunt
- Possible breed predisposition
- Clinical signs usually seen in young dogs <1 year

Microvascular portal dysplasia
- Breed predisposition
- Possibly inherited as a polygenic trait
- May be asymptomatic

Congenital polycystic liver disease
- Breed predisposition
- May be associated with polycystic kidney disease

Haematological conditions
Pyruvate kinase deficiency
- Inherited as an autosomal recessive trait

Haemophilia B
- Factor IX deficiency
- Also known as Christmas disease
- Inherited as a sex-linked trait
- Less common than haemophilia A

Musculoskeletal conditions
Craniomandibular osteopathy
- Aetiology unknown in this breed
- Usually affects dogs aged 3–8 months

Inguinal hernia

Neurological conditions
Lysosomal storage disease – globoid cell leukodystrophy (Krabbe's disease)
- Autosomal recessive inheritance
- Rare
- Signs seen at 6–12 months

Ocular conditions
Refractory corneal ulceration
- Breed predisposition
- Usually middle-aged

Ocular melanosis
- Familial
- Age of onset: 7–13 years
- Predisposes to glaucoma
- Schedule 3 of the BVA/KC/ISDS Eye Scheme

Lens luxation
- Autosomal dominant inheritance has been suggested
- Age of onset: 4–5 years

Cataract
- Inheritance suspected

DOGS

Retinal dysplasia
- Mode of inheritance unknown, but autosomal recessive suspected

Renal and urinary conditions
Polycystic kidney disease
- Autosomal recessive inheritance suggested
- Cysts are found throughout the liver and kidneys from an early age (6 weeks). Cases often present because of abdominal enlargement due to hepato- and renomegaly

Reproductive conditions
Cryptorchidism
- Developmental defect believed to be inherited as a sex-limited, autosomal recessive trait
- Believed to be a breed at increased risk of the condition

Respiratory conditions
Congenital bronchoesophageal fistula
- Possible breed predisposition

Pulmonary interstitial fibrosis
- Aetiology unknown
- Affects older dogs

CARNELIAN BEAR DOG

Endocrine conditions
Pituitary dwarfism
- Autosomal recessive mode of inheritance suggested
- Pituitary dwarfism occurs primarily in the German Shepherd Dog but has also been reported in this breed

CAVALIER KING CHARLES SPANIEL

Cardiovascular conditions
Endocardiosis
- Also known as chronic valvular disease
- Relative risk very high (20.1)
- In the UK, 59% of Cavaliers over 4 years of age had a heart murmur
- Increased prevalence with age
- Aetiology unknown but likely genetic basis

Patent ductus arteriosus
- Common congenital abnormality
- Females predisposed
- Mode of inheritance polygenic

Dermatological conditions
Ichthyosis
- Rare; congenital

Persistent scratching in Cavalier King Charles spaniels
- Young onset
- May be familial

Immunological conditions
Undefined immunodeficiency syndrome
- Involves a protozoal pneumonia *(Pneumocystis carinii)*
- Exact immunodeficiency uncertain

Infectious conditions
Pneumocystis carinii infection
- Reported in this breed
- May reflect a concurrent immunodeficiency syndrome (see Immunological conditions)

Musculoskeletal conditions
Myopathy associated with falling Cavaliers
- See episodic falling under Neurological conditions

Inguinal/scrotal herniation
- Females predisposed

Shoulder luxation
- Congenital

Neurological conditions
Episodic falling
- Seen in the UK
- Age of clinical onset: 3–4 months

Ocular conditions
Entropion (usually medial lids)
- Breed predisposition; polygenic inheritance likely

Distichiasis
- Breed predisposition; inheritance suspected

Keratoconjunctivitis sicca
- Breed predisposition

Corneal dystrophy
- Autosomal dominant or polygenic mode of inheritance has been suggested
- Stromal lipid dystrophy
- Age of onset: 2–4 years

Cataract
- Inheritance suspected
- Progressive cataracts which become complete in young adult
- Schedule 1 of the BVA/KC/ISDS Eye Scheme

Multifocal retinal dysplasia
- Congenital condition; inheritance as an autosomal recessive trait suspected
- Schedule 1 of the BVA/KC/ISDS Eye Scheme

Geographic retinal dysplasia
- Congenital condition; inheritance suspected
- Reported in the UK

Generalised progressive retinal atrophy (GPRA)
- Mode of inheritance unknown but presumed to be recessive
- Age of clinical onset may be delayed to 4–5 years

Multiple ocular defects
- Congenital condition; inheritance suspected
- Defects may include microphthalmia, persistence of the hyaloid system and congenital cataract
- Schedule 3 of the BVA/KC/ISDS Eye Scheme

Physiological conditions
Giant platelets and thrombocytopaenia
- Giant platelets may lead to reduced count of platelets if using automated methods
- Manual counts show normal or reduced platelet counts
- Inherited as an autosomal recessive trait

Respiratory conditions
Brachycephalic upper airway syndrome
- Complex of anatomical deformities
- Common in this breed
- A likely consequence of selective breeding for certain facial characteristics

Pneumonia due to *Pneumocystis carinii* infection
- Reported in this breed
- May reflect a concurrent immunodeficiency syndrome (see Immunological conditions)

CHESAPEAKE BAY RETRIEVER

Haematological conditions
Von Willebrand's disease
- This breed is affected by type III disease
- Inherited as an autosomal recessive trait

Musculoskeletal conditions
Cranial cruciate ligament rupture
- Neutered individuals may be predisposed
- Young animals may be predisposed in this breed

Neurological conditions
Distal symmetrical polyneuropathy
- Reported in this breed
- Age of clinical onset: >1 year

Ocular conditions
Entropion (usually lateral lower lid)
- Breed predisposition, polygenic inheritance likely

Distichiasis
- Breed predisposition inheritance suspected

Refractory corneal ulceration
- Breed predisposition
- Usually middle-aged

Uveal cysts
- Breed predisposition
- Age of clinical onset: 3–6 years

DOGS

Cataract

- Dominant mode of inheritance with incomplete penetration has been suggested
- Localisation: equator, posterior pole and lens sutures
- Age of onset: 1 year; may progress
- Schedule 1 of the BVA/KC/ISDS Eye Scheme

Multifocal retinal dysplasia

- Congenital condition; autosomal recessive inheritance suspected

Generalised progressive retinal atrophy (GPRA)

- Autosomal recessive inheritance suspected
- Early onset (ophthalmoscopically detectable at 8–12 months) and late onset (ophthalmoscopically detectable at 4–7 years) cases have been seen
- Schedule 1 BVA/KC/ISDS Eye Scheme

Reproductive conditions
Vaginal hyperplasia

- Possible breed predisposition

CHIHUAHUA

Cardiovascular conditions
Patent ductus arteriosus

- Common congenital abnormality
- Relative risk 2.8
- Females predisposed
- Mode of inheritance: polygenic

Endocardiosis

- Also known as chronic valvular disease
- Relative risk high (5.5)
- Increased prevalence with age
- Aetiology unknown but genetic basis likely

Pulmonic stenosis

- Third most frequent cause of canine congenital heart disease
- Possibly inherited as a polygenic trait
- Relative risk 3.7

Dermatological conditions
Malassezia dermatitis

- Any age
- May be seasonal

Pinnal alopecia

- Age of onset: usually >1 year

Pattern baldness

- Probably inherited

Colour-dilution alopecia

- Coat-colour genes significant in the pathogenesis

Anal sac disease

- No age or sex predispostition

Skin tumours

- See under Neoplastic conditions

Musculoskeletal conditions
Bilateral radial agenesis

- May be inherited as an autosomal recessive trait

Congenital elbow luxation

- Uncommon; accounts for 15% of non-traumatic elbow lameness
- Severe disability in this breed (type I)
- Present at birth or in first 3 months of life

Foramen magnum dysplasia

- Congenital

Medial patellar luxation

- Significant hereditary component suspected

Odontoid process dysplasia

- Congenital

Shoulder luxation

- Congenital

Delayed/non-union of fractures of the distal third of the radius and ulna in miniature and toy breeds

- May be associated with inadequate immobilisation

Inguinal/scrotal herniation

- Females predisposed

Neoplastic conditions
Melanoma

- Breed predisposition
- Average age 8–9 years

Testicular neoplasia
- Believed to be a breed at increased risk

Neurological conditions
Hydrocephalus
- Congenital
- Relatively common
- Age of clinical onset: <3 months

Lysosomal storage disease – ceroid lipofuscinosis
- Inheritance suspected
- Rare
- Signs seen at 6–12 months

Atlantoaxial subluxation
- Congenital
- Relatively common in this breed
- Age of clinical onset: <1 year

Ocular conditions
Corneal dystrophy
- Breed predisposition
- Endothelial dystrophy with progressive corneal oedema
- Age of onset: 6–13 years

Glaucoma
- Possible breed predisposition
- May be associated with goniodysgenesis in this breed

Lens luxation
- Breed predisposition; inheritance suspected
- Age of onset: 4–7 years

Neuronal ceroid lipofusinosis
- Inheritance suspected
- Rare condition

Renal and urinary conditions
Cystine urolithiasis
- Cystinuria results from an inherited defect in renal tubular transport of cystine and predisposes to cystine urolithiasis
- Higher incidence reported in this breed in some American surveys
- Average age at diagnosis is 1–8 years
- Males seem predisposed

Reproductive conditions
Cryptorchidism
- Developmental defect believed to be inherited as a sex-limited, autosomal recessive trait
- Believed to be a breed at increased risk of the condition

Testicular neoplasia
- Believed to be a breed at increased risk

Respiratory conditions
Collapsed trachea
- Lesion due to a deficiency in tracheal cartilage
- Usually acquired in older dogs but can be congenital

CHINESE CRESTED DOG

Dermatological conditions
Alopecia
- Chinese Crested is a hairless breed
- The breed is produced by a dominant gene for hypotrichosis being combined with the gene for long hair
- Homozygotes (HH) for hypotrichosis die prenatally
- All Cresteds are Hh if hairless
- hh are coated (called 'powder puffs')

CHOW CHOW

Cardiovascular conditions
Pulmonic stenosis
- Third most frequent cause of canine congenital heart disease
- Possibly inherited as a polygenic trait

Dermatological conditions
Flea bite hypersensitivity
- Most studies show no breed predisposition, but one French study showed Chow Chows were predisposed

Pemphigus foliaceous
- No age or sex predispositions noted

DOGS

Post-clipping alopecia

Colour-dilution alopecia
- Coat-colour genes significant in pathogenesis

Tyrosinase deficiency
- Extremely rare

Canine uveodermatological syndrome
- Also known as Vogt-Koyanagi-Harada-like syndrome
- See also under Ocular conditions

Adult-onset growth-hormone-responsive dermatosis
- See under Endocrine conditions

Endocrine conditions
Adult-onset growth-hormone-responsive dermatosis
- Breed predisposition
- Males maybe predisposed
- Clinical signs usually seen at 1–5 years

Hypothyroidism
- Reported in some texts to be at increased risk
- Often middle-aged (2–6 years)

Gastrointestinal conditions
Congenital (sliding) hiatal hernia
- Possible breed predisposition

Musculoskeletal conditions
Myotonia
- Condition described in this breed in the UK, Australia, New Zealand, Holland and the USA
- First seen in young puppies
- Familial, but mode of inheritance not known
- May have been bred into Chows when they were selected for being highly muscled, as they were previously bred for meat

Cranial cruciate ligament rupture
- Common cause of hind-limb lameness

Neoplastic conditions
Melanoma
- Breed predisposition
- Average age 8–9 years

Lymphosarcoma (malignant lymphoma)
- Higher incidence noted in this breed
- Most cases are seen in middle-aged dogs (mean 6–7 years)

Neurological conditions
Cerebellar malformation
- Congenital
- Uncommon
- Age of clinical onset: <3 months

Hypomyelination of the central nervous system
- Inheritance suspected
- Signs seen at 2–8 weeks

Ocular conditions
Micropalpebral fissure
- Breed predisposition

Entropion (usually lower lids)
- Breed predisposition; polygenic inheritance likely

Ectropion
- Breed predisposition; polygenic inheritance likely

Glaucoma
- Breed predisposition
- Age of onset: 3–6 years
- Usually associated in this breed with a narrow iridocorneal filtration angle

Persistent pupillary membranes
- Breed predisposition; inheritance suspected
- May be severe in this breed

Uveodermatologic syndrome
- Also known as Vogt-Koyanagi-Harada-like syndrome
- Breed predisposition
- Young adults affected (1.5–4 years)

Renal and urinary conditions
Familial renal disease (renal dysplasia)
- This condition was reported in six young related Chows
- Affected dogs presented with renal failure at 6 months to 1 year of age

CLUMBER SPANIEL

Musculoskeletal conditions
Mitochondrial myopathy
- Rare
- Primary defect is in mitochondrial function
- Can cause sudden death

Hip dysplasia
- This breed has the second worst breed mean score in the BVA/KC Hip Dysplasia Scheme as of October 2001
- Breed mean score 42

Ocular conditions
Entropion (may be associated with macropalpebral fissure)
- Breed predisposition; polygenic inheritance likely

Ectropion (may be associated with macropalpebral fissure)
- Breed predisposition; polygenic inheritance likely

Macropalpebral fissure resulting in combined entropion–ectropion ('diamond eye')
- Breed predisposition; genetic basis incompletely understood

Cataract
- Inheritance suspected

COCKER SPANIEL

Cardiovascular conditions
Patent ductus arteriosus
- Congenital
- Relative risk 2.6

Pulmonic stenosis
- Third most frequent cause of canine congenital heart disease
- Possibly inherited as a polygenic trait
- Relative risk of 1.6 not statistically significant

Endocardiosis
- Also known as chronic valvular disease
- Relative risk 2.0 (not statistically significant)
- Increased prevalence with age
- Aetiology unknown but a genetic basis is likely

Dilated cardiomyopathy (DCM) (American Cocker Spaniels)
- DCM in this breed is often related to taurine deficiency
- May respond to taurine and L-carnitine supplementation

Familial cardiomyopathy (English Cocker Spaniels)

Sick sinus syndrome
- Middle-aged to old dogs
- Relative risk 1.7
- No sex predisposition in this breed

Dermatological conditions
Atopy
- Common
- Possibly more common in females
- Age of onset variable, from 6 months to 7 years

Primary seborrhea (American Cocker Spaniels)
- Condition commonly recognised in this breed
- Probably inherited as an autosomal recessive trait
- Early onset; progresses with age

Congenital hypotrichosis (American Cocker Spaniels)
- Present at birth or occurs in first month
- May be sex linked

Black hair follicular dysplasia (American Cocker Spaniels)
- Familial
- Normal at birth; changes develop in the first month

Cryptococcosis
- See under Infectious conditions

Food hypersensitivity
- No age or sex predisposition reported

Vitamin-A-responsive dermatosis

Tail-dock neuroma
- Rare

DOGS

Intertrigo
- Spaniels are predisposed to lip fold pyoderma

Onychodystrophy
- May be related to seborrhoea in Cockers

Anal sac disease
- No age or sex predisposition

Skin tumours
- See under Neoplastic conditions

Endocrine conditions
Hypothyroidism
- Reported in some texts to be at increased risk
- Often middle-aged (2–6 years)

Musculoskeletal conditions
Brachyury
- Possibly inherited as an autosomal recessive trait

Chondrodysplasia
- Causes disproportionate dwarfism

Congenital elbow luxation
- Uncommon; accounts for 15% of non-traumatic elbow lameness
- Severe disability in this breed (type I)
- Present at birth or in first 3 months of life

Foramen magnum dysplasia
- Congenital

Incomplete ossification of the humeral condyle
- Cause unknown
- Polygenic recessive mode of inheritance
- Mean age of presentation is 6 years

Inguinal/scrotal herniation
- Females predisposed

Temporomandibular dysplasia
- Congenital
- Usually affects dogs from 6 months of age

Cranial cruciate ligament rupture (American Cocker Spaniels)
- Common cause of hind-limb lameness

Spondylosis deformans (American Cocker Spaniels)
- Usually clinically insignificant

Patellar luxation (American Cocker Spaniels)
- May be inherited as an autosomal recessive trait

Umbilical hernia (American Cocker Spaniels)

Prognathia (American Cocker Spaniels)
- Inherited as a recessive trait

Gastrointestinal diseases
Cricopharyngeal achalasia
- Possible breed predisposition
- Symptoms seen at or shortly after weaning

Oropharyngeal neoplasia
- Possible breed predisposition

Chronic hepatitis
- Breed predisposition

Alpha-1-antitrypsin-related hepatitis
- Breed predisposition, inheritance suspected

Haematological/immunological conditions
Immune-mediated haemolytic anaemia
- Common disease
- Usually affects young adult and middle-aged animals
- May be more common in bitches
- May be seasonal variations

Platelet storage-pool deficiency (American Cocker Spaniels)
- May cause severe haemorrhage

Haemophilia B (American Cocker Spaniels)
- Factor IX deficiency
- Also known as Christmas disease
- Inherited as a sex-linked trait
- Less common than haemophilia A

Factor X deficiency
- Familial
- May be inherited as an autosomal recessive trait

Immune-mediated thrombocytopaenia
- Common
- Inheritance likely
- Females more commonly affected than males

Immune-mediated cardiomyopathy
- Described in one colony
- Inherited
- Associated with anti-mitochondrial antibodies
- Other sporadic immune-mediated disease was seen in the same line

Infectious conditions
Coccidiomycosis
- Increased incidence in this breed, possibly due to an increased likelihood of exposure
- Seen mainly in young male dogs
- Geographic distribution: California, Arizona, Texas, New Mexico, Nevada, Utah, Mexico and parts of Central and South America. Not reported in the UK

Cryptococcosis (American Cocker Spaniels)
- Increased incidence in this breed, possibly due to an increased likelihood of exposure
- Usually seen in dogs under 4 years; no obvious sex predilection
- Worldwide distribution, but favoured by warm, humid climates

Infectious skin disease
- See under Dermatological conditions

Neoplastic conditions
Basal cell tumour
- Reported to be at increased risk

Sweat gland tumour
- Uncommon
- Reported to be at increased risk
- Average age reported as 9.5 years

Trichoepithelioma
- Possible breed predisposition
- Average age 9 years

Cutaneous papillomas
- Possible breed predisposition
- Seen in older dogs

Sebaceous gland tumours
- Possible breed predisposition to nodular sebaceous hyperplasia
- Seen in older dogs (average age 10 years)

Cutaneous plasmacytoma
- Occur at an average age of 10 years
- No sex predisposition

Canine cutaneous histiocytoma
- Possible breed predisposition
- More common in young dogs 1–2 years of age

Trichoblastoma
- Common
- No sex predisposition
- Usually older than 5 years

Fibrosarcoma
- Affects older dogs
- Females predisposed

Non-epitheliotropic lymphoma
- Affects older dogs
- No sex predisposition

Perianal (hepatoid) gland adenomas
- Breed predisposition suggested in one survey of 2700 cases
- Average age was 10.5 years
- Entire males were predisposed

Anal sac adenocarcinoma (English Cocker Spaniels)
- Breed predisposition suggested in one survey of 232 cases
- Average age was 10.5 years
- Some surveys suggest a predisposition for females

Melanoma
- Breed predisposition
- Average age 8–9 years

Lipoma
- Possible breed predisposition
- Most common in middle-aged, obese female dogs

Limbal melanoma
- Possible breed predisposition

Neurological conditions
Congenital deafness
- Signs seen from birth

Congenital vestibular disease (English Cocker Spaniels)
- Signs seen <3 months

Acquired vestibular disease secondary to otitis interna
- Breed predisposition to chronic otitis externa which may progress to otitis media/interna

Intervertebral disc disease (see figure 6)
- Breed predisposition
- Relatively common condition
- Age of clinical onset: 3–7 years

True epilepsy
- Inheritance suspected
- Age of onset: 6 months to 3 years

Lysosomal storage disease – ceroid lipofuscinosis
- Inheritance suspected
- Rare
- Signs seen at 1–2 years

Idiopathic facial paralysis
- Breed predisposition
- Acute onset in adults

Multisystem neuronal degeneration
- Reported in this breed; inheritance suspected
- Age of clinical onset: 10–14 months

Ocular conditions
Entropion (usually upper lateral eyelids) (American and English Cocker Spaniels)
- Breed predisposition
- Often seen as the dog ages

Ectropion (usually lower eyelids) (American and English Cocker Spaniels)
- Breed predisposition
- Often seen as the dog ages

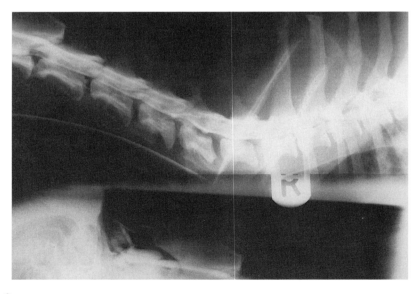

Figure 6
Myelogram of a nine-year-old male Cocker Spaniel with a disc herniation at C5–C6. There is a narrowed intervertebral space, compression of the spinal cord and evidence of disc material in the spinal canal at this site.

Distichiasis (American and English Cocker Spaniels)
- Breed predisposition; mode of inheritance unknown
- High incidence (>80% in some surveys)

Trichiasis (English Cocker Spaniels)
- Breed predisposition
- May be seen with upper eyelid entropion and lower eyelid ectropion in older dogs

Lacrimal punctal aplasia (usually lower duct) (American and English Cocker Spaniels)
- Breed predisposition

Limbal melanoma (American and English Cocker Spaniels)
- Possible breed predisposition

Refractory corneal ulceration (American Cocker Spaniels)
- Breed predisposition
- Usually middle-aged, may be a result of multiple eyelid defects

Keratoconjunctivitis sicca (American Cocker Spaniels)
- Breed predisposition

Corneal dystrophy (American Cocker Spaniels)
- Inheritance suspected; mode unknown
- Lipid dystrophy

Corneal (endothelial) dystrophy (American Cocker Spaniels)
- Dominant inheritance (complete or incomplete) has been suggested
- Posterior polymorphous dystrophy

Glaucoma

Primary glaucoma/goniodysgenesis (English Cocker Spaniels)
- Mode of inheritance unknown
- Mainly in the UK (less common in the USA)
- Schedule 1 of the BVA/KC/ISDS Eye Scheme

Primary glaucoma (American Cocker Spaniels)
- Mode of inheritance unknown
- Age of onset: 3.5–9 years

- Most cases are associated with a narrow iridocorneal filtration angle
- Schedule 1 of the BVA/KC/ISDS Eye Scheme

Lens luxation (English Cocker Spaniels)
- Possible breed predisposition in the UK

Persistent pupillary membranes (English Cocker Spaniels)
- Inheritance suspected
- Schedule 3 of the BVA/KC/ISDS Eye Scheme

Cataract (English Cocker Spaniels)
- Inheritance suspected
- Localisation: posterior suture lines
- Age of onset bimodal: 1.5–3 years and 8–9 years
- Females appear to be predisposed to later onset cataracts
- Nuclear cataracts also occur (at 2 years)

Cataract (American Cocker Spaniels)
- Autosomal recessive has been suggested in some cases
- Localisation: posterior and anterior cortex
- Age of onset: 1–5 years; progression is variable
- Schedule 1 of the BVA/KC/ISDS Eye Scheme
- Relatively common condition in this breed

Multifocal retinal dysplasia (American Cocker Spaniels)
- Simple autosomal recessive inheritance suspected
- Schedule 1 of the BVA/KC/ISDS Eye Scheme

Generalised progressive retinal atrophy (English Cocker Spaniels)
- Autosomal recessive inheritance
- Progressive rod-cone degeneration (PRCD)
- Ophthalmoscopic signs are visible by 4–8 years. May be associated with cataract formation
- Schedule 1 BVA/KC/ISDS Eye Scheme

Generalised progressive retinal atrophy (GPRA) (American Cocker Spaniels)
- Autosomal recessive inheritance
- Progressive rod-cone degeneration (PRCD)

- Ophthalmoscopic signs are visible by 2–3 years, night blindness is present at 3–5 years, progressing to total blindness at 5–7 years. May be associated with cataract formation
- Schedule 1 BVA/KC/ISDS Eye Scheme

Central progressive retinal atrophy (CPRA) or retinal pigment epithelial dystrophy (RPED) (English Cocker Spaniels)
- Breed predisposition; inheritance suspected
- More prevalent in the UK than in the USA
- Schedule 1 of the BVA/KC/ISDS Eye Scheme

Optic nerve coloboma (American Cocker Spaniels)
- Mode of inheritance unknown
- Seen occasionally in this breed, no effect on vision

Multiple ocular defects (English Cocker Spaniels)
- Mode of inheritance unknown
- Defects may include microphthalmia, persistent pupillary membranes and congenital cataract
- Schedule 3 of the BVA/KC/ISDS Eye Scheme

Neuronal ceroid lipofuscinosis
- Inheritance suspected
- See also under Neurological conditions

Renal and urinary conditions
Familial renal disease (English Cocker Spaniels)
- Autosomal recessive inheritance suggested
- The condition is believed to be a glomerular basement-membrane disorder
- Cases present at between 6 months and 2 years of age with proteinuria and chronic renal failure

Struvite (magnesium ammonium phosphate) urolithiasis
- Higher incidence has been reported in this breed in some surveys
- Average age at diagnosis is 2–8 years
- Females seem to be predisposed

Calcium phosphate urolithiasis (hydroxyapatite and carbonate apatite)
- Higher incidence has been reported in this breed in some surveys

Reproductive conditions
XX sex reversal
- Congenital condition reported to be an autosomal recessive trait in this breed

Penile hypoplasia
- Rare congenital condition that has been reported in this breed
- May be seen as part of some intersex states

Respiratory conditions
Spontaneous thymic haemorrhage
- Usually fatal
- Usually occurs in dogs less than two years old in association with thymic involution

Bronchiectasis (American Cocker Spaniels)
- Usually affects middle-aged to older dogs
- Usually occurs secondary to chronic pulmonary disease

COLLIES (ROUGH AND SMOOTH)

Dermatological conditions
Cutaneous histiocytosis
- No apparent age or sex predisposition

Superficial bacterial folliculitis
- Can resemble endocrine alopecia in this breed
- Relative risk 2.0

Muzzle folliculitis/furunculosis
- Also known as canine acne
- Local trauma, hormones and genetics may play a role in the pathogenesis

Malassezia dermatitis
- Often seasonal
- Affects any age

Protot’hecosis
- Rare
- Females predisposed

Food hypersensitivity
- No age or sex predisposition reported

Pemphigus erythematosus
- No age or sex predisposition

Systemic lupus erythematosus
- Uncommon (incidence approximately 0.03% of general canine population)
- No age or sex predisposition

Discoid lupus erythematosus
- No age or sex predisposition
- Accounted for 0.3% of skin diseases at one referral institution

Familial canine dermatomyositis
- Inherited as an autosomal dominant trait with incomplete penetrance
- No predispositions for sex, coat colour or coat length

Idiopathic ulcerative dermatosis in Shetland Sheepdogs and Collies
- Unknown cause
- No sex predisposition
- Affects middle-aged to older dogs

Vitiligo
- Presumed to be hereditary

Waardenburg-Klein syndrome
- Inherited as an autosomal dominant trait with incomplete penetrance

Idiopathic sterile granuloma and pyogranuloma
- Uncommon
- No age or sex predisposition

Skin tumours
- See under Neoplastic conditions

Drug reactions
Ivermectin and milbemycin (see figure 7)
- High doses can cause tremors, ataxia, coma and death

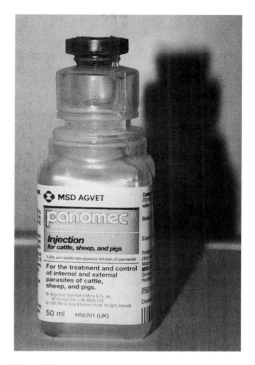

Figure 7
Collies can have severe reactions to ivermectin.

Gastrointestinal conditions
Gastric neoplasia (Rough Collies)
- Higher risk for this breed noted in one study
- Male dogs more commonly affected
- Mean age of occurrence: 8–10 years

Lymphocytic-plasmacytic colitis (Rough Collies)
- Possible breed predisposition

Pancreatic acinar atrophy (causing exocrine pancreatic insufficiency)
- Breed predisposition

Haematological/immunological conditions
Canine cyclic neutropaenia
- Inherited as an autosomal recessive trait
- Associated with grey Collies

DOGS

Immune-mediated haemolytic anaemia
- Common disease
- Usually affects young adult and middle-aged animals
- May be more common in bitches
- May be seasonal variations in incidence

Systemic lupus erythematosus
- Inherited, but not by a simple mechanism

Infectious conditions
Aspergillosis
- Breed predisposition
- Usually seen in young to middle-aged dogs

Infectious skin diseases
- See under Dermatological conditions

Musculoskeletal conditions
Carpal ligament weakening
- Affects older, obese dogs
- Tarsal ligaments may also be affected

Carpal soft tissue injuries
- Often caused by carpal hyperextension during exercise

Congenital elbow luxation
- Type II luxation occurs in this breed (proximal radius displaced caudolaterally)
- Usually 4–5 months old at presentation

Angular deformity of the tibia
- Uncommon
- Caused by injury to the distal tibial growth plate

Calcaneoquartal subluxation due to plantar tarsal ligament rupture
- Common hock injury
- Affects athletic dogs during exercising

Neoplastic conditions
Sweat gland tumour
- Reported to be at increased risk
- Average age reported as 9.5 years

Benign fibrous histiocytoma
- Occurs at an average age of 2–4 years
- No sex predisposition

Haemangiopericytoma
- Occurs at a mean age of 7–10 years
- No sex predisposition

Keratoacanthoma
- Usually affects dogs younger than 5 years
- Male dogs predisposed
- This breed is predisposed to the solitary form of the disease

Nasal cavity tumours
- Reported to be at increased risk
- Average age reported as 10.5–11 years
- Dogs in urban areas may be at increased risk

Colorectal neoplasia
- A higher incidence in this breed suggested in some reports
- Older dogs affected, with a mean age of 8.5 years

Neurological conditions
Congenital bilateral vestibular disease
- Reported in this breed

Congenital deafness
- Signs seen from birth

Cerebellar degeneration (seen in Rough Collies in Australia)
- Autosomal recessive inheritance
- Uncommon
- Signs seen at 1–2 months

Neuroaxonal dystrophy
- Autosomal recessive inheritance suspected
- Rare
- Age of clinical onset: 2–4 months

Ocular conditions
Micropalpebral fissure
- Breed predisposition

Entropion (usually lower lids, may be associated with micropalpebral fissure)
- Breed predisposition; polygenic inheritance likely

Distichiasis (Rough Collies)
- Breed predisposition

Medial canthal pocket syndrome
- Breed predisposition resulting from head shape

Nodular Episclerokeratitis
- Breed predisposition
- Usually presents at 2–5 years

Microcornea
- Breed predisposition
- Usually found associated with multiple ocular anomalies

Congenital, sub-epithelial, geographic corneal dystrophy
- Breed predisposition
- Occurs in young puppies (<10 weeks); transient condition

Corneal dystrophy (Rough Collies) (see plate 5)
- Autosomal dominant or polygenic mode of inheritance has been suggested
- Stromal lipid dystrophy
- Age of onset: 1–4 years

Cataract
- Inheritance suspected
- Several types and ages of onset exist

Collie eye anomaly
- Congenital disorder originally thought to be inherited as a simple autosomal recessive trait. More recently, polygenic inheritance has been suggested
- High incidence in this breed throughout the world (50–90% has been reported)
- Schedule 1 of the BVA/KC/ISDS Eye Scheme (Rough and Smooth Collies)

Multifocal retinal dysplasia
- Congenital condition; mode of inheritance not defined
- Schedule 3 of the BVA/KC/ISDS Eye Scheme (Rough Collies)

Generalised progressive retinal atrophy (GPRA)
- Autosomal recessive inheritance
- Rod-cone dysplasia type 2
- Ophthalmoscopic signs visible by 16 weeks; endstage and blindness reached at approximately 1 year

- Schedule 1 of the BVA/KC/ISDS Eye Scheme (Rough Collies)
- Rod-cone degeneration occurs less commonly; blindness occurs later at 5–7 years (mode of inheritance undefined)

Central progressive retinal atrophy (CPRA) or retinal pigment epithelial dystrophy (RPED)
- Breed predisposition; inheritance suspected
- More prevalent in the UK than in the USA. Becoming less prevalent following the introduction of control schemes
- Opthalmoscopic signs seen from 2 years of age; visual problems noticed at 4–5 years
- Schedule 1 of the BVA/KC/ISDS Eye Scheme (Rough and Smooth Collies)

Optic nerve hypoplasia
- Congenital condition; not known if inherited
- Seen occasionally in Collies

Optic nerve colobomas
- Congenital defect
- Usually seen as part of Collie eye anomaly

Multiple ocular defects
- Congenital condition, seen in homozygous merles (the result of merle to merle breeding) with predominantly white coats
- Defects may include microphthalmia, microcornea, congenital cataract and defects of the retina. Affected animals are also usually deaf
- Schedule 3 of the BVA/KC/ISDS Eye Scheme (Rough Collies)

Renal and urinary conditions
Ectopic ureters
- Congenital anomaly; higher incidence reported in Collies
- Usually presents <1 year of age
- More commonly diagnosed in females

Urethral sphincter mechanism incompetence (causing urinary incontinence)
- Possible breed predisposition in female dogs

Reproductive conditions
Penile hypoplasia
- Rare congenital condition which has been reported in this breed
- May be seen as part of some intersex states

DOGS

Respiratory conditions
Aspergillosis
- See under Infectious conditions

COONHOUND

Dermatological conditions
Blastomycosis
- See under Infectious conditions

Haematological conditions
Haemophilia B (Black and Tan Coonhounds)
- Factor IX deficiency
- Also known as Christmas disease
- Inherited as a sex-linked trait
- Less common than haemophilia A

Infectious conditions
Blastomycosis
- A breed predisposition due to increased likelihood of exposure has been suggested in Bluetick and Treeing Walker Coonhounds
- Seen mainly in young male dogs living near water
- Geographic distribution: around the Mississippi, Ohio, Missouri, Tennessee and St Lawrence Rivers, the southern Great Lakes and the southern mid-Atlantic states

Neurological conditions
Polyradiculoneuritis
- Breed predisposition, possibly due to exposure to raccoon bites whilst hunting

Ocular conditions
Entropion (Black and Tan Coonhounds)
- Breed predisposition; polygenic inheritance likely

Ectropion (Black and Tan Coonhounds)
- Breed predisposition; polygenic inheritance likely

Cataract (Black and Tan Coonhounds)
- Inheritance suspected

Generalised progressive retinal atrophy (GPRA) (Black and Tan Coonhounds)
- Mode of inheritance unknown but presumed to be recessive
- Clinically evident at 2 years of age

Central progressive retinal atrophy (CPRA) or retinal pigment epithelial dystrophy (RPED) (Black and Tan Coonhounds)
- Breed predisposition; inheritance suspected
- Reported in the USA
- Clinically evident at 2 years of age

CURLY-COATED RETRIEVER

Dermatological conditions
Canine follicular dysplasia
- A marked predilection in this breed implies a genetic basis for this group of diseases
- Hair loss begins at 2–4 years of age and occurs mainly on the flanks
- Hair loss is due to fracture of the hair in this breed
- Eventually the whole of the trunk is involved

Ocular conditions
Entropion (usually lateral lower lids)
- Breed predisposition; polygenic inheritance likely

Ectropion
- Breed predisposition; polygenic inheritance likely

Distichiasis
- Breed predisposition; mode of inheritance unknown

Cataract
- Inheritance suspected
- Anterior cortical subcapsular cataracts occur at 5–8 years and are slowly progressive
- Posterior subcapsular cataracts occur at 2–4 years and are slowly progressive

Generalised progressive retinal atrophy (GPRA)
- Autosomal recessive inheritance suspected
- Detected at 3–5 years; end stage by 6–7 years

DACHSHUND

Cardiovascular conditions
Sick sinus syndrome
- Affects old dogs of this breed
- No sex predisposition

Patent ductus arteriosus
- Common congenital abnormality
- Relative risk 2.5
- Females predisposed
- Mode of inheritance is polygenic

Dermatological conditions
Alopecia areata
- Uncommon
- No age or sex predisposition

Pododermatitis
- Front feet more commonly affected

Malassezia dermatitis
- May be seasonal

Food hypersensitivity
- No age or sex predisposition
- Not all studies confirm a breed predisposition

Pemphigus foliaceous
- Uncommon disease
- No sex predisposition
- Mean age of onset 4 years

Canine linear IgA dermatosis
- Very rare

Oestrogen-responsive dermatosis
- Affects spayed females
- Usually occurs in young adults
- Rare

Canine pinnal alopecia (pattern baldness)
- Onset from 6–9 months of age
- Males more commonly affected than females in this breed
- Alopecia of the pinnae is usually complete by 8–9 years of age

Primary seborrhoea
- Probably inherited as an autosomal recessive trait
- Signs occur early and worsen with age

Black hair follicular dysplasia
- Rare
- Early onset
- Familial

Idiopathic sterile nodular panniculitis
- Multiple lesions seen
- Females predisposed
- No age predisposition

Colour-dilution alopecia
- Coat-colour genes are involved in the pathogenesis

Acanthosis nigricans
- Uncommon
- Multiple causes, but primary form may be inherited
- Affects either sex, usually beginning at less than 1 year of age

Ehler-Danlos syndrome
- Also known as cutaneous asthenia
- Inherited group of diseases
- May be inherited as an autosomal dominant trait
- Probably lethal to homozygotes

Canine ear margin dermatosis

Callus dermatitis/pyoderma
- Sternal calluses are often seen in this breed

Canine juvenile cellulitis
- Familial; possibly inherited
- Usually 1–4 months of age at onset

Idiopathic chronic ulcerative blepharitis

Onychodystrophy

Vasculitis
- Uncommon
- Usually type III hypersensitivity reaction

Skin tumours
- See Neoplastic conditions

Endocrine conditions
Hypothyroidism
- Reported in some texts to be at increased risk
- Often middle-aged (2–6 years)

DOGS

Hyperadrenocorticism: pituitary-dependent (PDH) and adrenocortical tumour (AT)

- Possible breed predisposition (PDH and AT)
- Middle-aged/older
- AT: 60–65% female; PDH: 55–60% female

Diabetes mellitus

- Reported in some texts to be at increased risk
- Usual age range: 4–14 years; peak incidence: 7–9 years
- Old entire females are predisposed

Gastrointestinal conditions

Haemorrhagic gastroenteritis

- Possible breed predisposition
- Seen most commonly at 2–4 years of age

Immunological conditions

Undefined immunodeficiency syndrome

- Caused by a protozoal pneumonia (*Pneumocystis carinii*)
- Exact immunodeficiency uncertain

Immune-mediated thrombocytopaenia

- Common
- Familial in this breed; likely inherited
- Females more commonly affected than males

Infectious conditions

Pneumocystis carinii infection

- Reported in this breed
- May reflect a concurrent immunodeficiency syndrome (see Immunological conditions)

Musculoskeletal conditions

Inguinal/scrotal herniation

- Females predisposed

Pes varus

- A distal tibial deformity
- Seen from 5–6 months of age
- Possible autosomal recessive inheritance

Prognathia

- Possibly inherited as an autosomal recessive trait

Spondylosis deformans

- Usually clinically insignificant

Neoplastic conditions

Anal sac adenocarcinoma

- Breed predisposition suggested in one survey of 232 cases
- Average age was 10.5 years
- Some surveys suggest a predisposition for females

Lipoma

- Common
- Possible breed predisposition
- Most common in middle-aged, obese female dogs

Liposarcoma

- Average age of onset: 10 years
- Males may be predisposed

Mast cell tumours

- Possible breed predisposition
- May be seen at any age (from 4 months onwards), but usually seen in older animals

Squamous cell carcinoma of the digit

- Possible breed predisposition
- Older dogs

Canine cutaneous histiocytoma

- Possible breed predisposition
- More common in young dogs, 1–2 years of age

Pituitary tumour resulting in hyperadrenocorticism

- See under Endocrine diseases

Adrenocortical tumour resulting in hyperadrenocorticism

- See under Endocrine diseases

Limbal melanoma

- Possible breed predisposition

Neurological conditions

Congenital deafness (Dappled Dachshunds)

- Signs seen from birth

Intervertebral disc disease (see figures 8a and 8b)

- Breed predisposition
- Very common condition
- Age of clinical onset: 3–7 years

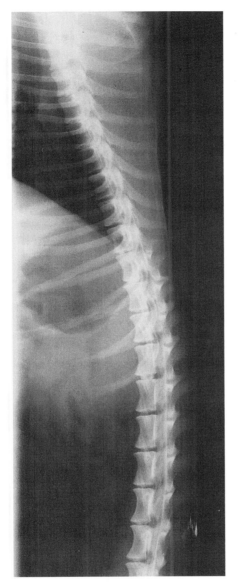

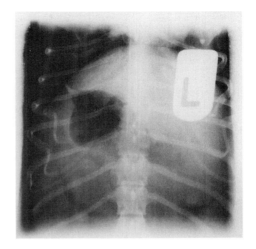

Figure 8b
Dorsoventral view.

Lysosomal storage disease – ceroid lipofuscinosis
- Inheritance suspected
- Rare
- Signs seen at 3–7 years

Sensory neuropathy (Long-haired Dachschunds)
- Autosomal recessive inheritance suspected
- Rare
- Signs seen at 8–12 weeks

Narcolepsy-cataplexy
- Inheritance suspected
- Age of clinical onset: <1 year

Atlantoaxial subluxation (Miniature Dachshunds)
- Congenital
- Relatively common in this breed
- Age of clinical onset: <1 year

Ocular conditions
Dermoid
- Breed predisposition, autosomal recessive inheritance suggested

Figure 8a
Myelogram demonstrating a disc herniation at T12–T13 in a four-year-old female Dachshund. There is loss of the contrast column in an area of the spinal cord centred over T12–T13 (lateral view).

Entropion (usually lower lids)
- Breed predisposition; polygenic inheritance likely
- Uncommon in the USA

Distichiasis (Miniature Long-haired Dachshund)
- Breed predisposition
- High incidence (>80% in the UK)

Chronic superficial keratitis (pannus)
- Breed predisposition; autosomal recessive inheritance suggested
- Age of onset: 2–4 years

Refractory corneal ulceration
- Breed predisposition
- Usually middle-aged

Corneal endothelial dystrophy
- Inheritance suspected
- Age of onset: 8–11 years
- Results in corneal oedema

Limbal melanoma
- Possible breed predisposition

Glaucoma
- Possible breed predisposition
- Age of onset: 4–9 years

Persistent pupillary membranes (PPM)
- Inheritance suspected
- Schedule 3 of the BVA/KC/ISDS Eye Scheme (Miniature Wire-haired)

Cataract (Miniature Smooth and Wire-haired)
- Inheritance suspected
- Localisation: posterior subcapsular cortex
- Age of onset: 1 year, slowly progressive

Retinal detachment with abnormal vitreous
- Breed predisposition; mode of inheritance unknown
- Occurs from 8 months

Generalised progressive retinal atrophy (GPRA) (Miniature Long-haired)
- Autosomal recessive inheritance suspected
- Clinically apparent at 6 months; rapidly progressive
- Schedule 1 of the BVA/KC/ISDS Eye Scheme

Generalised progressive retinal atrophy (GPRA) (Miniature Smooth-haired)
- Autosomal recessive inheritance suspected
- Schedule 3 of the BVA/KC/ISDS Eye Scheme

Optic nerve hypoplasia
- Congenital condition; not known if inherited
- Seen frequently in this breed
- Schedule 3 of the BVA/KC/ISDS Eye Scheme (Miniature Long-haired Dachshund)

Multiple ocular defects (associated with merling)
- Inherited; defects more severe in homozygous than heterozygous merles
- Defects include microphalmia, microcornea, cataract and colobomas

Neuronal ceroid lipofuscinosis
- Inheritance suspected
- See also under Neurological conditions

Physiological conditions
Hypochondroplasia
- Accepted as breed standard
- Short, bowed legs, but normal skulls seen

Renal and urinary conditions
Urethral sphincter mechanism incompetence (causing urinary incontinence)
- Possible breed predisposition in female dogs

Cystine urolithiasis
- Cystinuria results from an inherited defect in renal tubular transport of cystine and predisposes to cystine urolithiasis
- Higher incidence reported in this breed in some American surveys
- Average age at diagnosis is 1–8 years
- Males seem predisposed

Reproductive conditions
Cryptorchidism (Miniature Dachshund)
- Developmental defect believed to be inherited as a sex-limited, autosomal recessive trait
- Believed to be a breed at increased risk of the condition

Respiratory conditions
Pneumonia due to *Pneumocystis carinii* infection
- Reported in this breed
- May reflect a concurrent immunodeficiency syndrome (see Immunological conditions)

DALMATIAN

Dermatological conditions
Pododermatitis
- Front feet more commonly affected

Atopy
- Common
- Possibly more common in females
- Age of onset variable, from 6 months to 7 years

Food hypersensitivity
- No age or sex predisposition
- Some reports have not demonstrated a breed predisposition

Waardenburg-Klein syndrome
- Inherited as an autosomal dominant trait with incomplete penetrance

Canine solar dermatitis
- Sunnier climates predispose

Skin tumours
- See under Neoplastic conditions

Musculoskeletal conditions
Temporomandibular dysplasia/luxation
- Congenital dysplasia may predispose to luxation

Muscular cramping
- Condition similar to Scottie cramp reported in this breed

Neoplastic conditions
Actinic keratosis (solar keratosis)
- Reported to be at increased risk
- Seen more commonly in pale-skinned animals with the opportunity for long periods of intense sun exposure

Cutaneous haemangioma
- Reported breed predisposition
- Average age was 8.7 years in one study

Neurological conditions
Congenital deafness
- Signs seen from birth
- Overall incidence of approximately 30% in this breed

Dalmatian leukodystrophy
- Autosomal recessive inheritance suggested
- Rare
- Clinical signs at 3–6 months

Muscular cramping
- Condition similar to Scottie cramp reported in this breed

Lysosomal storage disease – ceroid lipofuscinosis
- Inheritance suspected
- Rare
- Signs seen at 1–2 year

Ocular conditions
Dermoid
- Breed predisposition

Entropion (usually lower lids)
- Breed predisposition; polygenic inheritance likely

Distichiasis
- Breed predisposition; mode of inheritance unknown
- Mild condition occurring from 6 months onwards

Chronic superficial keratitis (pannus)
- Breed predisposition, mode of inheritance unknown
- Age of onset: 2–3 years

Nodular episclerokeratitis
- Breed predisposition
- Usually presents at 2–5 years

Glaucoma
- Possible breed predisposition

Cataract
- Inheritance suspected

Generalised progressive retinal atrophy (GPRA)
- Autosomal recessive inheritance suspected
- End stage at 7 years

Neuronal ceroid Lipofuscinosis
- Inheritance suspected
- See also under Neurological conditions

Renal and urinary conditions
Hyperuricuria and urate urolithiasis
- Hyperuricuria is inherited recessively in this breed and predisposes to urate urolithiasis
- Average age at diagnosis is 5 years, although hyperuricuria is present at birth
- Males seem to be predisposed

Respiratory conditions
Laryngeal paralysis
- Associated with a polyneuropathy in this breed
- Affects young dogs
- Inheritance suspected

Adult respiratory distress syndrome
- Possibly inherited as an autosomal recessive

DANDIE DINMONT TERRIER

Neurological conditions
Intervertebral disc disease
- Breed predisposition
- Adults affected

Ocular conditions
Refractory corneal ulceration
- Breed predisposition
- Seen in older dogs

Glaucoma/goniodysgenesis
- Mode of inheritance unknown
- Age of onset: 6 years and older
- Schedule 3 of the BVA/KC/ISDS Eye Scheme

Physiological conditions
Hypochondroplasia
- Accepted as breed standard
- Short, bowed legs, but normal skulls seen

DOBERMANN

Cardiovascular conditions
Atrial septal defect
- Uncommon disease
- Congenital
- Not yet proven to be inherited
- Some studies do not demonstrate a predisposition for this condition in this breed

Dilated cardiomyopathy
- Very common in this breed (relative risk 33.7, prevalance 5.8%)
- This breed accounts for 50% of cases of this condition
- Increased prevalence with age
- Approximately twice as common in males as females
- Thought to be familial, possibly inherited
- Some cases in this breed exhibit bradydysrhythmias and syncope

Sudden death
- Uncommon
- Thought to be caused by fatal arrhythmias

Dermatological conditions
Muzzle folliculitis/furunculosis
- Also known as canine acne
- Local trauma, hormones and genetics may play a role in pathogenesis

Cryptococcosis
- See under Infectious conditions

Coccidiomycosis
- See under Infectious conditions

Blastomycosis
- See under Infectious conditions

Pemphigus foliaceous
- Uncommon disease
- No sex predisposition
- Mean age of onset 4 years

Bullous pemphigoid
- Very rare
- No age or sex predispositions

Seasonal flank alopecia
- Occurs in spring or autumn

Primary seborrhoea
- Probably inherited as an autosomal recessive trait
- Signs occur early and worsen with age

Ichthyosis
- Rare
- Congenital
- Possibly inherited as an autosomal recessive trait

Colour-dilution alopecia
- Reported in blue or fawn Dobermanns and Miniature Pinschers
- Coat-colour genes play a role in the inheritance of this condition

Follicular dysplasia
- Affects black or red Dobermanns
- Age of onset: 1–4 years
- Affects caudal dorsum and flanks

Hypopigmentary disorders
- Inheritance suspected

Vitiligo
- Presumed to be inherited

Nasal depigmentation
- Also known as Dudley nose
- Cause unknown

Mucocutaneous hypopigmentation
- Congenital in this breed
- Affects the lips and nose

Acral lick dermatitis (see plate 6)
- Occurs in males more commonly than females
- Can occur at any age, but usually over 5 years

Flank sucking

Callus dermatitis/pyoderma
- Usually affects the sternum in this breed

Zinc-responsive dermatosis
- Occurs in rapidly-growing dogs fed zinc-deficient diets

Follicular cyst
- No age or sex predisposition

Focal mucinosis

Skin tumours
- See under Neoplastic conditions

Drug reactions
Sulphonamides
- This breed has been known to suffer cutaneous reactions and polyarthropathy following the use of this drug

Endocrine conditions
Hypothyroidism
- Breed predisposition
- Often middle-aged (2–6 years)

Gastrointestinal conditions
Gastric dilatation-volvulus
- Breed predisposition

Parvovirus enteritis
- Breed predisposition
- Usually young dogs

Chronic hepatitis (see plate 7)
- Breed predisposition
- Middle-aged females are predisposed
- Very aggressive form of hepatitis in this breed. Copper accumulation may occur but is considered secondary to cholestasis

Congenital portosystemic shunt
- Breed predisposition reported in the USA
- Clinical signs usually seen in young dogs <1 year of age

DOGS

Haematological conditions
Neutrophil defect
- Related Dobermanns showed chronic rhinitis and pneumonia
- Only described in a single report from 1987

Von Willebrand's disease
- Possibly inherited as an autosomal recessive trait
- Common in this breed in both the USA and UK
- Mainly type I disease in this breed
- Most Dobermanns with clinical signs of bleeding have vWF <35%
- Most severe haemorrhage associated with vWF <20%
- Not all at-risk dogs will bleed

Infectious conditions
Parvovirus enteritis
- Possible breed predisposition

Coccidiomycosis
- Increased incidence in this breed possibly due to an increased likelihood of exposure
- Seen mainly in young male dogs
- Geographic distribution: California, Arizona, Texas, New Mexico, Nevada, Utah, Mexico and parts of Central and South America. Not reported in the UK

Cryptococcosis
- Increased incidence in this breed possibly due to an increased likelihood of exposure
- Usually seen in dogs under 4 years
- Worldwide distribution, but favoured by warm, humid climates

Blastomycosis
- Increased incidence in this breed possibly due to an increased likelihood of exposure
- Seen mainly in young male dogs living near water
- Geographic distribution: around the Mississippi, Ohio, Missouri, Tennessee and St Lawrence Rivers, the southern Great Lakes and the southern mid-Atlantic states. Not reported in the UK

Infectious skin diseases
- See under Dermatological conditions

Musculoskeletal conditions
Carpal ligament weakening
- Affects older obese dogs
- Tarsal ligaments may also be affected

Bone cyst
- Uncommon
- Usually affects young dogs
- Males are predisposed

Von Willebrand heterotopic osteochondrofibrosis in Dobermann Pinschers
- Young to middle-aged dogs affected
- Suspected that low levels of von Willebrand factor lead to microvascular bleeding which initiates the condition

Congenital elbow luxation
- Uncommon
- Severe disability in this breed (type I)
- Present at birth or in the first 3 months of life

Gastrocnemius tendon avulsion
- May lead to rupture and subsequent hyper-flexion of the hock and digits

Neoplastic conditions
Melanoma
- Breed predisposition
- Average age 8–9 years

Lipoma
- Possible breed predisposition
- Most common in middle-aged, obese female dogs
- Infiltrative lipomas can be seen in this breed

Canine cutaneous histiocytoma
- Possible breed predisposition
- More common in young dogs, 1–2 years of age

Fibroma
- Affects older dogs
- Females predisposed

Fibrosarcoma
- Affects older dogs
- Females predisposed

Myxoma/myxosarcoma
- Affects older dogs
- No sex predisposition

Primary brain tumour
- See under Neurological conditions

Neurological conditions
Congenital vestibular disease
- Signs seen <3 months
- Occasionally seen with congenital deafness

Congenital deafness
- Autosomal recessive inheritance suggested
- Signs seen from birth

Intervertebral disc disease
- Breed predisposition to cervical disc disease
- Common condition
- Age of clinical onset: 5–10 years

Narcolepsy-cataplexy
- Autosomal recessive inheritance suspected
- Age of clinical onset: <1 year

Atlantoaxial subluxation
- Congenital
- Has been reported in this breed
- Age of clinical onset: <1 year

Cervical vertebral malformation (wobbler syndrome)
- Breed predisposition
- Common in this breed
- Age of clinical onset: 3–9 years, occasionally before 1 year

Primary brain tumour
- Higher incidence noted in this breed
- Older dogs affected (mean 9–10 years)

Dancing Dobermann disease
- Seen occasionally
- Age of clinical onset: 6 months to 7 years

Arachnoid cysts
- Breed predisposition
- Age of clinical onset: <1 year

Hyperaesthesia syndrome
- Possible breed predisposition

Ocular conditions
Dermoid
- Breed predisposition

Entropion
- Breed predisposition; polygenic inheritance likely

Eversion of the cartilage of the nictitating membrane
- Breed predisposition

Medial canthal pocket syndrome
- Breed predisposition due to general head shape

Congenital tumours of the iris and ciliary body
- Breed predisposition
- Age of presentation 6 months to 2 years

Cataract
- Inheritance suspected
- Localisation: posterior sutures
- Age of onset: 1–2 years; slowly progressive

Persistent hyaloid artery
- Inheritance suspected

Persistent hyperplastic tunica vasculosa lentis and persistent hyperplastic primary vitreous
- Breed predisposition reported in the Netherlands but rare in the USA
- Dominant inheritance with incomplete penetration suggested
- Schedule 1 of the BVA/KC/ISDS Eye Scheme

Generalised progressive retinal atrophy (GPRA)
- Autosomal recessive inheritance suspected
- Clinical onset at 1 year; end stage at 3 years

Multiple ocular defects
- Autosomal recessive inheritance suspected
- May include microphthalmia, anterior segment dysgenesis, congenital cataract and retinal dysplasia
- Schedule 3 of the BVA/KC/ISDS Eye Scheme

DOGS

Physiological conditions
Gestation
- Mean gestation period reported as 61.4 days

Renal and urinary conditions
Familial renal disease
- Mode of inheritance unknown
- The condition is believed to be a glomerular basement-membrane disorder which may progress to glomerulonephritis
- The disease presents at 1–6 years with proteinuria and chronic renal failure

Urethral sphincter mechanism incompetence (causing urinary incontinence)
- Possible breed predisposition in female dogs

Reproductive conditions
XO syndrome
- Congenital abnormality of chromosomal sex which has been reported in this breed

Penile hypoplasia
- Rare congenital condition which has been reported in this breed
- May be seen as part of some intersex states

Respiratory conditions
Chronic rhinitis and pneumonia
- Thought to be due to a neutrophil deficiency
- See Haematological conditions

DOGUE DE BORDEAUX

Dermatological conditions
Footpad hyperkeratosis
- Familial in this breed
- Lesions appear by 6 months of age

DUTCH KOOIKER

Haematological conditions
Von Willebrand's disease
- Type III disease is seen in this breed
- Inherited as an autosomal recessive trait
- Precise genetic defect responsible identified

ENGLISH SETTER

Dermatological conditions
Atopy
- Females probably predisposed
- Age of onset from 6 months to 7 years
- May or may not be seasonal

Canine benign familial chronic pemphigus
- Inherited as an autosomal dominant trait
- Also affects English Setter crosses

Musculoskeletal conditions
Hip dysplasia
- Tenth worst mean-scoring breed in the BVA/KC Hip Dysplasia Scheme as of October 2001
- Breed mean score 19

Neurological conditions
Congenital deafness
- Signs seen from birth

Lysosomal storage disease – ceroid lipofuscinosis
- Autosomal recessive inheritance
- Rare
- Signs seen at 1–2 years

Ocular conditions
Ectropion
- Breed predisposition; polygenic inheritance likely

Eversion of the cartilage of the nictitating membrane
- Breed predisposition; inheritance suspected
- Usually occurs in young dogs

Generalised progressive retinal atrophy (GPRA)
- Mode of inheritance unknown, but autosomal recessive suspected

Neuronal ceroid lipofuscinosis
- Autosomal recessive inheritance

ESKIMO DOG

Ocular conditions
Cataract
- Inheritance suspected
- Schedule 3 of the BVA/KC/ISDS Eye Scheme

FIELD SPANIEL

Ocular conditions
Cataract
- Inheritance suspected
- Schedule 3 of the BVA/KC/ISDS Eye Scheme

Multifocal retinal dysplasia
- Congenital condition; inheritance as an autosomal recessive trait suspected
- May be seen with abnormal vitreous
- Schedule 3 of the BVA/KC/ISDS Eye Scheme

Generalised progressive retinal atrophy (GPRA)
- Mode of inheritance unknown but presumed to be recessive
- Clinically apparent at 5 years

FINNISH SPITZ

Dermatological conditions
Pemphigus foliaceous
- Uncommon disease
- No sex predisposition
- Mean age of onset: 4 years

Haematological/immunological conditions
Transient hypogammaglobulinaemia
- Congenital
- May cause a delay in the development of active immunity

Spitz dog thrombopathia
- Affects young dogs
- Causes chronic intermittent bleeding

FLAT-COATED RETRIEVER

Musculoskeletal conditions
Genu valgum
- High incidence seen in some strains

Neoplastic conditions
Canine cutaneous histiocytoma
- Possible breed predisposition
- More common in young dogs 1–2 years of age

Anaplastic sarcoma
- Possible breed predisposition
- Average age of onset for soft-tissue sarcomas is 8–9 years, but may be seen earlier in this breed

Ocular conditions
Entropion (usually lower lids)
- Breed predisposition; polygenic inheritance likely

Ectropion (mild, usually disappears with maturity)
- Breed predisposition; polygenic inheritance likely

Distichiasis
- Breed predisposition; mode of inheritance unknown

Ectopic cilia
- Breed predisposition

Primary glaucoma/goniodysgenesis
- Mode of inheritance unknown
- Mainly seen in the UK
- Schedule 1 of the BVA/KC/ISDS Eye Scheme

Cataract
- Not known if inherited
- Nuclear opacities from 4 years of age onwards; visual deficits unlikely

Micropapilla
- Congenital condition, seen commonly in this breed
- Not associated with visual problems

DOGS

Optic nerve colobomas
- Congenital defect; not known if inherited
- Seen occasionally in this breed

FOXHOUND

Haematological conditions
Pelger-Huet anomaly (American Foxhound)
- May not be clinically significant

Neurological conditions
Hound ataxia
- Reported in the UK
- Age of clinical onset: 2–7 years

FOX TERRIER

Cardiovascular conditions
Tetralogy of Fallot
- Congenital
- Rare
- Relative risk 22.0

Pulmonic stenosis
- Third most frequent cause of canine congenital heart disease
- Polygenic mode of inheritance likely
- Relative risk 10.5

Dermatological conditions
Atopy
- Females probably predisposed
- Age of onset from 6 months to 7 years
- May or may not be seasonal

Flea bite hypersensitivity
- Most studies show there is no breed predisposition, but one French study showed Fox Terriers to be predisposed

Skin tumours
- See under Neoplastic conditions

Endocrine conditions
Insulinoma
- Higher incidence seen in this breed
- Usually middle-aged/older dogs

Gastrointestinal conditions
Congenital idiopathic megaoesophagus (Wire-haired Fox Terrier)
- Autosomal recessive inheritance

Musculoskeletal conditions
Shoulder luxation
- Congenital

Myasthenia gravis
- See under Neurological conditions

Neoplastic conditions
Mast cell tumours
- Possible breed predisposition
- May be seen at any age (from 4 months onwards), but usually seen in older animals

Fibroma
- Females predisposed
- Affects older animals

Haemangiopericytoma
- Occurs at a mean age of 7–10 years
- No sex predisposition

Schwannoma
- No sex predisposition
- Affects older animals

Insulinoma
- See under Endocrine conditions

Neurological conditions
Cerebellar malformation (Wire-haired Fox Terrier)
- Congenital
- Uncommon
- Age of clinical onset: <3 months

Congenital vestibular disease (Smooth-haired Fox Terrier)
- Signs seen <3 months

Congenital deafness (Smooth-haired Fox Terrier)
- Signs seen from birth

True epilepsy (Wire-haired Fox Terrier)
- Inheritance suspected
- Age of onset: 6 months to 3 years

Lissencephaly (Wire-haired Fox Terrier)
- Rare developmental disease reported in this breed
- Age of clinical onset: <1 year

Hereditary Ataxia (Smooth-haired Fox Terrier)
- Autosomal recessive inheritance suspected
- Reported in Sweden
- Age of clinical onset: 2–6 months

Congenital myasthenia gravis (Smooth-haired Fox Terrier)
- Autosomal recessive inheritance suspected
- Rare
- Age of clinical onset: 6–8 weeks

Ocular conditions
Refractory corneal ulceration (Wire-haired Fox Terrier)
- Breed predisposition
- Usually middle-aged

Glaucoma (Smooth-haired and Wire-haired Fox Terriers)
- Possible breed predisposition

Primary lens luxation (Smooth-haired and Wire-haired Fox Terriers)
- Autosomal dominant inheritance has been suggested in Smooth-haired Fox Terriers
- Age of onset: 4–7 years
- Often followed by glaucoma
- Schedule 1 of the BVA/KC/ISDS Eye Scheme

Cataract (Smooth-haired and Wire-haired Fox Terriers)
- Inheritance suspected

Generalised progressive retinal atrophy (Smooth-haired and Wire-haired Fox Terriers)
- Mode of inheritance unknown, but presumed to be recessive
- Age of clinical onset: 2 years

Renal and urinary conditions
Ectopic ureters
- Congenital defect; higher incidence reported in this breed
- Usually presents <1 year of age

FRENCH BULLDOG

Dermatological conditions
Canine follicular dysplasia
- A marked predilection in this breed implies a genetic basis for this group of diseases

Seasonal flank alopecia
- Tends to occur in spring or autumn

Congenital hypotrichosis
- Present at birth or develops in the first month of life
- Predisposition for males suggests sex linkage

Gastrointestinal conditions
Histiocytic colitis
- Breed predisposition
- Most common in young dogs

Haematological conditions
Haemophilia B
- Factor IX deficiency
- Also known as Christmas disease
- Inherited as a sex-linked trait
- In one family, concurrent haemophilia A was seen

Musculoskeletal conditions
Hemivertebrae
- Mode of inheritance not known

Sacrocaudal dysgenesis
- Congenital
- See also under Neurological conditions

Neoplastic conditions
Primary brain tumours
- See under Neurological conditions

Neurological conditions
Primary brain tumours
- Higher incidence seen in this breed
- Older dogs affected (mean 9–10 years)

Hemivertebrae
- Congenital
- Occasionally reported

DOGS

Sacrocaudal dysgenesis
- Congenital
- Occasionally reported

Ocular conditions
Entropion (upper and lower lids)
- Breed predisposition; polygenic inheritance likely

Distichiasis (usually with entropion)
- Breed predisposition

Trichiasis
- Breed predisposition

Cataract
- Inheritance suspected
- Localisation: posterior cortex and equatorial region
- Age of onset: 6 months to 3 years; rapid progression; visual deficiencies common
- Schedule 3 of the BVA/KC/ISDS Eye Scheme

Renal and urinary conditions
Cystine urolithiasis
- Cystinuria results from an inherited defect in renal tubular transport of cystine and predisposes to cystine urolithiasis
- Higher incidence reported in this breed in some American surveys
- Average age at diagnosis is 1–8 years
- Males seem predisposed

GERMAN SHEPHERD DOG (GSD)

Cardiovascular conditions
Aortic stenosis
- Congenital
- Relative risk 2.6
- No sex predilection
- Inheritance possibly autosomal dominant with modifying genes, or polygenic

Mitral dysplasia
- Congenital
- Relative risk 2.7
- Males predisposed
- Inheritance suspected

Pericardial effusion
- Acquired
- Relative risk 2.3
- Haemangiosarcoma of the right atrium is a common cause in this breed

Persistent left cranial vena cava
- Congenital
- Only of clinical significance during thoracic surgery

Persistent right aortic arch
- Congenital
- Relative risk 4.5
- See also vascular ring anomaly under Gastrointestinal conditions

Tricuspid dysplasia
- Congenital
- Relative risk 3.1
- Males predisposed

Ventricular ectopy
- Reported to be familial
- Genetic predisposition
- Seen in the USA and UK, but possibly geographically widespread

Dermatological conditions
Mucocutaneous pyoderma
- No age or sex predisposition

Nasal folliculitis/furunculosis
- Uncommon
- Unknown cause

Pododermatitis
- Males predisposed
- Front feet more commonly affected

German Shepherd Dog folliculitis, furunculosis and cellulitis
- Familial
- Probably an inherited immunodeficiency
- May be inherited as an autosomal recessive trait
- Affects middle-aged dogs
- No sex predisposition
- Relative risk for recurrent folliculitis/furunculosis in this breed 3.7

Malassezia dermatitis
- Often seasonal
- Affects any age

Pythiosis
- Most common in tropical and sub-tropical regions
- Male dogs more commonly affected

Contact hypersensitivity
- A Danish study showed that 50% of affected dogs were GSDs (the general population of pedigree dogs is composed of 16% GSDs)
- No age or sex predisposition

Food hypersensitivity
- No age or sex predisposition reported
- Relative risk 2.1

Pemphigus erythematosus
- No age or sex predisposition

Systemic lupus erythematosus
- Uncommon (incidence approximately 0.03% of general canine population)
- No age or sex predisposition

Discoid lupus erythematosus
- No age or sex predisposition
- Accounted for 0.3% of skin diseases at one referral institution

Primary seborrhoea
- Probably inherited as an autosomal recessive trait
- Signs first appear in young dogs and get worse with age

Hypopigmentary disorders
- Possibly inherited

Ehler-Danlos syndrome
- Also known as cutaneous asthenia
- Inherited group of diseases
- May be inherited as an autosomal dominant trait
- Probably lethal to homozygotes

Disorder of the footpads in German Shepherd Dogs
- Unknown cause
- Often familial
- No sex predisposition
- Usually early onset of symptoms

Focal metatarsal fistulation of German Shepherd Dogs
- Uncommon
- Most common in dogs descended directly from German ancestors
- Age of onset usually 2.5–4 years

Multiple collagenous naevi
- Age of onset: 3–5 years
- May be a cutaneous marker for renal cystadenocarcinomas or uterine leiomyomas (See under Renal and urinary conditions)
- Probably autosomal dominant inheritance

Familial vasculopathy
- Occurs early in life, often triggered by first vaccination
- No sex predisposition
- Autosomal recessive inheritance

Primary lymphoedema
- No apparent sex predisposition
- Usually occurs within first 12 weeks of life

Vitiligo
- Presumed to be hereditary

Nasal depigmentation
- Also known as Dudley nose
- Unknown cause
- Affects white German Shepherd Dogs

Acral lick dermatitis
- Occurs in males more commonly than females
- Can occur at any age, but usually over 5 years

Zinc-responsive dermatosis
- Occurs in rapidly-growing dogs fed zinc-deficient diets

Idiopathic chronic ulcerative blepharitis

Symmetric lupoid onchodystrophy
- Age range of dogs affected 3–8 years

Idiopathic onychomadesis

Fibropruritic nodule
- Usually older than 8 years at onset

Calcinosis circumscripta
- Uncommon
- Usually affects dogs less than 2 years of age
- No sex predisposition

Vasculitis
- Uncommon
- Usually type III hypersensitivity reaction

Greying
- May occur at a young age in this breed

Pyotraumatic folliculitis
- Young dogs predisposed
- Also known as hot spot; wet eczema

Skin tumours
- See Neoplastic conditions

Endocrine conditions
Pituitary dwarfism
- Autosomal recessive mode of inheritance suggested
- Clinical signs (failure to grow) seen at 2–3 months

Hyperadrenocorticism: pituitary-dependent (PDH) and adrenocortical tumour (AT)
- Possible breed predisposition (PDH and AT)
- Middle-aged/older
- AT: 60–65% female; PDH: 55–60% female

Insulinoma
- Higher incidence seen in this breed
- Usually middle aged/older dogs

Primary hyperparathyroidism
- Hereditary neonatal primary hyperparathyroidism has been reported in two German Shepherd Dogs
- Autosomal recessive inheritance likely

Primary hypoparathyroidism
- Uncommon condition
- Frequently affected breed according to some surveys
- Occurs at any age

Gastrointestinal conditions
Oropharyngeal neoplasia
- Possible breed predisposition

Congenital idiopathic megaoesophagus (see figure 9)
- Breed predisposition

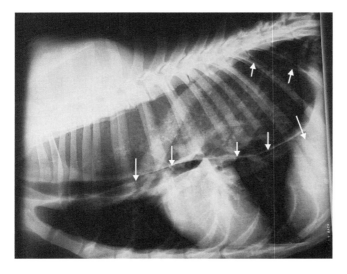

Figure 9
Lateral thoracic radiograph of a three-year-old German Shepherd dog with idiopathic megaoesophagus. The dilated oesophagus may be seen dorsal to the heart (arrows).

Secondary megaoesophagus
- A breed predisposition to myasthenia gravis exists, which may be an underlying cause of megaoesophagus

Vascular ring anomaly
- Breed predisposition; inheritance suspected

Gastro-oesophageal intussusception
- Breed predisposition
- Usually seen in dogs <3 months old
- Males may be predisposed

Gastric dilatation-volvulus
- Possible breed predisposition

Small intestinal bacterial overgrowth (SIBO)
- Possible breed predisposition
- May be associated with impaired intestinal immunity due to reduced intestinal IgA secretion in this breed

Lymphocytic-plasmacytic enteritis
- Possible breed predisposition
- Most common in middle-aged and older dogs

Small intestinal volvulus
- Possible breed predisposition
- Presence of exocrine pancreatic insufficiency may be a predisposing factor

Eosinophilic gastroenteritis, enteritis and enterocolitis
- Breed predisposition
- Most common in dogs 5 years and younger

Chronic idiopathic (lymphocytic-plasmacytic) colitis
- Possible breed predisposition
- Most common in young to middle-aged dogs

Perianal fistula (see plate 8)
- Breed predisposition
- Most common in middle-aged to older dogs

Idiopathic hepatic fibrosis
- Breed predisposition
- Usually seen in young dogs

Congenital portosystemic shunt
- Breed predisposition reported in the USA
- Clinical signs usually seen in young dogs (<1 year)

Hepatic haemangiosarcoma
- Breed predisposition
- Usually metastases from the spleen or heart; occasionally the tumour originates in the liver

Pancreatic acinar atrophy (causing exocrine pancreatic insufficiency)
- Breed predisposition; possibly inherited as an autosomal recessive trait

Haematological/immunological conditions
Selective IgA deficiency
- Often asymptomatic
- May be increased susceptibility to enteric infection

Haemophilia A
- A moderately severe form of the disease in this breed allows survival to adulthood

Haemophilia B
- Reported in a family of German Shepherd Dog pups

Immune-mediated thrombocytopaenia
- Common
- Inheritance likely
- Females more commonly affected than males

Von Willebrand's disease
- Possibly inherited as an autosomal recessive trait

Systemic lupus erythematosus
- Inherited, but not by a simple mechanism

Infectious conditions
Aspergillosis
- Possible breed predisposition
- Usually seen in young to middle-aged dogs

Infectious skin disease
- See Dermatological conditions

Musculoskeletal conditions
Spondylosis deformans
- Usually clinically insignificant

Cartilaginous exostosis

Elbow dysplasia
- Also known as osteochondrosis
- Genetically determined in this breed
- Medial coronoid process disease and ununited anconeal process are common in this breed

Hip dysplasia (see figure 10)
- Thirteenth worst mean-scoring breed in the BVA/KC Hip Dysplasia Scheme as of October 2001
- Breed mean score 19

Lumbosacral disease
- Affected by age and body weight
- Facet geometry influenced congenitally

Panosteitis
- Also known as enostosis, eosinophilic panosteitis
- Common
- Young males predisposed

Bone cyst
- Uncommon
- Usually affects young dogs
- Males predisposed

Glycogen storage disease type III
- Also known as Cori's disease
- Only reported in females so far
- Signs first seen at two months of age
- Rare disease
- Poor prognosis

Hypotrophy of the pectineus muscle
- Developmental myopathy

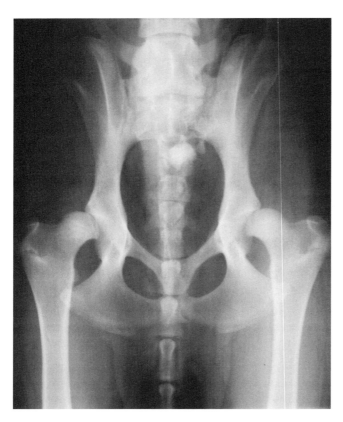

Figure 10
Ventrodorsal radiograph of a dog showing dysplastic hips. Photo courtesy of Andy Moores.

Masticatory myopathy
- Also known as eosinophilic myositis
- Common muscle disease

Fibrotic myopathy of semitendinosus
- Dogs affected age 2–7 years

Gracilis contracture
- Especially occurs in athletic individuals

Canine idiopathic polyarthritis
- Usually affects dogs at 1–3 years, but any age can be affected

Transitional lumbosacral vertebra
- Thought to be inherited
- This breed is greatly over-represented

Myasthenia gravis
- See under Neurological conditions

Neoplastic conditions
Sweat gland tumour
- Reported to be at increased risk
- Average age reported as 9.5 years

Trichoepithelioma
- Possible breed predisposition
- Average age reported as 9 years

Anal sac adenocarcinoma
- Breed predisposition suggested in one survey of 232 cases
- Average age was 10.5 years
- Some surveys suggest a predisposition for females

Cutaneous haemangioma
- Possible breed predisposition
- Average age was 8.7 years in one study

Cutaneous haemangiosarcoma
- Possible breed predisposition
- Average age 9–10 years

Haemangiopericytoma (see plate 9)
- Occurs at a mean age of 7–10 years

Non-epitheliotropic lymphoma
- Affects older dogs

Keratoacanthoma
- Possibly inherited
- Uncommon
- Affects dogs of 5 years or younger

Myxoma/myxosarcoma
- Affects older individuals

Nasal cavity tumours
- Reported to be at increased risk for nasal carcinoma
- Usually older dogs
- Dogs in urban areas may be at increased risk

Haemangiosarcoma (e.g. cardiac, splenic, hepatic)
- Higher incidence has been reported in this breed
- Possible predisposition for males

Colorectal neoplasia
- A higher incidence in this breed suggested in some reports
- Older dogs affected, with a mean age of 8.5 years

Renal cystadenocarcinomas
- See under Renal and urinary conditions

Insulinoma
- See under Endocrine conditions

Pituitary tumour resulting in hyperadrenocorticism
- See under Endocrine conditions

Adrenocortical tumour resulting in hyperadrenocorticism
- See under Endocrine conditions

Lymphosarcoma (malignant lymphoma)
- Higher incidence noted in this breed
- Most cases are seen in middle-aged dogs (mean 6–7 years)

Limbal melanoma
- Breed predisposition

Canine anterior uveal melanoma
- Breed predisposition suggested due to dark pigmentation

DOGS

Testicular neoplasia
- Believed to be a breed at increased risk

Thymoma
- Uncommon tumour
- High incidence reported in this breed in one study
- Mean age 7.5 years
- Possible predisposition for females

Neurological conditions
Congenital vestibular disease
- Signs seen <3 months

Congenital deafness
- Signs seen from birth

Glycogenosis (glycogen storage disease)
- Rare
- Age of clinical onset: <3 months

Intervertebral disc disease
- Breed predisposition to thoracolumbar disc disease
- Relatively common condition
- Age of clinical onset: 7–9 years

Discospondylitis
- Breed predisposition; possibly due to concurrent immunodeficiency
- Young/middle-aged dogs affected
- Males may be predisposed

True epilepsy
- Inherited
- Age of onset: 6 months to 3 years

Acquired myasthenia gravis
- Breed predisposition
- Adults affected

Giant axonal neuropathy
- Autosomal recessive inheritance suggested
- Rare
- Age of clinical onset: 14–16 months

Lumbosacral stenosis
- Breed predisposition
- Adults affected

Degenerative myelopathy
- Breed predisposition
- Common in this breed
- Age of clinical onset: >5 years

Hyperaesthesia syndrome
- Possible breed predisposition

Ocular conditions
Dermoid
- Congenital defect

Eversion of the cartilage of the nictitating membrane
- Breed predisposition; possibly inherited as a recessive trait
- Usually occurs in young dogs

Plasma cell infiltration of the nictitating membrane (plasmoma) (see plates 10–12)
- Breed predisposition
- May be associated with pannus

Chronic superficial keratitis (pannus)
- Recessive inheritance with variable expression has been suggested. Highest incidence in this breed
- Age of onset: 1–6 years
- Rapidly progressive in this breed

Refractory corneal ulceration
- Breed predisposition
- Usually middle-aged

Corneal dystrophy
- Breed predisposition; not known if inherited
- Stromal lipid dystrophy
- Age of onset: 1–6 years
- May be associated with pannus

Limbal melanoma
- Breed predisposition

Canine anterior uveal melanoma
- Breed predisposition suggested due to dark pigmentation
- Age of onset: 8–10 years

Cataract
- Autosomal recessive inheritance
- Initial localisation: posterior sutures
- Age of onset: 8–12 weeks; slowly progressive
- Seen in England
- Schedule 1 of the BVA/KC/ISDS Eye Scheme

Congenital cataract
- Autosomal dominant inheritance suggested
- A rare non-progressive cataract found in the anterior capsule

Lens luxation
- Possible breed predisposition
- Age of onset: 10–11 years

Multifocal retinal dysplasia
- Congenital condition; mode of inheritance not known
- Schedule 3 of the BVA/KC/ISDS Eye Scheme

Micropapilla
- Congenital condition
- Seen occasionally in this breed

Optic nerve hypoplasia
- Congenital condition; not known if inherited
- Seen occasionally in this breed

Optic nerve coloboma
- Congenital defect; not known if inherited
- Seen occasionally in this breed

Pseudopapilloedema
- Congenital condition; no evidence of inheritance
- Seen occasionally in this breed

Physiological conditions
Pronounced eosinophilic response
- May be normal in this breed
- Individuals with eosinophilia should still be evaluated for underlying causes of the condition

Blood group
- This breed is often DEA 1.1 and 1.2 negative

Gestation
- Mean gestation period reported as 60.4 days

Renal and urinary conditions
Renal cystadenocarcinomas
- Autosomal dominant inheritance suggested
- Age of presentation: 5–11 years
- Multiple, bilateral tumours are seen, with generalised nodular dermatofibrosis, and (in female dogs) multiple uterine leiomyomas

Urethral sphincter mechanism incompetence (causing urinary incontinence)
- Possible breed predisposition in female dogs

Silica urolithiasis
- Higher incidence reported in this breed in some surveys
- Males seem to be predisposed

Reproductive conditions
Vaginal hyperplasia
- Possible breed predisposition

Testicular neoplasia
- Believed to be a breed at increased risk

Variation in the interoestrus interval
- Fertile cycles may occur as often as every 4–5 months

Respiratory conditions
Spontaneous thymic haemorrhage
- Usually fatal
- Usually occurs in dogs less than 2 years old in association with thymic involution

Nasal dermoid sinus cyst
- Newly identified condition

GOLDEN RETRIEVER

Cardiovascular conditions
Aortic stenosis
- Congenital
- Relative risk 6.8
- No sex predilection
- Inheritance possibly autosomal dominant with modifying genes, or polygenic

DOGS

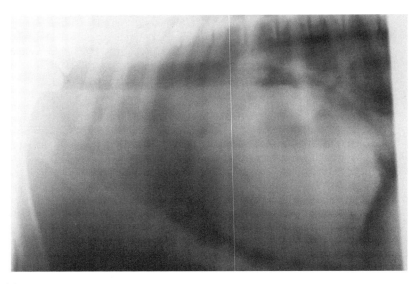

Figure 11
Pericardial effusion in a Golden Retriever.

Tricuspid dysplasia
- Congenital
- Males predisposed

Duchenne's X-linked muscular dystrophy cardiomyopathy
- Also known as Golden Retriever muscular dystrophy
- Rare
- Genetically determined

Pericardial effusion (see figure 11)
- Acquired
- Relative risk 7.4
- Haemangiosarcoma of the right atrium common in this breed

Mitral valve dysplasia
- Congenital

Dermatological conditions
Pyotraumatic folliculitis
- Young dogs predisposed
- Also known as hot spot; wet eczema
- Relative risk 2.3

Pododermatitis
- Front feet more commonly affected

Grass awn migration
- Common in the summer months

Atopy
- Females probably predisposed
- Age of onset from 6 months to 7 years
- May or may not be seasonal
- Relative risk 2.3

Food hypersensitivity
- No age or sex predisposition reported

Nasal depigmentation
- Also known as Dudley nose
- Unknown cause
- Seasonal depigmentation (snow nose) also seen in this breed

Mucocutaneous hypopigmentation
- Nasal form common in this breed

Acral lick dermatitis
- Occurs in males more commonly than females
- Can occur at any age, but usually over 5 years

Idiopathic sterile granuloma and pyogranuloma
- Uncommon
- No age or sex predisposition

Canine juvenile cellulitis
- Familial; possibly inherited
- Usually 1–4 months of age at onset

Skin tumours
- See Neoplastic conditions

Endocrine diseases
Hypothyroidism
- Breed predisposition
- Often middle-aged (2–6 years)

Thyroid neoplasia (may be associated with hyper- or hypothyroidism, but most cases are euthyroid)
- Possible breed predisposition
- Average age 10 years

Insulinoma
- Higher incidence seen in this breed
- Usually middle-aged/older dogs

Gastrointestinal conditions
Oropharyngeal neoplasia
- Possible breed predisposition

Secondary megaoesophagus
- A breed predisposition exists to myasthenia gravis, which may be an underlying cause of megaoesophagus

Congenital portosystemic shunt
- Breed predisposition reported in the USA
- Clinical signs usually seen in young dogs (<1 year)

Musculoskeletal conditions
Muscular dystrophy
- X-linked recessive inheritance in this breed
- Similar to Duchenne's muscular dystrophy in man

Myasthenia gravis
- See under Neurological conditions

Shoulder osteochondrosis
- Male:female ratio 2.24:1
- 50% bilateral
- Age of onset usually 4–7 months but can be older

Elbow dysplasia
- Also known as osteochondrosis
- Osteochondritis of the medial condyle of the humerus is common in this breed

Hip dysplasia
- Eleventh worst mean-scoring breed in the BVA/KC Hip Dysplasia Scheme as of October 2001
- Breed mean score 19
- A large 1989 study showed a prevalence of 25.9% in this breed

Hock osteochondrosis
- Common disease
- Mainly affects the proximal medial trochlear ridge

Temporomandibular dysplasia
- Congenital
- Uncommon

Neoplastic conditions
Mast cell tumours
- Possible breed predisposition
- May be seen at any age (from 4 months onwards), but usually seen in older animals

Sweat gland tumour
- Reported to be at increased risk
- Average age reported as 9.5 years

Trichoepithelioma
- Possible breed predisposition
- Average age reported as 9 years

Melanoma
- Breed predisposition
- Average age 8–9 years

Cutaneous haemangioma
- Possible breed predisposition
- Average age was 8.7 years in one study

Cutaneous haemangiosarcoma
- Uncommon
- Possible breed predisposition
- Average age 9–10 years

Benign fibrous histiocytoma
- Occur at an average age of 2–4 years

DOGS

DOGS

Fibroma
- Females predisposed
- Affects older animals

Non-epitheliotropic lymphoma
- Affects older dogs

Nasal cavity tumours
- Reported to be at increased risk for nasal carcinoma
- Average age reported as 10.5–11 years
- Dogs in urban areas may be at increased risk

Thyroid neoplasia
- See under Endocrine conditions

Insulinoma
- See under Endocrine conditions

Primary brain tumour
- See under Neurological conditions

Lymphosarcoma (malignant lymphoma)
- Higher incidence noted in this breed
- Most cases are seen in middle-aged dogs (mean 6–7 years)

Fibrosarcoma (oral and soft tissue)
- High incidence in this breed reported by some authors
- Males may be predisposed to oral fibrosarcomas
- Mean age of onset is 7.5 years but up to 25% of cases have been seen <5 years

Neurological conditions
True epilepsy
- Inheritance suspected
- Age of onset: 6 months to 3 years

Hypomyelination of the peripheral nervous system
- Inheritance suspected
- Rare
- Age of clinical onset: 5–7 weeks

Acquired myasthenia gravis
- Breed predisposition
- Adults affected

Eosinophilic meningoencephalitis
- 3 of 6 dogs were Golden Retrievers in a report of this condition
- Age of onset: 4 months to 5.5 years

Primary brain tumour
- Higher incidence noted in this breed
- Older dogs affected (mean 9–10 years)

Ocular conditions
Entropion (usually lower lids)
- Breed predisposition; polygenic inheritance likely

Ectropion (mild, usually disappears with maturity)
- Breed predisposition; polygenic inheritance likely

Distichiasis
- Breed predisposition
- Common in this breed

Lacrimal punctal aplasia
- Congenital condition; predisposed breed

Medial canthal pocket syndrome
- Breed predisposition due to head shape

Refractory corneal ulceration
- Breed predisposition
- Usually middle-aged

Corneal dystrophy
- Mode of inheritance unknown
- Progressive, bilateral degeneration, with lipid and calcium salt deposition seen first at the periphery of the cornea
- Age of onset: <2 years

Primary glaucoma/goniodysgenesis
- Mode of inheritance unknown
- Mainly in the UK
- Schedule 3 of the BVA/KC/ISDS Eye Scheme

Uveal cysts
- Breed predisposition
- Age of clinical onset: 2 years
- May be associated with anterior uveitis and secondary glaucoma in this breed

Pigmentary uveitis
- Breed predisposition
- May be associated with uveal cysts

Congenital tumours of the iris and ciliary body
- Breed predisposition suggested
- Present at a young age (2 years)

Cataract
- Dominant inheritance with incomplete penetration suggested
- Localisation: posterior subcapsular cortex
- Age of onset: 6–18 months; slowly progressive
- Schedule 1 of the BVA/KC/ISDS Eye Scheme

Congenital hereditary cataract
- Inheritance suspected
- Schedule 3 of the BVA/KC/ISDS Eye Scheme

Multifocal retinal dysplasia
- Congenital condition; autosomal recessive inheritance suspected
- Schedule 1 of the BVA/KC/ISDS Eye Scheme

Geographic retinal dysplasia
- Congenital condition, inheritance suspected
- Reported in the UK

Generalised progressive retinal atrophy
- Mode of inheritance unknown but presumed recessive
- There may be two types, one occurring in the first 2 years, the other later at 5–7 years
- Schedule 1 BVA/KC/ISDS Eye Scheme

Central progressive retinal atrophy (CPRA) or retinal pigment epithelial dystrophy (RPED)
- Breed predisposition; inheritance suspected
- More prevalent in the UK than in the USA. Becoming less prevalent following the introduction of control schemes
- Dogs affected from 3 years of age; visual problems noticed at 4–5 years
- Schedule 1 of the BVA/KC/ISDS Eye Scheme

Optic nerve colobomas
- Congenital defect; not known if inherited
- Seen occasionally in this breed

Pseudopapilloedema
- Congenital condition
- Reported in this breed

Multiple ocular defects
- Congenital defects; inheritance suspected
- Defects may include cataract, retinal detachment and microphthalmia
- Schedule 3 of the BVA/KC/ISDS Eye Scheme

Renal and urinary conditions
Familial renal disease (renal dysplasia)
- Reported in young dogs <3 years
- Cases present in renal failure

Ectopic ureters
- Congenital defect; higher incidence reported in this breed
- Usually presents <1 year of age
- More commonly diagnosed in females

Silica urolithiasis
- Higher incidence has been noted in this breed in some surveys
- Males seem to be predisposed

Reproductive conditions
Congenital preputial stenosis
- Reports of familial occurrence in this breed

Respiratory conditions
Laryngeal paralysis
- Idiopathic

GORDON SETTER

Dermatological conditions
Atopy
- Females probably predisposed
- Age of onset from 6 months to 7 years
- May or may not be seasonal

Callus dermatitis/pyoderma
- Often sternal calluses in this breed

Black hair follicular dysplasia
- Rare
- Early onset
- Familial

Canine juvenile cellulitis
- Familial; possibly inherited
- Usually 1–4 months of age at onset

Vitamin-A responsive dermatosis
- In this breed the condition presents with pruritus rather than seborrhoea

Gastrointestinal conditions
Gastric dilatation-volvulus
- Possible breed predisposition

Musculoskeletal conditions
Hip dysplasia
- Sixth worst mean-scoring breed in the BVA/KC Hip Dysplasia Scheme as of October 2001
- Breed mean score 25

Neurological conditions
Cerebellar degeneration (late-onset)
- Autosomal recessive inheritance
- Uncommon
- Signs seen at 6–30 months

Ocular conditions
Combined entropion-ectropion ('diamond eye')
- Breed predisposition; genetic basis incompletely understood
- May be seen with medial canthal pocket syndrome

Medial canthal pocket syndrome
- Breed predisposition due to head shape

Cataract
- Inheritance suspected
- Localisation: posterior lens capsule and sub-capsular cortex
- Age of onset: 2–3 years

Generalised progressive retinal atrophy
- Mode of inheritance unknown but presumed recessive
- Age of onset varies

Micropapilla
- Congenital condition
- Seen occasionally in this breed

Respiratory conditions
Primary ciliary dyskinesia
- Signs usually seen early in life

GREAT DANE

Cardiovascular conditions
Aortic stenosis
- Congenital
- No sex predilection
- Inheritance possibly autosomal dominant with modifying genes, or polygenic

Persistent right aortic arch
- Congenital

Tricuspid dysplasia
- Congenital
- Males predisposed

Mitral valve dysplasia
- Congenital

Dilated cardiomyopathy
- Prevalence of 3.9% in this breed compared to 0.16% in mixed breeds and 0.65% in pure breeds
- Increased prevalence with age
- Approximately twice as common in males as females
- Thought to be familial or genetic

Dermatological conditions
Muzzle folliculitis/furunculosis
- Also known as canine acne
- Local trauma, hormones and genetics may play a role in pathogenesis

Pododermatitis
- Males predisposed
- Front feet more commonly affected

Generalised demodicosis
- Great Danes are in the ten breeds at highest statistical risk of this disease in the Cornell, USA population

Cryptococcosis
- See under Infectious conditions

Colour-dilution alopecia
- Coat-colour genes involved in the pathogenesis

Primary lymphoedema
- No apparent sex predisposition
- Usually occurs within first 12 weeks of life

Acral lick dermatitis
- Occurs in males more commonly than females
- Can occur at any age, but usually over 5 years

Callus dermatitis/pyoderma
- Most common over hock and elbow joints of this breed

Zinc-responsive dermatosis
- Occurs in rapidly-growing dogs fed zinc-deficient diets

Idiopathic sterile granuloma and pyogranuloma
- Uncommon
- No age or sex predisposition

Skin tumours
- See under Neoplastic conditions

Endocrine conditions
Hypothyroidism
- Reported in some texts to be at increased risk
- Often middle-aged (2–6 years)

Gastrointestinal conditions
Congenital idiopathic megaoesophagus
- Breed predisposition

Gastric dilatation-volvulus
- Breed predisposition

Lymphocytic-plasmacytic colitis
- Possible breed predisposition

Infectious conditions
Cryptococcosis
- Increased incidence seen in this breed possibly due to an increased likelihood of exposure

- Usually seen in dogs under 4 years; no obvious sex predilection
- Worldwide distribution, but favoured by warm, humid climates

Musculoskeletal conditions
Central core myopathy
- Very rare
- Young adults affected

Shoulder osteochondrosis
- Male:female ratio 2.24:1
- 50% bilateral
- Age of onset usually 4–7 months, but can be older

Lateral patellar luxation
- Also known as genu valgum
- May be inherited

Neoplastic conditions
Canine cutaneous histiocytoma
- Possible breed predisposition
- More common in young dogs 1–2 years of age

Primary bone tumours (most commonly osteosarcoma) (see figure 12)
- Breed predisposition
- Males may be predisposed

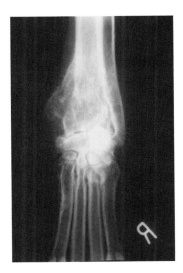

Figure 12
Radiograph of a dog with osteosarcoma.
Photo courtesy of Andy Moores.

Neurological conditions

Congenital deafness (Harlequin Great Danes)
- Signs seen from birth

Cervical vertebral malformation (wobbler syndrome)
- Breed predisposition
- Common in this breed
- Age of clinical onset: 1–2 years

Distal polyneuropathy
- Age of clinical onset: 1.5–5 years

Hyperaesthesia syndrome
- Possible breed predisposition

Ocular conditions

Entropion (usually lateral lower lids, occasionally lateral upper lids)
- Breed predisposition; polygenic inheritance likely

Ectropion (may be associated with 'diamond eye')
- Breed predisposition; polygenic inheritance likely

Combined entropion-ectropion ('diamond eye')
- Breed predisposition; genetic basis incompletely understood

Medial canthal pocket syndrome
- Breed predisposition due to head shape

Eversion of the cartilage of the nictitating membrane
- Breed predisposition; possibly inherited as a recessive trait
- Usually occurs in young dogs

Primary glaucoma/goniodysgenesis
- Inheritance suspected
- Age of onset: 1–9 years
- Mainly in the UK
- Schedule 3 of the BVA/KC/ISDS Eye Scheme

Cataract
- Inheritance suspected
- Localisation: posterior subcapsular cortex

- Age of onset: 2 years; may progress to completion and blindness

Generalised progressive retinal atrophy (GPRA)
- Mode of inheritance unknown but presumed recessive

Multiple ocular defects
- Autosomal dominant inheritance with variable expression has been suggested
- Seen in homozygous merles (the result of merle to merle breeding) with predominantly white coats
- Defects may include microphthalmia, microcornea, cataract, equatorial staphylomas and retinal dysplasia. These dogs may also be deaf

Reproductive conditions

Penile hypoplasia
- Rare congenital condition which has been reported in this breed
- May be seen as part of some intersex states

GREYHOUND

Dermatological conditions

Idiopathic cutaneous and renal glomerular vasculopathy
- Seen in kenneled and racing Greyhounds
- No age or sex predilection

Pattern baldness
- Affects almost exclusively females
- Ventral neck and ventrum affected

Ehler-Danlos syndrome
- Also known as cutaneous asthenia
- Inherited group of diseases
- May be inherited as an autosomal dominant trait
- Probably lethal to homozygotes

Ventral comedone syndrome
- Common

Vasculitis
- Uncommon
- Usually type III hypersensitivity reaction

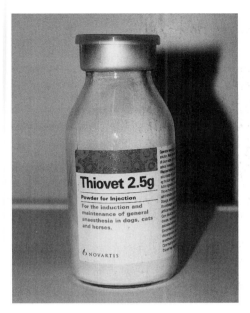

Figure 13
Greyhounds are very sensitive to the effects of thiopentone anaesthesia.

Drug reactions
Thiopentone (see figure 13)
- This breed has a greatly increased susceptibility to thiopentone
- Use of this drug is not recommended in this breed

Haematological conditions
Haemolytic uraemic syndrome
- A disorder of platelet hyperaggregability

Musculoskeletal conditions
Polyarthritis of Greyhounds
- Affects animals aged 3–30 months

Exertional myopathy
- Lack of fitness, over-excitement and hot humid conditions predispose

Medial displacement of biceps brachii tendon
- Uncommon

Accessory carpal-bone fracture
- Usually affects right carpus
- Sprain-avulsion type fractures due to carpal hyperextension occur during racing

Carpal soft-tissue injuries
- Often caused by carpal hyperextension during racing

Chronic sesamoiditis
- Common
- May be asymptomatic

Avulsion of tibial tuberosity
- Growth-plate fracture

Spontaneous tibial fracture
- Fractures of caudal distal articular margin of the tibia reported in racing Greyhounds

Calcaneoquartal subluxation due to plantar tarsal ligament rupture
- Common hock injury
- Affects athletic dogs during racing

Calcaneus fracture
- Common in racing Greyhounds
- May be associated with central-tarsal-bone fracture or extreme tension along plantar aspect of bone

Central-tarsal-bone fracture
- Very common in racing Greyhound
- Usually affects right hock due to stresses of cornering to the left

Superficial digital flexor tendon luxation
- Uncommon
- Usually lateral luxation

Neurological conditions
Congenital deafness
- Signs seen from birth

Ocular conditions
Chronic superficial keratitis (pannus)
- Breed predisposition
- Age of onset: 2–5 years

DOGS

Lens luxation
- Breed predisposition; inheritance suspected
- Age of onset: 3–5 years

Generalised progressive retinal atrophy
- Mode of inheritance unknown but presumed recessive
- Condition occurs early and may progress to blindness by 2 years

Physiological conditions
Hypertension
- Greyhounds have higher blood pressures than other breeds, even if not trained for racing

Cardiac hypertrophy
- Cardiac output is higher and total peripheral resistance is lower in this breed than others
- Blood volume is also higher than in other breeds

Prominent cytoplasmic vacuolation of eosinophils

Short red blood cell lifespan
- It is not known if the survival of red cells after transfusion is shorter than for other breeds
- Erythrocytes are larger in this breed than in others

Packed cell volume
- Greyhounds have a higher packed cell volume than other breeds
- Mean cellular haemoglobin concentration and mean cell volume is higher than for other breeds
- Red blood cell count is lower than for other breeds

Thrombocytopaenia
- Platelet counts are lower in this breed than others

Blood group
- This breed tends to be DEA 1.1 and 1.2 negative

Thyroid hormones
- T4 and free T4 are lower in healthy Greyhounds than other breeds
- Mean cTSH is the same as for other breeds

Supernumerary teeth
- Present in 36.4% of Greyhounds surveyed
- Usually first premolar
- Usually occurs in the upper arcade

GRIFFON BRUXELLOIS

Ocular conditions
Refractory corneal ulceration
- Breed predisposition
- Usually middle-aged
- May be associated with distichiasis or trichiasis

Cataract
- Inheritance suspected
- Schedule 3 of the BVA/KC/ISDS Eye Scheme

HARRIER HOUND

Neurological conditions
Hound ataxia
- Reported in the UK
- Age of clinical onset: 2–7 years

HAVANESE

Ocular conditions
Cataract
- Inheritance suspected

HUNGARIAN PULI

Endocrine diseases
Diabetes mellitus
- Possible breed predisposition
- Usual age range: 4–14 years; peak incidence: 7–9 years
- Old entire females are predisposed

Musculoskeletal conditions
Hip dysplasia
- This breed has the twentieth worst breed mean score in the BVA/KC Hip Dysplasia Scheme as of October 2001
- Breed mean score 17

Ocular conditions
Cataract
- Inheritance suspected
- Localisation: posterior sutures and cortex
- Likely to progress and may cause visual deficiencies

Multifocal retinal dysplasia
- Congenital condition; autosomal recessive inheritance suspected
- Schedule 1 of the BVA/KC/ISDS Eye Scheme

Micropapilla
- Congenital condition
- Seen occasionally in this breed

HUNGARIAN VIZSLA

Dermatological conditions
Granulomatous sebaceous adenitis
- No sex predisposition
- Annular scaling and alopecia occurs in this breed

Immunological conditions
Immune-mediated thrombocytopaenia
- Common
- Familial in this breed; likely inherited
- Females more commonly affected than males

Ocular conditions
Entropion (usually lateral lower lids)
- Breed predisposition; polygenic inheritance likely

Cataract
- Inheritance suspected

Primary glaucoma/goniodysgenesis
- Schedule 3 of the BVA/KC/ISDS Eye Scheme

Generalised progressive retinal atrophy (GPRA)
- Mode of inheritance unknown but presumed recessive
- Clinically apparent by 3 years

IBIZAN HOUND

Neurological conditions
Congenital deafness
- Signs seen from birth

Ocular conditions
Medial canthal pocket syndrome
- Breed predisposition due to general head shape

Cataract 1
- Autosomal recessive inheritance has been suggested
- Cortical cataract seen in young dogs which progresses rapidly to completion with vision loss

Cataract 2
- Breed predisposition
- Nuclear fibrillar cataract in older dogs (5–8 years); little effect on vision

IRISH RED AND WHITE SETTER

Haematological conditions
Canine leucocyte adhesion deficiency (CLAD)
- Seen in the UK and Sweden
- A molecular diagnostic test is available

Ocular conditions
Cataract
- Inheritance suspected
- Schedule 1 of the BVA/KC/ISDS Eye Scheme

IRISH SETTER

Cardiovascular conditions
Persistent right aortic arch (vascular ring anomaly)
- Congenital
- Not all studies confirm predisposition in this breed
- See also vascular ring anomaly under Gastro-intestinal conditions

DOGS

Dermatological conditions

Pododermatitis
- Males predisposed
- Front feet more commonly affected

Atopy
- Females probably predisposed
- Age of onset from 6 months to 7 years
- May or may not be seasonal

Primary seborrhoea
- Probably inherited as autosomal recessive
- Signs first appear at early age and get worse with age

Ichthyosis
- Rare
- Congenital
- Possibly inherited as autosomal recessive

Ehler-Danlos syndrome
- Also known as cutaneous asthenia
- Inherited group of diseases
- May be inherited as an autosomal dominant trait
- Probably lethal to homozygotes

Nasal depigmentation
- Also known as Dudley nose
- Unknown cause

Acral lick dermatitis
- Occurs in males more commonly than females
- Can occur at any age, but usually over 5 years

Callus dermatitis/pyoderma
- Usually affects the sternum in this breed

Greying
- May occur at a young age in this breed

Skin tumours
- See under Neoplastic conditions

Endocrine conditions

Hypothyroidism
- Probable breed predisposition
- Often middle-aged (2–6 years)

Insulinoma
- Higher incidence seen in this breed
- Usually middle-aged/older dogs

Gastrointestinal conditions

Congenital idiopathic megaoesophagus
- Breed predisposition

Vascular ring anomaly
- Breed predisposition; inheritance suspected

Gastric dilatation-volvulus
- Breed predisposition

Gluten-sensitive enteropathy
- Breed predisposition

Perianal fistula
- Possible breed predisposition

Musculoskeletal conditions

Temporomandibular dysplasia/luxation
- Congenital dysplasia may predispose to luxation

Irish Setter hypochondroplasia
- Mildly short limbs seen
- Inherited as autosomal recessive

Canine idiopathic polyarthritis
- Usually affects dogs at 1–3 years, but any age can be affected
- Males predisposed

Neoplastic conditions

Trichoepithelioma
- Possible breed predisposition
- Average age reported as 9 years

Sebaceous gland tumours
- Possible breed predisposition to sebaceous epithelioma
- Seen in older dogs (average age 10 years)

Haemangiopericytoma
- Occurs at a mean age of 7–10 years

Non-epitheliotropic lymphoma
- Affects older dogs

Melanoma
- Breed predisposition
- Average age 8–9 years

Melanoma of the digit
- Possible breed predisposition
- Average age 10–11 years

Insulinoma
- See under Endocrine conditions

Haematological conditions
Granulocytopathy of Irish Setters
- Inherited as an autosomal recessive trait

Canine leucocyte adhesion deficiency (CLAD)
- Seen in the UK and Sweden
- A molecular diagnostic test is available

Neurological conditions
Cerebellar malformation
- Congenital
- Uncommon
- Age of clinical onset: <3 months

True epilepsy
- Inherited
- Age of onset: 6 months to 3 years

Lissencephaly
- Rare developmental disease
- Age of onset: <1 year

Ambylopia and quadriplegia
- Autosomal recessive inheritance
- Congenital paralysis and blindness with no visible ocular cause (ambylopia)

Hyperaesthesia syndrome
- Possible breed predisposition

Ocular conditions
Entropion (usually lower lids)
- Breed predisposition; polygenic inheritance likely

Eversion of the cartilage of the nictitating membrane
- Breed predisposition; possibly inherited as a recessive trait
- Usually occurs in young dogs

Refractory corneal ulceration
- Breed predisposition
- Usually middle-aged

Glaucoma
- Possible breed predisposition

Cataract
- Inheritance suspected
- Localisation: posterior subcapsular cortex
- Age of onset: 6–18 months; slowly progressive

Generalised progressive retinal atrophy (GPRA)
- Autosomal recessive inheritance
- Rod-cone dysplasia type I
- Ophthalmoscopic signs visible by 16 weeks, endstage reached at approximately 1 year
- Schedule 1 BVA/KC/ISDS Eye Scheme
- A second form of PRA, occurring at 4–5 years, may be seen in this breed

Micropapilla
- Congenital condition
- Seen occasionally in this breed

Optic nerve colobomas
- Congenital defect; not known if inherited
- Seen occasionally in this breed

Ambylopia and quadriplegia
- Autosomal recessive inheritance
- Congenital paralysis and blindness with no visible ocular cause (ambylopia)

Renal and urinary conditions
Urethral sphincter mechanism incompetence (causing urinary incontinence)
- Possible breed predisposition in female dogs

Respiratory conditions
Laryngeal paralysis
- Idiopathic

IRISH TERRIER

Dermatological conditions
Footpad hyperkeratosis
- Familial in this breed

Skin tumours
- See under Neoplastic conditions

Musculoskeletal conditions
Muscular dystrophy
- X-linked degenerative myopathy described in a litter of Irish Terrier puppies

Neoplastic conditions
Melanoma
- Breed predisposition
- Average age 8–9 years

Ocular conditions
Multiple ocular defects
- Autosomal recessive inheritance has been suggested
- Defects may include microphthalmia, cataract, persistent pupillary membranes and retinal dysplasia

IRISH WATER SPANIEL

Dermatological conditions
Canine follicular dysplasia
- A marked predilection in this breed implies a genetic basis for this group of diseases
- Hair loss begins at 2–4 years of age, and occurs mainly on the flanks
- Hair loss is due to fracture of the hair in this breed
- Eventually the whole of the trunk is involved

Musculoskeletal conditions
Hip dysplasia
- This breed has the seventeenth worst breed mean score in the BVA/KC Hip Dysplasia Scheme as of October 2001
- Breed mean score 18

Ocular conditions
Cataract
- Inheritance suspected
- Localisation: posterior subcapsular cortex
- Age of onset: 5 years; slowly progressive

IRISH WOLFHOUND

Cardiovascular conditions
Dilated cardiomyopathy
- Prevalence of 5.6% in this breed compared to 0.16% in mixed breeds and 0.65% in pure breeds
- Increased prevalence with age
- Approximately twice as common in males as females
- Thought to be familial or genetic

Atrial fibrillation (see figure 14)
- High frequency (10.5%) in this breed
- Often asymptomatic
- Ventricular premature complexes may also be seen in this breed

Dermatological conditions
Callus dermatitis/pyoderma
- Most common over hock and elbow joints of this breed

Endocrine conditions
Hypothyroidism
- Reported in some texts to be at increased risk
- Often middle-aged (2–6 years)

Gastrointestinal conditions
Gastric dilatation-volvulus
- Possible breed predisposition

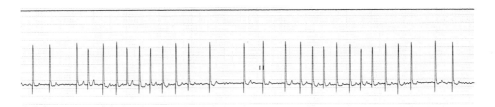

Figure 14
Atrial fibrillation (Lead II trace, 10mm/mV, 25mm/s).

Congenital portosystemic shunt
- Breed predisposition
- Clinical signs usually seen in young dogs <1 year

Haematological/immunological conditions

Immunodeficiency syndrome of Irish Wolfhounds
- Seen in different geographical regions
- Variously reported as a defect in cell-mediated immunity or a deficiency in IgA

Von Willebrand's disease
- Possibly inherited as an autosomal recessive trait
- Common in this breed in the UK

Musculoskeletal conditions

Increased anteversion of the femoral head and neck
- Conformational abnormality

Shoulder osteochondrosis
- Male:female ratio 2.24:1
- 50% bilateral
- Age of onset usually 4–7 months but can be older

Lateral patellar luxation
- Also known as genu valgum
- May be inherited

Neoplastic conditions

Primary bone tumours (most commonly osteosarcoma)
- Breed predisposition
- Males may be predisposed

Neurological conditions

Cervical vertebral malformation (wobbler syndrome)
- Breed predisposition
- Seen occasionally in this breed
- Age of clinical onset: >1 year

Ocular conditions

Entropion (usually lateral lower lids)
- Breed predisposition; polygenic inheritance likely

Eversion of the cartilage of the nictitating membrane
- Breed predisposition; possibly inherited as a recessive trait
- Usually occurs in young dogs

Cataract
- Inheritance suspected
- Localisation: posterior subcapsular cortex
- Age of onset: 1–2 years (with rapid progression), or 5–7 years (with slower progression)

Multifocal retinal dysplasia with liquefied vitreous
- Autosomal recessive inheritance suggested

Generalised progressive retinal atrophy (GPRA)
- Inheritance suspected
- Schedule 1 BVA/KC/ISDS Eye Scheme

Micropapilla
- Congenital condition
- Seen occasionally in this breed

ITALIAN GREYHOUND

Dermatological conditions

Pinnal alopecia
- Age of onset usually greater than 1 year

Pattern baldness
- Affects almost exclusively females
- Ventral neck and ventrum affected

Colour-dilution alopecia
- Coat-colour genes are involved in the pathogenesis

Drug reactions

Thiopentone
- This breed has a greatly increased susceptibility to thiopentone
- Use of this drug is not recommended in this breed

Ocular conditions

Corneal dystrophy
- Breed predisposition
- Focal opacity at Descemet's membrane
- Occurs in young dogs

DOGS

DOGS

Glaucoma
- Mode of inheritance unknown
- Age of onset: 2 years
- Vitreal degeneration is believed to be a common cause of glaucoma in this breed

Cataract
- Inheritance suspected
- Localisation: posterior subcapsular cortex
- Age of onset: 2–3 years; may progress to interfere with vision

Optic nerve hypoplasia
- Congenital condition; not known if inherited
- Seen occasionally in this breed

JACK RUSSELL TERRIER

Dermatological conditions
Malassezia dermatitis
- Often seasonal
- Affects any age

Ichthyosis
- Rare
- Congenital
- Possibly inherited as an autosomal recessive trait

Vasculitis
- Uncommon
- Usually type III hypersensitivity reaction

Endocrine conditions
Diabetes mellitus
- Possible breed predisposition
- Usual age range: 4–14 years; peak incidence: 7–9 years
- Old entire females are predisposed

Hyperadrenocorticism: pituitary-dependent (PDH)
- Possible breed predisposition
- Middle-aged/older
- 55–60% female

Musculoskeletal conditions
Congenital myasthenia gravis
- See under Neurological conditions

Avascular necrosis of the femoral head
- Mechanism of inheritance not known

Patellar luxation
- May be inherited as an autosomal recessive trait

Neoplastic conditions
Pituitary tumour resulting in hyperadrenocorticism
- See under Endocrine diseases

Neurological conditions
Hereditary ataxia
- Reported in Britain
- Age of clinical onset: 2–6 months

Congenital myasthenia gravis
- Autosomal recessive inheritance suspected
- Rare
- Age of clinical onset: 2–6 months

Ocular conditions
Lens luxation
- Autosomal dominant inheritance suggested
- Age of onset: 3–6 years
- High incidence with females predisposed

Cataract
- Inheritance suspected

JAPANESE AKITA

Cardiovascular conditions
Ventricular septal defect
- Relative risk 3 to 4.9
- No sex predilection
- Not known to be inherited in this breed

Pericardial effusion
- Relative risk 6.5
- Usually affects middle-aged dogs

Dermatological conditions
Pemphigus foliaceous
- Uncommon disease
- No sex predisposition
- Mean age of onset 4 years

Canine uveodermatological syndrome
- Also known as Vogt-Koyanagi-Harada-like syndrome
- See also under Ocular conditions

Granulomatous sebaceous adenitis
- Young to middle-aged dogs affected
- No sex predisposition
- Tends to involve generalised, greasy changes in Akitas
- Some animals may show systemic signs

Gastrointestinal conditions
Gastric dilatation-volvulus
- Possible breed predisposition

Musculoskeletal conditions
Polyarthritis/meningitis
- Idiopathic
- This breed is prone to a more severe form of the disease

Cranial cruciate ligament rupture
- Neutered individuals may be predisposed
- Young animals may be predisposed in this breed

Neurological conditions
Congenital vestibular disease
- Signs seen <3 months
- May be seen with congenital deafness

Congenital deafness
- Signs seen from birth

Meningitis and polyarteritis
- Reported in this breed
- Age of onset: <1 year

Glycogenosis (glycogen storage disease)
- Rare
- Age of clinical onset: <3 months

Ocular conditions
Entropion (usually lower lids)
- Breed predisposition; polygenic inheritance likely

Uveodermatologic syndrome
- Also known as Vogt-Koyanagi-Harada-like syndrome
- Breed predisposition
- Young adults (1.5–4 years)

Glaucoma
- Breed predisposition
- May be associated with a narrow iridocorneal filtration angle
- Age of onset: 2–4 years

Multifocal retinal dysplasia
- Congenital condition; inheritance as an autosomal recessive trait suspected

Generalised progressive retinal atrophy (GPRA)
- Autosomal recessive inheritance suspected
- Night blindness is present at 1–3 years, complete blindness at 3–5 years
- Schedule 3 BVA/KC/ISDS Eye Scheme

Multiple ocular defects
- Congenital defects; autosomal recessive inheritance suggested
- May include microphthalmia, cataract and retinal dysplasia

Physiological conditions
Red blood cell microcytosis
- Red blood cells may be small in this breed without disease
- MCV may be as low as 55–64 fl (normal 85–95)
- Red blood cells contain more potassium than other breeds, therefore haemolysis can cause false findings of hyperkalaemia

JAPANESE CHIN

Neurological conditions
Atlantoaxial subluxation
- Congenital
- Relatively common in this breed
- Age of clinical onset: <1 year

DOGS

Ocular conditions
Distichiasis
- Breed predisposition

Refractory corneal ulceration
- Breed predisposition

Cataract
- Inheritance suspected
- May be seen with progressive retinal atrophy and retinal detachment

KEESHOND

Cardiovascular conditions
Patent ductus arteriosus
- Common congenital abnormality
- Relative risk 5.9
- Females predisposed
- Mode of inheritance is polygenic

Tetralogy of Fallot
- Congenital
- Uncommon

Ventricular septal defect
- Congenital
- Uncommon

Dermatological conditions
Ehler-Danlos syndrome
- Also known as cutaneous asthenia
- Inherited group of diseases
- May be inherited as an autosomal dominant trait
- Probably lethal to homozygotes

Adult-onset growth-hormone-responsive dermatosis
- See under Endocrine conditions

Skin tumours
- See under Neoplastic conditions

Endocrine conditions
Adult-onset growth-hormone-responsive dermatosis
- Breed predisposition
- Males may be predisposed
- Clinical signs usually seen at 1–5 years

Diabetes mellitus
- Possible breed predisposition
- Usual age range: 4–14 years; peak incidence: 7–9 years
- Old entire females are predisposed

Primary hyperparathyroidism
- Uncommon condition
- Suspected breed predisposition
- Older dogs affected

Neoplastic conditions
Keratoacanthoma
- Usually affects dogs younger than 5 years
- Male dogs predisposed
- This breed is predisposed to the generalised form of the disease

Nasal cavity tumours
- Reported to be at increased risk for nasal carcinoma
- Usually older dogs
- Dogs in urban areas may be at increased risk

Parathyroid tumours (resulting in primary hyperparathyroidism)
- See under Endocrine conditions

Neurological conditions
True epilepsy
- Inherited
- Age of onset: 6 months to 3 years

Ocular conditions
Glaucoma
- Possible breed predisposition

Cataract
- Inheritance suspected
- 3 types: rapidly progressive posterior cortical cataracts are seen in young dogs (5 months); slowly progressive posterior cortical cataracts seen at 6–24 months; slowly progressive anterior cortical cataracts seen at 6 years

KERRY BLUE TERRIER

Cardiovascular conditions
Patent ductus arteriosus
- Common congenital abnormality
- Females predisposed

Dermatological conditions
Footpad hyperkeratosis
- Reported in several related Kerry Blues

Spiculosis
- Rare
- Affects young, entire male Kerry Blues

Dermoid cyst
- Rare
- Solitary or multiple
- Occur on dorsal midline

Scrotal vascular naevus
- More common in older dogs

Skin tumours
- See under Neoplastic conditions

Haematological conditions
Factor XI deficiency
- Inherited as an autosomal dominant trait
- Only heterozygotes asymptomatic

Neoplastic conditions
Basal cell tumour
- Reported to be at increased risk

Pilomatrixoma
- Possible breed predisposition
- Rare
- Average age reported as 6.6 years

Cutaneous papillomas
- Possible breed predisposition
- Seen in older dogs

Neurological conditions
Cerebellar degeneration
- Autosomal recessive inheritance
- Uncommon
- Signs seen at 3–6 months

Ocular conditions
Entropion (usually lower lids)
- Breed predisposition, polygenic inheritance likely

Cataract
- Inheritance suspected

- Localisation: posterior cortex
- Early onset and progress rapidly to cause visual difficulties at 2 years

Optic nerve hypoplasia
- Congenital condition; not known if inherited
- Seen occasionally in this breed

Reproductive conditions
XX sex reversal
- Congenital condition reported in this breed

KING CHARLES SPANIEL (ENGLISH TOY SPANIEL)

Gastrointestinal conditions
Haemorrhagic gastroenteritis
- Possible breed predisposition
- Seen most commonly at 2–4 years of age

Neurological conditions
Partial seizures ('fly-biting' and 'star-gazing')
- Reported in this breed

Ocular conditions
Corneal dystrophy
- Breed predisposition; not known if inherited
- Stromal lipid dystrophy
- Age of onset: 2–5 years

Cataract
- Inheritance suspected
- Localisation: posterior cortex and nucleus
- Age of onset: 6 months; rapidly progressive to completion and blindness

Persistence of the hyaloid system and posterior lenticonus
- Breed predisposition

Pseudopapilloedema
- Congenital condition
- Seen occasionally in this breed

Microphthalmia
- Autosomal recessive inheritance suspected
- May be accompanied by cataract

KOMONDOR

Ocular conditions
Entropion
- Breed predisposition; polygenic inheritance likely

Cataract
- Inheritance suspected
- Localisation: posterior subcapsular cortex
- Age of onset: 2–3 years; slowly progressive

KUVASZ

Neurological conditions
Congenital deafness
- Signs seen from birth

Ocular conditions
Entropion
- Breed predisposition; polygenic inheritance likely

Cataract
- Inheritance suspected
- Cataracts in this breed seem to be slowly progressive

LABRADOR RETRIEVER

Cardiovascular conditions
Tricuspid dysplasia
- Congenital
- Males predisposed
- Marked risk in this breed (relative risk >5)

Patent ductus arteriosus
- Generally this breed is at lower risk of this condition than other breeds
- May be predisposed in some areas

Pericardial effusion
- Acquired
- Relative risk 2.2

Pulmonic stenosis
- Third most frequent cause of canine congenital heart disease
- Polygenic mode of inheritance likely

Bypass tract macro re-entrant tachycardia in Labrador Retrievers
- Abnormal conduction leading to dysrhythmia

Dermatological conditions
Pyotraumatic folliculitis
- Young dogs predisposed
- Also known as hot spot, wet eczema

Eosinophilic dermatitis and oedema
- Rare

Pododermatitis
- Males predisposed
- Front feet more commonly affected

Blastomycosis
- See under Infectious conditions

Cryptococcosis
- See under Infectious conditions

Atopy
- Females probably predisposed
- Age of onset from 6 months to 7 years
- May or may not be seasonal

Contact hypersensitivity
- One study found 20% of cases occurred in yellow Labradors

Food hypersensitivity
- No age or sex predisposition reported

Pemphigus foliaceous
- Usually drug induced in this breed

Cyclic follicular dysplasia
- Seems to be a particular problem in Alaska, so duration of daylight exposure may be important

Primary seborrhoea
- Autosomal recessive inheritance likely
- Signs first appear at early age and get worse with age

Ichthyosis
- Rare
- Congenital
- Possibly inherited as an autosomal recessive trait

Congenital hypotrichosis
- Present at birth or develops in the first month of life
- Predisposition for males suggests sex linkage

Primary lymphoedema
- No apparent sex predisposition
- Usually occurs within the first 12 weeks of life

Nasal depigmentation
- Affects yellow Labradors
- Also known as Dudley nose
- Cause unknown
- Seasonal depigmentation also seen in this breed; also known as snow nose

Nasal hyperkeratosis
- Possibly inherited as an autosomal recessive trait
- Affects males and females 6–12 months of age

Mucocutaneous hypopigmentation
- Nasal form is common in this breed

Acral lick dermatitis
- Occurs in males more commonly than females
- Can occur at any age, but usually over 5 years

Zinc-responsive dermatosis
- Occurs in rapidly-growing dogs fed zinc-deficient diets

Waterline disease of black Labrador Retrievers
- Affects either sex

Scrotal vascular naevus
- More common in older dogs

Greying
- May occur at a young age in this breed

Skin tumours
- See under Neoplastic conditions

Endocrine conditions
Hyperadrenocorticism: adrenocortical tumour (AT)
- Possible breed predisposition
- Middle-aged/older
- 60–65% female

Diabetes mellitus
- Frequently affected breed in some surveys
- Usual age range: 4–14 years; peak incidence: 7–9 years
- Old entire females are predisposed

Primary hypoparathyroidism
- Frequently affected breed in some surveys
- Uncommon condition
- Occurs at any age

Insulinoma
- Higher incidence seen in this breed
- Usually middle-aged/older dogs

Gastrointestinal conditions
Congenital idiopathic megaoesophagus
- Possible breed predisposition

Secondary megaoesophagus
- Familial reflex myoclonus may be associated with megaoesophagus

Lymphocytic-plasmacytic colitis
- Possible breed predisposition

Perianal fistula
- Possible breed predisposition

Chronic hepatitis
- Possible breed predisposition

Congenital portosystemic shunt
- Breed predisposition
- Clinical signs usually seen <1 year

Haematological conditions
Haemophilia B
- Factor IX defiency
- Also known as Christmas disease
- Inherited as a sex-linked trait
- Less common than haemophilia A

Infectious conditions
Cryptococcosis
- Increased incidence in this breed possibly due to an increased likelihood of exposure
- Usually seen in dogs under 4 years; no obvious sex predilection
- Worldwide distribution, but favoured by warm, humid climates

DOGS

DOGS

Blastomycosis
- Increased incidence in this breed possibly due to an increased likelihood of exposure
- Seen mainly in young male dogs living near water
- Geographic distribution: around the Mississippi, Ohio, Missouri, Tennessee, and St Lawrence Rivers, the southern Great Lakes and the southern mid-Atlantic states. Not reported in the UK

Infectious skin disease
- See under Dermatological conditions

Musculoskeletal conditions
Carpal ligament weakening
- Affects older obese dogs
- Tarsal ligaments may also be affected

Elbow dysplasia
- Also known as osteochondrosis
- Genetically determined in this breed
- Medial coronoid process disease is common in this breed
- A 1999 study estimated the prevalence in this breed as 17.8%
- Osteochondritis dissecans and fragmented coronoid processes are inherited independently as polygenic traits in this breed

Hip dysplasia
- A 1999 study estimated the prevalence in this breed as 12.6%

Ocular-skeletal dysplasia
- Defect of growth of tubular bone
- See retinal dysplasia with skeletal abnormalities under Ocular conditions

Labrador Retriever myopathy
- Common in the UK
- Onset of signs usually 8–12 weeks

Myasthenia gravis
- See under Neurological conditions

Shoulder osteochondrosis
- Male:female ratio 2.24:1
- 50% of cases are bilateral
- Age of onset is usually 4–7 months but can be older

Hock osteochondrosis
- Common disease
- Mainly affects the proximal medial trochlear ridge

Temporomandibular dysplasia
- Congenital
- Uncommon

Cranial cruciate ligament rupture
- Common cause of hind-limb lameness
- Neutered individuals may be predisposed
- Young animals may be predisposed in this breed

Transitional vertebral segments
- Females are predisposed
- Thought to be inherited

Neoplastic conditions
Mast cell tumours
- Possible breed predisposition
- May be seen at any age (from 4 months onwards), but usually seen in older animals

Canine cutaneous histiocytoma
- Possible breed predisposition
- More common in young dogs 1–2 years of age

Lipoma
- Possible breed predisposition
- Most common in middle-aged, obese female dogs
- Infiltrative lipomas can be seen in this breed

Squamous cell carcinoma of the digit
- Possible breed predisposition
- Older dogs
- Dogs with black coats seem to be more frequently affected

Nasal cavity tumours
- Reported to be at increased risk
- Average age reported as 10.5–11 years
- Dogs in urban areas may be at increased risk

Insulinoma
- See under Endocrine conditions

Adrenocortical tumour resulting in hyperadrenocorticism
- See under Endocrine conditions

Lymphosarcoma (malignant lymphoma)
- Higher incidence noted in this breed
- Most cases are seen in middle-aged dogs (mean 6–7 years)

Limbal melanoma
- Breed predisposition

Oral fibrosarcoma
- High incidence in this breed reported by some authors
- Males may be predisposed
- Mean age of onset is 7.5 years but up to 25% of cases have been seen <5 years

Thymoma
- Uncommon tumour
- High incidence reported in this breed in one study
- Mean age 7.5 years
- Possible predisposition for females

Neurological conditions
Cerebellar degeneration
- Has been reported
- Signs seen at 12 weeks

True epilepsy
- Inheritance suspected
- Age of onset: 6 months to 3 years

Narcolepsy-cataplexy
- Autosomal recessive inheritance suspected
- Age of clinical onset: <1 year

Acquired myasthenia gravis
- Possible breed predisposition
- Adults affected

Spongiform degeneration
- Inheritance suspected
- Rare
- Age of clinical onset: 3–6 months

Distal polyneuropathy
- Age of clinical onset: >1 year

Ocular conditions
Entropion (usually lower lids)
- Breed predisposition; polygenic inheritance likely

Ectropion (mild, usually disappears with maturity)
- Breed predisposition; polygenic inheritance likely

Medial canthal pocket syndrome
- Breed predisposition due to general head shape

Limbal melanoma
- Breed predisposition

Uveal cysts
- Breed predisposition
- Age of clinical onset: 3–6 years

Canine anterior uveal melanoma
- Breed predisposition

Cataract
- Dominant inheritance with incomplete penetrance suggested
- Localisation: posterior polar subcapsular
- Age of onset: 6–18 months; slowly progressive; rarely proceeds to blindness
- Schedule 1 of the BVA/KC/ISDS Eye Scheme
- Other types: anterior subcapsular occurring at about 5 years and progressing slowly (mode of inheritance unknown); peripheral cortical cataract occurring at 3 years and progressing slowly (mode of inheritance unknown)

Primary glaucoma
- Breed predisposition
- An association with goniodysgenesis has been suggested in this breed

Total retinal dysplasia with retinal detachment
- Congenital condition inherited as a simple autosomal recessive trait
- Retinal dysplasia without skeletal deformity is seen more commonly in Europe than the US
- Schedule 1 of the BVA/KC/ISDS Eye Scheme

DOGS

Multifocal retinal dysplasia
- Congenital condition; dominant inheritance with incomplete penetrance has been proposed
- Schedule 3 of the BVA/KC/ISDS Eye Scheme

Geographic retinal dysplasia
- Congenital condition; inheritance suspected
- Reported in the UK

Retinal dysplasia with skeletal abnormalities
- Dogs may be affected with retinal dysplasias (total, geographic or multifocal) and varying degrees of developmental skeletal abnormalities (short-limbed dwarfism)
- It has been suggested that this condition is inherited as one autosomal gene which has recessive effects on the skeleton and incomplete dominant effects on the eye

Generalised progressive retinal atrophy (GPRA)
- Autosomal recessive inheritance
- Progressive rod-cone degeneration (PRCD)
- Age of clinical onset and rate of progression vary; may be associated with cataract formation
- Schedule 1 BVA/KC/ISDS Eye Scheme

Central progressive retinal atrophy (CPRA) or retinal pigment epithelial dystrophy (RPED)
- Dominant inheritance with incomplete penetrance has been suggested
- More prevalent in the UK than in the USA
- Becoming less prevalent following the introduction of control schemes
- Ophthalmoscopic signs seen at 2–3 years of age; visual problems noticed at 4–5 years
- Schedule 1 of the BVA/KC/ISDS Eye Scheme

Micropapilla
- Congenital condition
- Seen occasionally in this breed

Optic nerve colobomas
- Congenital defect; not known if inherited
- Seen occasionally in this breed

Pseudopapilloedema
- Seen occasionally in this breed

Physiological conditions
Blood group
- This breed is usually DEA 1.1 or DEA 1.2 positive

Gestation
- Mean gestation reported as 60.9 days

Vertebral heart score
- The healthy dog has a higher mean score than most other breeds

Renal and urinary conditions
Ectopic ureters
- Congenital anomaly; higher incidence reported in this breed
- Usually presents <1 year of age
- More commonly diagnosed in females

Silica urolithiasis
- Higher incidence has been noted in this breed in some surveys
- Males seem to be predisposed

Reproductive conditions
Vaginal hyperplasia
- Possible breed predisposition

Azoospermia with spermatogenic arrest
- Reported in this breed

Respiratory conditions
Laryngeal paralysis
- Idiopathic

LAKELAND TERRIER

Cardiovascular conditions
Ventricular septal defect
- Congenital
- Uncommon

Ocular conditions
Glaucoma
- Possible breed predisposition

Lens luxation
- Possible breed predisposition; inheritance suspected

Cataract
- Inheritance suspected
- Localisation: posterior subcapsular cortex
- Age of onset: 1–3 years; slowly progressive

Microphthalmia and persistent pupillary membranes
- Autosomal recessive inheritance has been suggested
- May be seen with cataract formation and focal retinal dysplasia

LANCASHIRE HEELER

Ocular conditions
Persistent pupillary membranes
- Inheritance suspected
- Schedule 3 of the BVA/KC/ISDS Eye Scheme

Cataract
- Inheritance suspected
- Schedule 3 of the BVA/KC/ISDS Eye Scheme

Primary lens luxation
- Inheritance suspected
- Often followed by glaucoma
- Schedule 3 of the BVA/KC/ISDS Eye Scheme

Collie eye anomaly
- Congenital condition; inheritance suspected
- Schedule 3 of the BVA/KC/ISDS Eye Scheme

LAPLAND DOG

Musculoskeletal conditions
Glycogen storage disease type II
- Also known as Pompe's disease
- Seen in four related Lapland dogs
- Age of onset from 6 months

LEONBERGER

Endocrine conditions
Hypoadrenocorticism
- Possible genetic predisposition suggested by familial occurrence

Ocular conditions
Cataract
- Inheritance suspected
- Schedule 3 of the BVA/KC/ISDS Eye Scheme

LHASA APSO

Cardiovascular conditions
Endocardiosis
- Also known as chronic valvular disease
- Relative risk 2.4 (not statistically significant)
- Increased prevalence with age
- Aetiology unknown but likely genetic basis

Dermatological conditions
Atopy
- Females probably predisposed
- Age of onset is from 6 months to 7 years
- May or may not be seasonal

Food hypersensitivity
- No age or sex predisposition reported

Congenital hypotrichosis
- Present at birth or develops in the first month of life
- Predisposition for males suggests sex linkage

Skin tumours
- See under Neoplastic conditions

Drug reactions
Glucocorticoids
- Subcutaneous injections in this breed may cause local areas of alopecia

Gastrointestinal conditions
Pyloric stenosis (antral pyloric hypertrophy syndrome)
- Breed predisposition to adult-onset pyloric hypertrophy syndrome
- Males may be predisposed

DOGS

Neoplastic conditions
Sebaceous gland tumours
- Possible breed predisposition to sebaceous epithelioma
- Seen in older dogs (average age 10 years)

Keratoacanthoma
- Usually affects dogs younger than 5 years
- Male dogs predisposed
- This breed is predisposed to the solitary form of the disease

Perianal (hepatoid) gland adenomas
- Breed predisposition suggested in one survey of 2700 cases
- Average age was 10.5 years
- Entire males were predisposed

Neurological conditions
Hydrocephalus
- Congenital
- Relatively common
- Onset of signs: usually 4–5 months

Lissencephaly
- Rare developmental disease
- Age of onset: <1 year

Intervertebral disc disease
- Breed predisposition

Ocular conditions
Entropion (usually lower lids)
- Breed predisposition; polygenic inheritance likely

Distichiasis
- Breed predisposition

Ectopic cilia
- Breed predisposition

Caruncular trichiasis
- Breed predisposition

Keratoconjunctivitis sicca
- Breed predisposition

Prolapse of the gland of the nictitating membrane
- Breed predisposition; possibly inherited
- Usually presents before 2 years of age

Pigmentary keratitis
- Breed predisposition

Refractory corneal ulceration
- Breed predisposition

Corneal dystrophy
- Not known if inherited
- Subepithelial lipid dystrophy

Cataract
- Inheritance suspected
- Localisation: posterior cortex
- Age of onset: 3–6 years; progressive, with visual deficiencies likely

Vitreous syneresis
- Breed predisposition
- Age of onset: 2 years and older
- May result in glaucoma

Generalised progressive retinal atrophy (GPRA)
- Autosomal recessive inheritance suspected
- Clinically detected at 3 years
- Schedule 1 BVA/KC/ISDS Eye Scheme

Renal and urinary conditions
Familial renal disease (renal dysplasia)
- Mode of inheritance unknown
- Cases present with chronic renal failure from a few months to 5 years of age

Renal glucosuria
- May be seen with familial renal disease

Calcium oxalate urolithiasis
- Higher incidence has been noted in this breed
- Average age at diagnosis is 5–12 years
- Males may be predisposed

Struvite (magnesium ammonium phosphate) urolithiasis
- Higher incidence has been noted in this breed
- Average age at diagnosis is 2–8 years
- Females seem to be predisposed

Silica urolithiasis
- Higher incidence has been noted in this breed in some surveys
- Males seem to be predisposed

Respiratory conditions
Tracheal collapse
- Aetiology unknown
- Usually affects middle-aged to old dogs

LOWCHEN

Ocular conditions
Cataract
- Inheritance suspected

LUNDEHUND

Gastrointestinal conditions
Primary congenital lymphangiectasia (resulting in protein-losing enteropathy)
- Breed predisposition

Diarrheal syndrome (in Lundehunds)
- Specific disease of Lundehunds

LURCHER

Musculoskeletal conditions
Accessory carpal bone fracture
- Sprain/avulsion-type fractures due to carpal hyperextension during exercise

Neurological conditions
Hypomyelination of the central nervous system
- Reported
- Signs seen at 2–8 weeks

MALTESE

Cardiovascular conditions
Patent ductus arteriosus
- Common congenital abnormality
- Females predisposed
- Relative risk 12.4

Endocardiosis
- Also known as chronic valvular disease
- Relative risk 4.2
- Increased prevalence with age
- Aetiology unknown but likely genetic basis

Dermatological conditions
Malassezia dermatitis
- Often seasonal
- Affects any age

Gastrointestinal conditions
Pyloric Stenosis (antral pyloric hypertrophy syndrome)
- Possible breed predisposition to adult-onset pyloric hypertrophy syndrome
- Males may be predisposed

Congenital portosystemic shunt
- Possible breed predisposition
- Clinical signs usually seen <1 year

Musculoskeletal conditions
Inguinal/scrotal herniation
- Females predisposed

Neurological conditions
Hydrocephalus
- Congenital
- Relatively common
- Onset of signs: usually 4–5 months

Hypoglycaemia (as a possible cause of seizures)
- Breed predisposition
- Seen in dogs <1 year

Shaker dog disease
- Breed predisposition
- Age of clinical onset: 9 months to 2 years

Ocular conditions
Entropion (usually medial lower lid)
- Breed predisposition; polygenic inheritance likely

Distichiasis
- Breed predisposition

Caruncular trichiasis
- Breed predisposition

Glaucoma
- Breed predisposition
- Age of onset: 6–16 years

DOGS

Multifocal retinal dysplasia
- Congenital condition; autosomal recessive inheritance suspected

Generalised progressive retinal atrophy (GPRA)
- Autosomal recessive inheritance suspected
- Clinically detected at 4–7 years

Reproductive conditions
Cryptorchidism
- Developmental defect believed to be inherited as a sex-limited, autosomal recessive trait
- Believed to be a breed at increased risk of the condition

MANCHESTER TERRIER

Dermatological conditions
Pattern baldness
- Almost exclusively affects females
- Ventral neck and ventrum affected

Ehler-Danlos syndrome
- Also known as cutaneous asthenia
- Inherited group of diseases
- May be inherited as an autosomal dominant trait
- Probably lethal to homozygotes

Haematological conditions
Von Willebrand's disease
- Possibly inherited as an autosomal recessive trait
- Common in this breed in both the USA and UK
- Mainly type I disease seen in this breed

Ocular conditions
Lens luxation
- Breed predisposition
- Age of onset: 2–4 years
- Often results in glaucoma

Cataract
- Inheritance suspected
- Localisation: posterior subcapsular
- Age of onset: 5 years; progression and visual deficiencies likely

Generalised progressive retinal atrophy (GPRA)
- Autosomal recessive inheritance suspected
- Clinically detected at 5–6 years

MASTIFF

Cardiovascular conditions
Pulmonic stenosis
- Third most frequent type of canine congenital heart disease
- May be polygenic mode of inheritance

Mitral dysplasia
- Congenital
- Males predisposed
- Genetic basis suspected

Gastrointestinal conditions
Gastric dilatation-volvulus
- Possible breed predisposition

Musculoskeletal conditions
Hip dysplasia
- This breed has the eighteenth worst breed mean score in the BVA/KC Hip Dysplasia Scheme as of October 2001
- Breed mean score 18

Cranial cruciate ligament rupture
- Neutered individuals may be predisposed
- Young animals may be predisposed in this breed

Ocular conditions
Entropion (may be associated with macropalpebral fissure)
- Breed predisposition; polygenic inheritance likely

Ectropion (may be associated with macropalpebral fissure)
- Breed predisposition; polygenic inheritance likely

Macropalpebral fissure resulting in combined entropion-ectropion ('diamond eye')
- Breed predisposition; genetic basis incompletely understood

Eversion of the cartilage of the nictitating membrane
- Breed predisposition; inheritance suspected
- Usually occurs in young dogs

Prolapse of the gland of the nictitating membrane ('cherry eye')
- Breed predisposition
- Usually presents before 2 years of age

Corneal dystrophy
- Breed predisposition; not known if inherited
- Subepithelial, lipid dystrophy

Persistent pupillary membranes and microphthalmia
- Recessive inheritance has been suggested
- Multifocal retinal dysplasia may be present

Cataract
- Inheritance suspected

Renal and urinary conditions
Cystine urolithiasis
- Cystinuria results from an inherited defect in renal tubular transport of cystine predisposing to cystine urolithiasis
- Higher incidence reported in this breed in some American surveys
- Average age at diagnosis is 1–8 years
- Males seem predisposed

Reproductive conditions
Vaginal hyperplasia
- Breed predisposition

MEXICAN HAIRLESS

Immunological conditions
Perinatal mortality
- May be associated with impaired antibody responses and lymphoid depletion of thymus and spleen

MINIATURE BULL TERRIER

Ocular conditions
Entropion
- Breed predisposition; polygenic inheritance likely

Primary lens luxation
- Inheritance suspected
- Often followed by glaucoma
- Schedule 1 of the BVA/KC/ISDS Eye Scheme

MINIATURE PINSCHER

Dermatological conditions
Pattern baldness
- May be inherited

Colour-dilution alopecia
- Reported in blue or fawn Dobermanns and Miniature Pinschers
- Coat-colour genes play a role in inheritance

Endocrine conditions
Diabetes mellitus
- Possible breed predisposition
- Usual age range 4–14 years; peak incidence: 7–9 years
- Old entire females are predisposed

Musculoskeletal conditions
Shoulder luxation
- Congenital

Ocular conditions
Chronic superficial keratitis (pannus)
- Breed predisposition
- Age of onset: 7–8 years

Corneal dystrophy
- Mode of inheritance unknown
- Subepithelial lipid dystrophy
- Age of onset: 1–2 years

Glaucoma
- Possible breed predisposition
- Age of onset: 3–4 years

Cataract
- Inheritance suspected
- Localisation: cortex
- Age of onset: 1.5–3 years

DOGS

Generalised progressive retinal atrophy (GPRA)
- Mode of inheritance unknown but presumed recessive
- Cases presented from 7 years

Renal and urinary conditions
Cystine urolithiasis
- Cystinuria results from an inherited defect in renal tubular transport of cystine and predisposes to cystine urolithiasis
- Higher incidence reported in this breed in some American surveys
- Average age at diagnosis is 1–8 years
- Males seem predisposed

MUNSTERLANDER

Dermatological conditions
Black hair follicular dysplasia
- Coat changes seen from 4 weeks of age

Ocular conditions
Cataract
- Inheritance suspected
- Localisation: posterior polar subcapsular
- Schedule 1 of the BVA/KC/ISDS Eye Scheme

NEAPOLITAN MASTIFF

Musculoskeletal conditions
Cranial cruciate ligament rupture
- Neutered individuals may be predisposed
- May occur at a young age in this breed

Ocular conditions
Entropion (may be associated with macropalpebral fissure)
- Breed predisposition; polygenic inheritance likely

Ectropion (may be associated with macropalpebral fissure)
- Breed predisposition; polygenic inheritance likely

Macropalpebral fissure resulting in combined entropion-ectropion ('diamond eye')
- Breed predisposition; genetic basis incompletely understood

Eversion of the cartilage of the nictitating membrane
- Breed predisposition; possibly inherited as a recessive trait
- Usually occurs in young dogs

Prolapse of the gland of the nictitating membrane ('cherry eye')
- Breed predisposition

Cataract
- Inheritance suspected

Reproductive conditions
Vaginal hyperplasia
- Breed predisposition

NEWFOUNDLAND

Cardiovascular conditions
Aortic stenosis
- Common congenital disease
- Relative risk 19.9
- Males strongly predisposed in this breed
- Inheritance possibly autosomal dominant with modifying genes or polygenic

Atrial septal defect
- Uncommon congenital disease
- Relative risk 24

Dilated cardiomyopathy
- Prevalence of 1.3% in this breed compared to 0.16% in mixed breeds and 0.65% in pure breeds
- Increased prevalence with age
- Approximately twice as common in males as females
- Thought to be familial or genetic

Pulmonic stenosis
- Third most frequent cause of canine congenital heart disease
- May be polygenic mode of inheritance

DOGS

Patent ductus arteriosus
- Common congenital abnormality
- Females predisposed
- This breed predisposed in some areas

Dermatological conditions
Pyotraumatic folliculitis
- Young dogs predisposed
- Also known as hot spot, wet eczema
- Relative risk 5.1

Pemphigus foliaceous
- Uncommon disease
- No sex predisposition
- Mean age of onset: 4 years

Colour-dilution alopecia
- Coat-colour genes are involved in the pathogenesis

Acquired depigmentation
- Affects normal black Newfoundlands around 18 months of age
- Depigmenatation affects the nose, lips and eyelids and may progress to affect hair colour

Callus dermatitis/pyoderma
- Most common over hock and elbow joints of this breed

Endocrine diseases
Hypothyroidism
- Reported in some texts to be at increased risk
- Often middle-aged (2–6 years)

Gastrointestinal conditions
Congenital idiopathic megaoesophagus
- Breed predisposition

Neurological conditions
Distal polyneuropathy
- Reported in this breed
- Age of clinical onset: >1 year

Ocular conditions
Entropion (may be associated with macropalpebral fissure)
- Breed predisposition; polygenic inheritance likely

Ectropion (may be associated with macropalpebral fissure)
- Breed predisposition; polygenic inheritance likely

Macropalpebral fissure resulting in combined entropion-ectropion ('diamond eye')
- Breed predisposition; genetic basis incompletely understood

Eversion of the cartilage of the nictitating membrane
- Breed predisposition
- Usually occurs in young dogs

Medial canthal pocket syndrome
- Breed predisposition

Cataract
- Inheritance suspected

Renal and urinary conditions
Ectopic ureters
- Congenital anomaly; higher incidence reported in this breed
- Usually presents <1 year of age
- More commonly diagnosed in females

Cystine urolithiasis
- Cystinuria results from an inherited defect in renal tubular transport of cystine and predisposes to cystine urolithiasis. The defect seems to be more severe than in other breeds, leading to earlier formation of uroliths (<1 year) and a higher incidence in this breed
- Autosomal recessive inheritance suggested
- Males and females both affected

Respiratory conditions
Primary ciliary dyskinesia
- Thought to be inherited as an autosomal recessive trait in this breed

NORFOLK TERRIER

Ocular conditions
Glaucoma
- Possible breed predisposition

DOGS

Lens luxation
- Breed predisposition

Cataract
- Inheritance suspected
- Localisation: posterior polar subcapsular
- Age of onset: 5 years; usually progressive with visual deficiencies likely

Micropapilla
- Congenital condition
- Seen occasionally in this breed

Optic nerve colobomas
- Congenital defect; not known if inherited
- Seen occasionally in this breed

NORWEGIAN BUHUND

Ocular conditions
Cataract
- Autosomal dominant inheritance suggested
- Localisation: posterior polar
- Age of onset: 3–4 months
- Schedule 1 of the BVA/KC/ISDS Eye Scheme

NORWEGIAN ELKHOUND

Musculoskeletal conditions
Norwegian Elkhound chondrodysplasia
- Inherited as an autosomal recessive trait
- Shortened body and disproportionately short limbs
- May be associated with glucosuria

Osteogenesis imperfecta
- Mechanism of inheritance unknown

Neoplastic conditions
Keratoacanthoma
- Breed predisposition to multiple tumours

Squamous cell carcinoma of the skin
- Occurs at an average of 9 years of age

Ocular conditions
Entropion (usually lower lids)
- Breed predisposition; polygenic inheritance likely

Primary glaucoma
- Mode of inheritance unknown
- Most primary cases appear to be open angle, however cases with a narrow iridocorneal filtration angle have been seen
- Age of onset: 4–7 years
- Schedule 3 of the BVA/KC/ISDS Eye Scheme

Lens luxation
- Breed predisposition; inheritance suspected
- Secondary glaucoma occurs
- Age of onset: 2–6 years

Cataract
- Inheritance suspected
- Localisation: posterior sutures and cortex
- Age of onset: 1–3 years; slowly progressive

Multifocal retinal dysplasia
- Congenital condition
- Schedule 3 of the BVA/KC/ISDS Eye Scheme

Generalised progressive retinal atrophy
(early retinal degeneration)
- Autosomal recessive inheritance
- Night blindness at 6 weeks followed by total vision loss at 12–18 months
- A recessively-inherited rod dysplasia used to be seen in this breed
- Schedule 1 BVA/KC/ISDS Eye Scheme

Renal and urinary conditions
Familial renal disease
- Mode of inheritance unknown
- Periglomerular fibrosis and later generalised interstitial fibrosis occur
- Dogs may present in renal failure from a few months to 5 years of age; Fanconi's syndrome is present in some cases

Primary renal glucosuria
- Cases have been seen with normal renal function

NORWICH TERRIER

Musculoskeletal conditions
Muscular cramping
- Condition similar to Scottie cramp reported in this breed

Neurological conditions
Muscular cramping
- Condition similar to Scottie cramp reported in this breed

Ocular conditions
Corneal dystrophy
- Not known if inherited
- Paralimbal lipid dystrophy

Glaucoma
- Possible breed predisposition

Lens luxation
- Breed predisposition
- Age of onset: 3 years

Cataract
- Inheritance suspected
- Localisation: posterior polar
- Age of onset: 6 months to 2.5 years; progression and visual deficiencies likely

NOVA SCOTIA DUCK TOLLING RETRIEVER

Endocrine diseases
Hypoadrenocorticism
- Possible genetic predisposition suggested by familial occurrence

Ocular conditions
Cataract
- Inheritance suspected
- May be associated with progressive retinal atrophy

Generalised progressive retinal atrophy (GPRA)
- Mode of inheritance not known but presumed to be recessive
- Clinical onset at 5–6 years

OLD ENGLISH SHEEPDOG

Cardiovascular conditions
Dilated cardiomyopathy
- Prevalence of 0.9% in this breed compared to 0.16% in mixed breeds and 0.65% in pure breeds
- Increased prevalence with age
- Approximately twice as common in males as females
- Thought to be familial or genetic

Persistent atrial standstill
- Rare condition

Tricuspid dysplasia
- Congenital
- Males predisposed

Dermatological conditions
Pododemodicosis
- Lesions may be confined to the paws in Old English Sheepdogs
- Relative risk 28.9

Primary lymphoedema
- No apparent sex predisposition
- Usually occurs within first 12 weeks of life

Melanotrichia
- Often following healing of deep inflammation

Vitiligo
- Presumed to be hereditary

Skin tumours
- See under Neoplastic conditions

Drug reactions
Ivermectin and milbemycin
- High doses can cause tremors, ataxia, coma and death

Endocrine conditions
Hypothyroidism
- Reported in some texts to be at increased risk
- Often middle-aged (2–6 years)

Haematological/immunological conditions

Immune-mediated haemolytic anaemia
- Common disease
- Usually affects young adult and middle-aged animals
- May be more common in bitches
- May be seasonal variations in incidence

Immune-mediated thrombocytopenia
- Common
- Inheritance likely
- Females more commonly affected than males

Haemophilia B
- Factor IX defiency
- Also known as Christmas disease
- Inherited as a sex-linked trait
- Less common than haemophilia A

Musculoskeletal conditions

Congenital elbow luxation
- Type II luxation is seen in this breed (proximal radius displaced caudolaterally)
- Usually 4–5 months old at presentation

Sacrocaudal dysgenesis
- Congenital
- See also under Neurological conditions

Hip dysplasia
- Ninth worst mean-scoring breed in the BVA/KC Hip Dysplasia Scheme as of October 2001
- Breed mean score 20
- Breed mean score is currently decreasing

Neoplastic conditions

Sweat gland tumour
- Reported to be at increased risk
- Average age reported as 9.5 years

Pilomatrixoma
- Possible breed predisposition
- Average age reported as 6.6 years

Keratoacanthoma
- Usually affects dogs younger than 5 years
- Male dogs predisposed

- This breed is predisposed to the generalised form of the disease

Nasal cavity tumours
- Reported to be at increased risk for nasal carcinoma
- Usually older dogs
- Dogs in urban areas may be at increased risk

Primary brain tumours
- See under Neurological conditions

Neurological conditions

Congenital deafness
- Signs seen from birth

Primary brain tumours
- Higher incidence noted in this breed by some authors
- Older dogs affected (9–10 years)

Sacrocaudal dysgenesis
- Congenital
- Occasionally reported

Ocular conditions

Microcornea
- Congenital
- Usually found associated with multiple ocular defects (see below)

Cataract
- Mode of inheritance unknown
- Localisation: nuclear or cortical
- Age of onset: 9 months to 6 years; generally progressive; some become complete cataracts
- May be seen with retinal detachment
- Schedule 1 of the BVA/KC/ISDS Eye Scheme

Congenital hereditary cataract
- Inheritance suspected
- Localisation: nuclear or cortical
- Schedule 3 of the BVA/KC/ISDS Eye Scheme

Generalised progressive retinal atrophy (GPRA)
- Autosomal recessive inheritance suspected
- Clinical onset at 4 years

Micropapilla
- Congenital condition
- Seen occasionally in this breed

Optic nerve hypoplasia
- Congenital condition; not known if inherited
- Seen occasionally in this breed

Multiple ocular defects
- Congenital; not known if inherited
- Defects may include congenital cataract, persistent pupillary membranes, retinal defects and microphthalmia
- Schedule 3 of the BVA/KC/ISDS Eye Scheme

Renal and urinary conditions
Urethral sphincter mechanism incompetence (causing urinary incontinence)
- Possible breed predisposition in female dogs

Silica urolithiasis
- Higher incidence reported in this breed in some surveys
- Males seem predisposed

Reproductive conditions
Cryptorchidism
- Developmental defect believed to be inherited as a sex-limited, autosomal recessive trait
- Believed to be a breed at increased risk of the condition

Respiratory conditions
Primary ciliary dyskinesia
- Signs usually seen early in life

OTTERHOUND

Haematological conditions
Glanzmann's thrombasthenia
- Due to a genetic platelet defect
- Inherited as an autosomal recessive trait

Musculoskeletal conditions
Hip dysplasia
- Worst mean scoring breed in the BVA/KC Hip Dysplasia Scheme as of October 2001
- Breed mean score 43

PAPILLON

Dermatological conditions
Black hair follicular dysplasia
- Familial
- Early age of onset

Neurological conditions
Congenital deafness
- Signs seen from birth

Ocular conditions
Entropion
- Breed predisposition; polygenic inheritance likely

Cataract
- Inheritance suspected
- Localisation: nuclear and posterior cortical
- Age of onset: 1.5–3 years; slowly progressive; visual deficiencies rare

Generalised progressive retinal atrophy (GPRA)
- Autosomal recessive inheritance suspected
- Late onset, with night blindness found in middle-aged dogs; blindness is not usually present until 7–8 years
- Schedule 3 BVA/KC/ISDS Eye Scheme

PARSON RUSSELL TERRIER

Ocular conditions
Primary lens luxation
- Inheritance suspected
- Often followed by glaucoma
- Schedule 1 of the BVA/KC/ISDS Eye Scheme

PEKINGESE

Cardiovascular conditions
Endocardiosis
- Also known as chronic valvular disease
- Relative risk 4.1
- Increased prevalence with age
- Aetiology unknown but likely genetic basis

DOGS

Dermatological conditions
Dermatophytosis
- Common fungal condition

Pododermatitis
- Can affect any age or sex
- Males predisposed
- Front feet more commonly affected

Flea bite hypersensitivity
- Most studies show no breed predisposition, but one French study showed Pekingese were predisposed

Intertrigo
- Facial fold intertrigo common in this breed
- May lead to corneal ulceration

Rabies-vaccine-associated vasculitis and alopecia
- Lesions appear at the site of the vaccine, 3–6 months after administration

Skin tumours
- See under Neoplastic conditions

Gastrointestinal conditions
Pyloric stenosis (antral pyloric hypertrophy syndrome)
- Breed predisposition to adult-onset pyloric hypertrophy syndrome
- Males may be predisposed

Haemorrhagic gastroenteritis
- Possible breed predisposition
- Seen most commonly at 2–4 years of age

Musculoskeletal conditions
Congenital elbow luxation
- Type I and type II luxation are seen in this breed
- Type I (90° rotation of proximal ulna) causes severe disability in this breed from birth or in the first 3 months of life
- Type II (proximal radius displaced caudolaterally) is usually seen at 4–5 months of age

Inguinal/scrotal herniation
- Females predisposed

Odontoid process dysplasia
- Congenital

Perineal hernia
- Intact males predisposed

Retrognathia
- Mode of inheritance not known

Umbilical hernia

Neoplastic conditions
Squamous cell carcinoma of the skin
- No sex predilection
- Occurs at an average of 9 years of age

Neurological conditions
Intervertebral disc disease
- Breed predisposition
- Relatively common
- Age of clinical onset: 3–7 years

Hydrocephalus
- Congenital
- Relatively common
- Onset of signs: usually 4–5 months

Hemivertebrae
- Congenital
- Occasionally seen

Atlantoaxial subluxation
- Congenital
- Relatively common
- Age of clinical onset: <1 year

Ocular conditions
Entropion
- Breed predisposition; polygenic inheritance likely

Distichiasis
- Breed predisposition; mode of inheritance unclear

Caruncular trichiasis
- Breed predisposition

Nasal fold trichiasis
- Breed predisposition

Keratoconjunctivitis sicca
- Breed predisposition

Refractory corneal ulceration
- Breed predisposition

Pigmentary keratitis
- Breed predisposition

Proptosis
- Occurs more easily in this breed due to head shape

Cataract
- Inheritance suspected

Generalised progressive retinal atrophy (GPRA)
- Mode of inheritance unknown but presumed recessive
- Clinically apparent at 8 years

Physiological conditions
Achondroplasia
- Genetic dwarfism
- Skull and limbs affected
- Accepted as a breed standard

Reproductive conditions
Cryptorchidism
- Developmental defect believed to be inherited as a sex-limited, autosomal recessive trait
- Believed to be a breed at increased risk of the condition

Male pseudohermaphroditism
- Congenital abnormality of phenotypic sex
- Reported in this breed

Respiratory conditions
Brachycephalic upper airway syndrome
- Complex of anatomical deformities
- Common in this breed
- Probably a consequence of selective breeding for certain facial characteristics

Bronchial cartilage hypoplasia
- Congenital

PETIT BASSET GRIFFON VENDEEN

Ocular conditions
Persistent pupillary membranes
- Inheritance suspected
- Schedule 3 of the BVA/KC/ISDS Eye Scheme

POINTERS

Cardiovascular conditions
Aortic stenosis
- Congenital
- No sex predilection
- Mode of inheritance may be autosomal dominant with modifying genes or polygenic

Hypertrophic cardiomyopathy
- Rare
- Inherited in this breed

Pericardial effusion
- Acquired
- Relative risk 9.5

Dermatological conditions
Nasal folliculitis/furunculosis
- Uncommon
- Cause unknown

Muzzle folliculitis/furunculosis
- Also known as canine acne
- Local trauma, hormones and genetics may play a role in the pathogenesis

Pododermatitis
- Can affect any age or sex
- Males predisposed
- Front feet more commonly affected

Blastomycosis
- See under Infectious conditions

Coccidiomycosis
- See under Infectious conditions

Histoplasmosis
- See under Infectious conditions

Discoid lupus erythematosus
- No age or sex predisposition
- Accounted for 0.3% of skin diseases at one referral institution

Hereditary lupoid dermatosis of German Short-haired Pointers
- Familial
- Cause unknown
- Age of onset 6 months

Black hair follicular dysplasia
- Rare
- Early onset
- Familial

Acral mutilation syndrome
- Probably inherited as an autosomal recessive trait
- No sex predisposition
- Age of onset: 3–5 months

Nasal depigmentation
- Also known as Dudley nose
- Cause unknown

Truncal solar dermatitis
- Sunnier climates predispose

Zinc-responsive dermatosis
- Occurs in rapidly-growing dogs fed zinc-deficient diets

Skin tumours
- See under Neoplastic conditions

Endocrine conditions

Central diabetes insipidus (CDI)
(German Short-haired Pointers)
- One report of CDI diagnosed in a litter of five 8-week-old pups suggesting a possible familial basis

Gastrointestinal conditions

Cleft palate
- Congenital disorder with inheritance suspected in this breed

Oropharyngeal neoplasia (German Short-haired Pointers)
- Possible breed predisposition

Haematological conditions

Von Willebrand's disease
- Affects German Short-haired and German Wire-haired Pointers
- This breed is predisposed to type II disease

Infectious conditions

Blastomycosis
- Increased incidence in this breed possibly due to an increased likelihood of exposure
- Seen mainly in young male dogs living near water
- Geographic distribution: around the Mississippi, Ohio, Missouri, Tennessee, and St Lawrence Rivers, the southern Great Lakes and the southern mid-Atlantic states; not reported in the UK

Coccidiomycosis
- Increased incidence in this breed possibly due to an increased likelihood of exposure
- Seen mainly in young male dogs
- Geographic distribution: California, Arizona, Texas, New Mexico, Nevada, Utah, Mexico and parts of Central and South America; not reported in the UK

Histoplasmosis
- Uncommon
- Mainly restricted to the central United States
- Usually affects dogs less than 4 years old

Infectious skin diseases
- See under Dermatological conditions

Musculoskeletal conditions

Polyarthritis/meningitis
- Idiopathic
- Affects dogs from 6 months of age onwards

English Pointer enchondrodystrophy
- Short limbs
- Probably inherited as an autosomal recessive trait

Cranial cruciate ligament rupture
- Common cause of hind-limb lameness
- More common in German Short-haired Pointers

Umbilical hernia

Hemivertebrae
• See under Neurological conditions

Neoplastic conditions
Mast cell tumours
• Possible breed predisposition
• May be seen at any age (from 4 months onwards), but usually seen in older animals

Cutaneous haemangioma (English Pointers)
• Possible breed predisposition
• Average age was 8.7 years in one study

Oropharyngeal neoplasia (German Short-haired Pointers)
• Possible breed predisposition

Nasal cavity tumours (German Short-haired Pointers)
• Reported to be at increased risk for nasal carcinoma
• Usually older dogs
• Dogs in urban areas may be at increased risk

Neurological conditions
Congenital deafness
• Signs seen from birth

Spinal muscular atrophy (English Pointers)
• Inheritance suspected
• Reported in Japan
• Age of clinical onset: 5 months

Sensory neuropathy (English and German Short-haired Pointers)
• Autosomal recessive inheritance
• Rare
• Signs seen at 3–6 months

Lysosomal storage disease – GM_2 gangliosidosis (Japanese and German Short-haired Pointers)
• Autosomal recessive inheritance
• Rare
• Signs seen at 6–12 months

Meningitis and polyarteritis (German Short-haired Pointers)
• Has been reported
• Age of clinical onset: <1 year

Pyogranulomatous meningoencephalomyelitis
• Reported in this breed
• Age of clinical onset: >1 year

Hemivertebrae (of the thoracic vertebrae in German Short-haired Pointers)
• Autosomal recessive inheritance reported in some lines
• Occasionally seen

Ocular conditions
Entropion (usually lateral lower lids)
• Breed predisposition; polygenic inheritance likely

Chronic superficial keratitis (pannus) (English Pointers)
• Breed predisposition

Eversion of the cartilage of the nictitating membrane (German Short-haired Pointers)
• Breed predisposition; believed to be inherited as a recessive trait
• Usually occurs in young dogs

Corneal dystrophy (English Pointers)
• Mode of inheritance unknown
• Lipid dystrophy
• Age of onset: 6 years

Cataract (English Pointers)
• Dominant inheritance suspected
• Localisation: lens periphery
• Age of onset: 2–3 years; progression resulting in visual deficiencies may occur

Cataract (German Short-haired and German Wire-haired Pointers)
• Inheritance suspected
• Localisation: posterior subcapsular cortex
• Age of onset: 6–18 months of age; slowly progressive

Generalised progressive retinal atrophy (GPRA) (German Short-haired and English Pointers)
• Autosomal recessive inheritance suspected
• Clinically apparent at 5–6 years in English Pointers

DOGS

DOGS

Reproductive conditions
XX sex reversal (German Short-haired Pointers)
- Congenital condition reported in this breed

Respiratory conditions
Primary ciliary dyskinesia
- Signs usually seen early in life
- Affects English Pointers

POLISH LOWLAND SHEEPDOG

Ocular conditions
Central progressive retinal atrophy (CPRA) or retinal pigment epithelial dystrophy (RPED)
- Breed predisposition; inheritance suspected
- Schedule 3 of the BVA/KC/ISDS Eye Scheme

POMERANIAN

Cardiovascular conditions
Patent ductus arteriosus
- Common congenital abnormality
- Relative risk 4.6
- Females predisposed
- Mode of inheritance polygenic

Sick sinus syndrome
- Middle-aged to old dogs
- Relative risk 3.5 in this breed
- No sex predisposition in this breed

Dermatological conditions
Adult-onset growth-hormone-responsive dermatosis
- See under Endocrine conditions

Endocrine conditions
Adult-onset growth-hormone-responsive dermatosis
- Breed predisposition
- Males maybe predisposed
- Clinical signs usually seen at 1–5 years

Hypothyroidism
- Reported in some texts to be at increased risk
- Often middle-aged (2–6 years)

Musculoskeletal conditions
Congenital elbow luxation
- Type II luxation is seen in this breed (proximal radius displaced caudolaterally)
- Usually 4–5 months old at presentation

Medial patellar luxation
- Significant hereditary component suspected

Shoulder luxation
- Congenital

Inguinal/scrotal herniation
- Females predisposed

Odontoid process dysplasia
- Congenital

Neoplastic conditions
Testicular neoplasia
- Believed to be a breed at increased risk

Neurological conditions
Hydrocephalus
- Congenital
- Relatively common
- Onset of signs: usually 4–5 months

Atlantoaxial subluxation
- Congenital
- Relatively common in this breed
- Age of clinical onset: <1 year

Ocular conditions
Entropion (usually medial canthal area of the lower lid)
- Breed predisposition; polygenic inheritance likely

Cataract
- Inheritance suspected
- Localisation: posterior cortical
- Age of onset: 4 years; may progress to completion

Generalised progressive retinal atrophy (GPRA)
- Autosomal recessive inheritance suspected
- Clinically apparent by 6 years

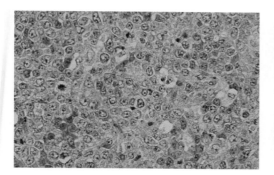

Plate 1
Section of a popliteal lymph node from a
ten-year-old male Basset Hound: malignant
lymphoma (H&E stain, × 132).

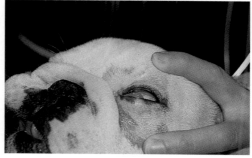

Plate 4
Prolapse of the gland of the nictitating membrane
('cherry eye') in a bulldog pup.

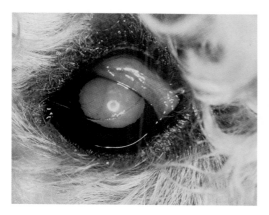

Plate 2
Mature cataract in a nine-year-old neutered male
Bichon Frise. Photo courtesy of Mark Bossley.

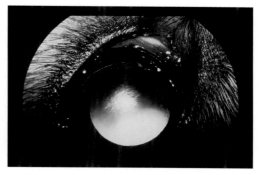

Plate 5
Corneal lipid dystrophy in a two-year-old entire
female Rough Collie. Photo courtesy of Mark
Bossley.

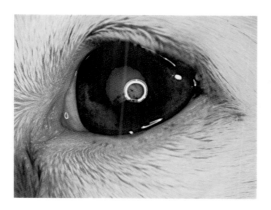

Plate 3
Iris cyst. Photo courtesy of Mark Bossley.

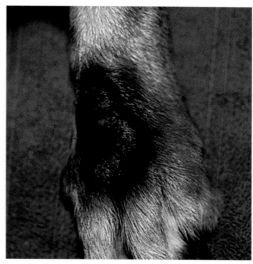

Plate 6
Acral lick granuloma. Courtesy of A. Foster,
University of Bristol.

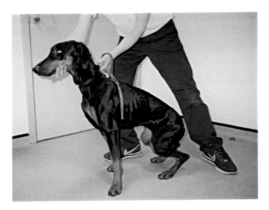

Plate 7
Severe weight loss in a three-year-old neutered
female Doberman with chronic hepatitis.

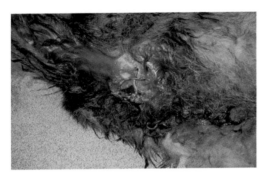

Plate 8
Severe perianal fistulation (anal furunculosis) in an
eight-year-old German Shepherd dog.

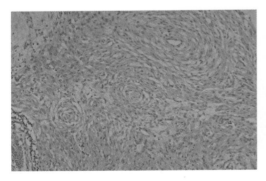

Plate 9
Haemangiopericytoma in a ten-year-old female
German Shepherd dog. Spindle cells are seen in
a whorl configuration, some are around blood
capillaries (H&E stain, × 132).

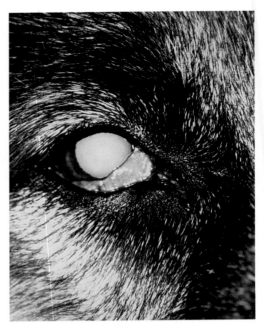

Plate 10
Plasmoma in a ten-year-old entire male German
Shepherd dog. Photo courtesy of Mark Bossley.

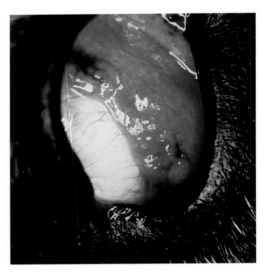

Plate 11
Plasmoma in a ten-year-old entire male German
Shepherd dog. Photo courtesy of Mark Bossley.

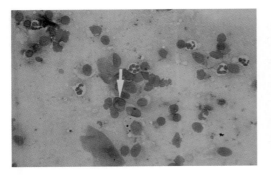

Plate 12
Plasmoma in a ten-year-old entire male German
Shepherd dog: conjunctival scraping. Photo
courtesy of Mark Bossley.

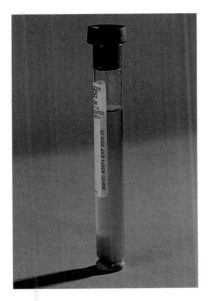

Plate 13
Urate crystals sedimented in a urine sample.
Courtesy of E. Hall, University of Bristol.

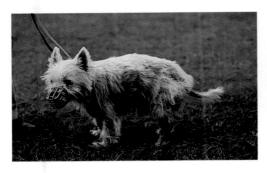

Plate 14
Atopy in a West Highland White terrier. Courtesy
of A. Foster, University of Bristol.

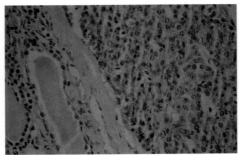

Plate 15
Parathyroid adenoma × 400 magnification.

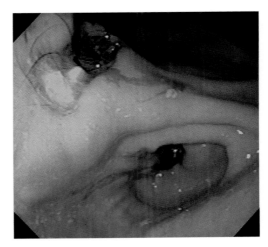

Plate 16
Gastric adenocarcinoma. Courtesy of E. Hall,
University of Bristol.

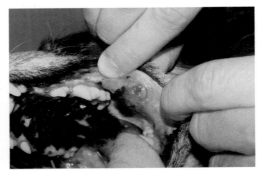

Plate 17
Oral malignant melanoma in a ten-year-old
crossbreed.

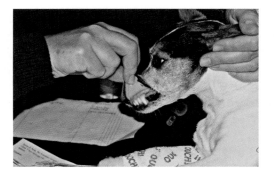

Plate 18
Jaundice is one of the symptoms of acute haemolytic anaemia.

Plate 21
Lipoma in an eleven-year-old neutered female Boxer (H&E stain, × 132).

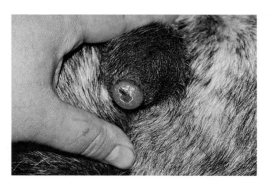

Plate 19
Scrotal histiocytoma in a two-year-old crossbreed dog.

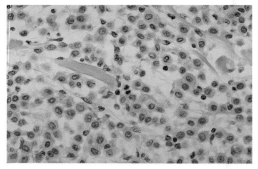

Plate 22
Mast cell tumour (skin) in a six-year-old female Staffordshire Bull Terrier. Mast cells have round nucleii with granular cytoplasm. Some eosinophils are present (H&E stain, × 132).

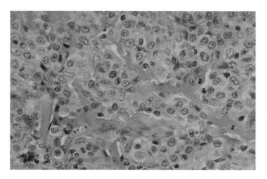

Plate 20
Cutaneous histiocytoma in an eight-month-old male Rottweiler (H&E stain, × 132).

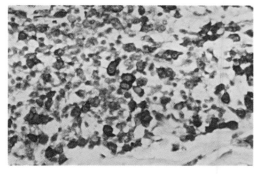

Plate 23
Mast cell tumour (skin): metachromatic granules are visible in the cytoplasm with a toluidine blue stain (toluidine blue, × 132).

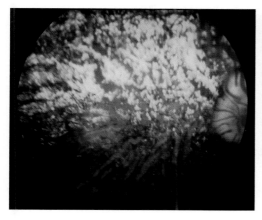

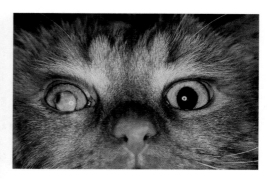

Plate 24
Choroidal hypoplasia and increased blood vessel tortuosity in a two-year-old entire female Rough Collie with collie eye anomaly. Photo courtesy of Mark Bossley.

Plate 25
Corneal sequestrum and secondary lower lid entropion in a five-year-old neutered male Domestic Short Hair cat. Photo courtesy of Mark Bossley.

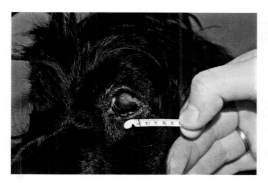

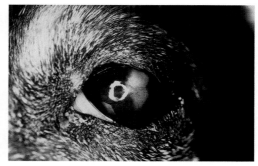

Plate 26
This crossbreed dog is showing signs of dry eye and the Schirmer tear test strip is reading '0' indicating lack of tear production.

Plate 27
Corneal pigmentation, neovascularisation and oedema secondary to keratoconjunctivitis sicca in a Jack Russell Terrier. Photo courtesy of Mark Bossley.

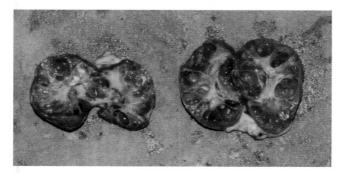

Plate 28
Polycystic kidney disease in a seven-year-old Persian cat at post mortem.

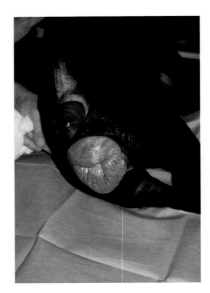

Plate 29
Vaginal hyperplasia. Note there is
also a rectal prolapse. Author:
Andy Moores.

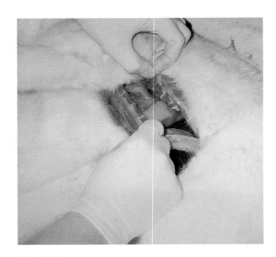

Plate 30
Chylothorax is seen in this post mortem
examination of a cat.

Reproductive conditions

Cryptorchidism
- Developmental defect believed to be inherited as a sex-limited, autosomal recessive trait
- Believed to be a breed at increased risk of the condition

Testicular neoplasia
- Believed to be a breed at increased risk

Respiratory conditions

Tracheal collapse
- Aetiology unknown
- Usually affects middle-aged to old dogs

POODLE

Cardiovascular conditions

Patent ductus arteriosus
- Common congenital abnormality
- Relative risk 6.7 for Toy Poodles and 5.9 for Miniature Poodles
- Females predisposed
- Mode of inheritance polygenic

Endocardiosis
- Also known as chronic valvular disease
- Relative risk 3.1 for Toy Poodles and 2.8 for Miniature Poodles
- Increased prevalence with age
- Aetiology unknown but genetic basis likely

Dilated cardiomyopathy
- Increased prevalence with age
- Approximately twice as common in males as females
- Thought to be familial or genetic
- Standard Poodles over-represented in one study

Dermatological conditions

Malassezia dermatitis
- Often seasonal
- Affects any age

Rabies-vaccine-associated vasculitis and alopecia
- Lesions appear at site of vaccine, 3–6 months after administration

Seasonal flank alopecia
- Miniature Poodles predisposed
- Occurs in spring or autumn

Adult-onset growth-hormone-responsive dermatosis (Toy and Miniature Poodles)
- See under Endocrine conditions

Congenital hypotrichosis (Toy and Miniature Poodles)
- Present at birth or develops in the first month of life
- Predisposition for males suggests sex linkage

Colour-dilution alopecia
- Coat-colour genes are involved in the pathogenesis
- Standard Poodles predisposed

Post-injectional calcinosis circumscripta
- Lesions usually occur within 5 months of injections

Primary lymphoedema
- No apparent sex predisposition
- Usually occurs within first 12 weeks of life

Melanotrichia
- Often following healing of deep inflammation

Nasal depigmentation
- Also known as Dudley nose
- Unknown cause

Anal sac disease (Toy and Miniature Poodles)
- May be caused by infection, impaction or *Malassezia*, or may be psychogenic

Zinc-responsive dermatosis (Standard Poodles)
- Occurs in rapidly-growing dogs fed zinc-deficient diets

Granulomatous sebaceous adenitis
- No sex predisposition
- In Standard Poodles, inherited as an autosomal recessive trait with variable expression
- In Standard Poodles, hyperkeratosis is followed by alopecia
- Affects the face and ears, progressing to the neck and dorsal trunk

Idiopathic chronic ulcerative blepharitis

Idiopathic sterile nodular panniculitis
- Multiple lesions seen
- Females predisposed
- No age predisposition

Skin tumours
- See under Neoplastic conditions

Drug reactions
Glucocorticoids
- Subcutaneous injections in this breed may cause local areas of alopecia

Endocrine conditions
Adult-onset growth-hormone-responsive dermatosis (Toy and Miniature Poodles)
- Breed predisposition
- Males maybe predisposed
- Clinical signs usually seen at 1–5 years

Hypothyroidism
- Breed reported in some texts to be at increased risk
- Often middle-aged (2–6 years)

Hypoadrenocorticism (Standard Poodles)
- Possible genetic predisposition suggested by familial occurrence

Hyperadrenocorticism: pituitary-dependent (PDH) and adrenocortical tumour (AT)
- Possible breed predisposition (PDH and AT)
- Middle-aged/older
- AT: 60–65% female; PDH 55–60% female

Diabetes mellitus
- Possible breed predisposition
- Usual age range: 4–14 years; peak incidence: 7–9 years
- Old entire females are predisposed

Insulinoma (Standard Poodles)
- Higher incidence seen in this breed
- Usually middle-aged/older dogs

Primary hypoparathyroidism (Miniature Poodles)
- Uncommon condition
- Breed at increased risk in some surveys
- Occurs at any age

Gastrointestinal conditions
Salivary mucocoele
- Possible breed predisposition

Cricopharyngeal achalasia
- Possible breed predisposition
- Symptoms seen at or shortly after weaning

Gastric dilatation-volvulus (Standard Poodles)
- Possible breed predisposition

Haemorrhagic gastroenteritis (Toy and Miniature Poodles)
- Breed predisposition
- Seen most commonly at 2–4 years of age

Lobular dissecting hepatitis (Standard Poodles)
- Possible breed predisposition
- Seen primarily in young dogs (7 months or younger)

Cholelithiasis
- Possible breed predisposition
- Older female dogs may be predisposed

Haematological/immunological conditions
Non-spherocytic haemolytic anaemia (Miniature Poodles)
- Rare
- Chronic haemolysis leads to myelofibrosis

Immune-mediated haemolytic anaemia
- Common disease
- Usually affects young adult and middle-aged animals
- May be more common in bitches
- May be seasonal variations in the incidence

Immune-mediated thrombocytopaenia (Miniature and Toy Poodles)
- Common
- Inheritance likely
- Females more commonly affected than males

Von Willebrand's disease
- Possibly inherited as autosomal recessive
- Mainly type I disease is seen in this breed

Systemic lupus erythematosus
- Inherited, but not by a simple mechanism

Musculoskeletal conditions
Inguinal/scrotal herniation
- Females predisposed

Perineal hernia
- Intact males predisposed

Medial patellar luxation
- Significant hereditary component suspected (Miniature and Toy Poodles)

Aseptic necrosis of the femoral head
(Miniature and Toy Poodles)
- Also known as Legg-Calve-Perthe's disease
- Mean age of onset: 7 months
- Unknown aetiology

Miniature Poodle multiple enchondromatosis
- Short, bowed limbs and femoral neck fractures
- Probably an autosomal recessive trait

Miniature Poodle multiple epiphyseal
dysplasia
- Rare
- Mode of inheritance unknown

Miniature Poodle pseudoachondroplasia
- Poor growth and short bowed legs
- Probably inherited as an autosomal recessive trait

Shoulder luxation (Miniature Poodles)
- Congenital

Congenital scapulohumeral luxation
- Rare condition
- Age of onset: usually 3–10 months

Delayed/non-union of fractures of the distal
third of the radius and ulna in miniature and
toy breeds (Toy and Miniature Poodles)
- May be associated with inadequate immobilization

Neoplastic conditions
Basal cell tumour (Miniature Poodles)
- Reported to be at increased risk

Trichoepithelioma (Standard Poodles)
- Possible breed predisposition
- Average age reported as 9 years

Pilomatrixoma (Miniature and Standard
Poodles)
- Rare
- Possible breed predisposition
- Average age reported as 6.6 years

Sebaceous gland tumours
- Possible breed predisposition to nodular sebaceous hyperplasia
- Seen in older dogs (average age 10 years)

Squamous cell carcinoma of the digit
(Standard Poodles)
- Possible breed predisposition
- Older dogs
- Dogs with black coats seem to be more frequently affected

Insulinoma (Standard Poodle)
- See under Endocrine conditions

Pituitary tumour resulting in
hyperadrenocorticism
- See under Endocrine conditions

Adrenocortical tumour resulting in
hyperadrenocorticism
- See under Endocrine conditions

Lymphosarcoma (malignant lymphoma)
- Higher incidence noted in this breed
- Most cases are seen in middle-aged dogs (mean 6–7 years)

Limbal melanoma
- Possible breed predisposition

Oral melanoma
- Possible breed predisposition
- Generally seen in older dogs (mean 9–12 years)
- Males may be predisposed

Testicular neoplasia (Miniature and
Standard Poodles)
- Believed to be a breed at increased risk

Neurological conditions

Acquired vestibular disease secondary to otitis interna
- Breed predisposition to chronic otitis externa which may progress to otitis media/interna

Congenital deafness (Miniature Poodles)
- Signs seen from birth

Intervertebral disc disease
- Breed predisposition
- Relatively common condition
- Age of clinical onset: 3–7 years

Lysosomal storage disease – globoid cell leukodystrophy (Krabbe's disease)
- Inheritance suspected
- Rare
- Signs seen at 6–12 months

Lysosomal storage disease – neuronal glycoproteinosis (Lafora's disease)
- Inheritance suspected
- Rare
- Signs seen at 5–12 months

Lysosomal storage disease – sphingomyelinosis (Niemann-Pick disease) (Miniature and Toy Poodles)
- Inheritance suspected
- Rare
- Signs seen at 3–6 months

Cerebellar degeneration (Miniature Poodles)
- Has been reported
- Signs seen at 3–4 weeks

True epilepsy (Miniature and Standard Poodles)
- Inheritance suspected
- Age of onset: 6 months to 3 years

Hydrocephalus (Toy Poodles)
- Congenital
- Relatively common
- Onset of signs: usually 4–5 months

Narcolepsy-cataplexy (Miniature and Standard Poodles)
- Inheritance suspected
- Age of clinical onset: <1 year

Hypoglycaemia (as a possible cause of seizures in Miniature and Toy Poodles)
- Breed predisposition
- Seen in dogs <1 year

Demyelinating myelopathy (Miniature Poodles)
- Inheritance suspected
- Rare
- Age of onset: 2–4 months

Atlantoaxial subluxation (Miniature and Toy Poodles)
- Congenital
- Relatively common in these breeds
- Age of clinical onset: <1 year

Granulomatous meningoencephalitis (GME) (Miniature and Toy Poodles)
- Breed predisposition
- Age of clinical onset: >1 year

Ocular conditions

Entropion (usually medial lower lids)
- Breed predisposition; polygenic inheritance likely

Distichiasis (Toy and Miniature Poodles)
- Breed predisposition; mode of inheritance unclear

Caruncular trichiasis
- Breed predisposition

Lacrimal punctal aplasia (Toy and Miniature Poodles)
- Congenital condition; mode of inheritance unknown

Medial canthal pocket syndrome (Standard Poodles)
- Breed predisposition; resulting from head shape

Pigmentary keratitis (Miniature Poodles)
- Breed predisposition

Microcornea
- Congenital
- Usually found associated with multiple ocular defects

Refractory corneal ulceration (Miniature and Toy Poodles)
- Breed predisposition
- Usually middle-aged

Congenital, sub-epithelial, geographic corneal dystrophy
- Congenital condition; predisposed breed
- Occurs in young puppies (<10 weeks); transient condition

Limbal melanoma
- Possible breed predisposition

Glaucoma (Miniature and Toy Poodles)
- Breed predisposition
- Age of onset: 6–16 years

Degeneration of the vitreous body (Miniature Poodles)
- Mode of inheritance is unknown
- Age of onset: 2 years
- Glaucoma is a common sequel

Lens luxation (Toy Poodles)
- Breed predisposition
- Seen in older dogs

Cataract (Standard Poodles)
- Autosomal recessive inheritance
- Age of onset: 1 year
- Localisation: equatorial progressing to involve the cortex resulting in blindness
- Schedule 1 of the BVA/KC/ISDS Eye Scheme

Cataract (Toy and Miniature Poodles)
- Inheritance suspected
- Localisation: anterior cortical and posterior polar subcapsular
- Age of onset: 4–5 years; both types progress and cause visual deficiencies

Generalised progressive retinal atrophy (GPRA) (Toy and Miniature Poodles)
- Autosomal recessive inheritance
- Progressive rod-cone degeneration (PRCD)
- Ophthalmoscopic signs are visible by 3–5 years, night blindness is present at 3–5 years,

total blindness at 5–7 years; may be associated with cataract formation
- Schedule 1 of the BVA/KC/ISDS Eye Scheme

Micropapilla (Miniature and Toy Poodles)
- Congenital condition
- Seen occasionally in this breed

Optic nerve hypoplasia (Miniature and Toy Poodles)
- Congenital condition; inheritance suspected
- Schedule 3 BVA/KC/ISDS Eye Scheme

Pseudopapilloedema (Miniature Poodles)
- Reported in this breed

Multiple ocular defects (Standard Poodles)
- Inheritance suspected
- Defects may include microphthalmia, congenital cataract, persistence of the hyaloid system and retinal defects
- Schedule 3 of the BVA/KC/ISDS Eye Scheme

Physiological conditions
Red blood cell macrocytosis
- Occurs rarely in Toy and Miniature Poodles
- Does not require treatment

Renal and urinary conditions
Familial renal disease (renal dysplasia) (Standard Poodle)
- Mode of inheritance unknown
- Cases present from a few months with renal failure

Ectopic ureters (Toy and Miniature Poodles)
- Congenital anomaly, higher incidence reported in this breed
- Usually presents <1 year of age
- More commonly diagnosed in females

Calcium oxalate urolithiasis (Miniature Poodles)
- Higher incidence has been noted in this breed in some surveys
- Average age at diagnosis is 5–12 years
- Males may be predisposed

Struvite (magnesium ammonium phosphate) urolithiasis (Miniature Poodles)
- Higher incidence has been noted in this breed in some surveys
- Average age at diagnosis is 2–8 years
- Females seem to be predisposed

Calcium phosphate urolithiasis (hydroxyapatite and carbonate apatite) (Miniature Poodles)
- Higher incidence has been noted in this breed in some surveys
- Average age at diagnosis is 7–11 years

Calcium phosphate urolithiasis (brushite) (Miniature Poodles)
- Higher incidence has been noted in this breed in some surveys
- Average age at diagnosis is 7–11 years
- Males seem to be predisposed

Reproductive conditions
Male pseudohermaphroditism
- Congenital abnormality reported in this breed

Cryptorchidism (Toy and Miniature Poodles)
- Developmental defect believed to be inherited as a sex-limited, autosomal recessive trait
- Believed to be a breed at increased risk

Testicular neoplasia (Miniature and Standard Poodles)
- Believed to be a breed at increased risk

Respiratory conditions
Tracheal collapse (Miniature and Toy Poodles)
- Aetiology unknown
- Usually affects middle-aged to old dogs

PORTUGUESE WATER DOG

Cardiovascular conditions
Dilated cardiomyopathy
- Can be juvenile onset in this breed
- 10 out of 124 surveyed puppies were affected

Dermatological conditions
Canine follicular dysplasia
- A marked predilection in this breed implies a genetic basis for this group of diseases

- Hair loss begins at 2–4 years of age and occurs mainly on the flank
- Hair loss is due to fracture of the hair in this breed
- Eventually the whole of the trunk is involved

Pattern baldness
- Hair loss occurs at about 6 months of age
- Ventral neck, thighs and tail

Neurological conditions
Lysosomal storage disease – GM$_1$ gangliosidosis
- Autosomal recessive inheritance
- Rare
- Signs seen at 3–6 months

Ocular conditions
Distichiasis
- Breed predisposition; mode of inheritance unclear

Cataract
- Inheritance suspected

Generalised progressive retinal atrophy (GPRA)
- Autosomal recessive inheritance
- Progressive rod-cone degeneration (PRCD)
- Ophthalmoscopic signs are visible by 3–6 years

Multiple ocular defects
- Inheritance suspected
- Defects may include microphthalmia, persistent pupillary membranes, cataract and retinal defects

PUG

Cardiovascular conditions
Hereditary stenosis of the bundle of His

Dermatological conditions
Atopy
- Females probably predisposed
- Age of onset from 6 months to 7 years
- May or may not be seasonal

Lentiginosis profusa
- Hereditary in pugs, probably inherited as an autosomal dominant trait

Intertrigo
- This breed is predisposed to facial-fold intertrigo

Papilloma-virus-associated pigmented lesions
- May have a genetic basis

Epidermal naevi
- Uncommon

Skin tumours
- See under Neoplastic conditions

Musculoskeletal conditions
Aseptic necrosis of the femoral head
- Mode of inheritance not known

Congenital elbow luxation
- Uncommon; accounts for 15% of non-traumatic elbow lameness
- Severe disability in this breed (type I)
- Present at birth or in the first 3 months of life

Hemivertebrae
- See under Neurological conditions

Neoplastic conditions
Oral melanoma
- Possible breed predisposition
- Generally seen in older dogs (mean 9–12 years)
- Males may be predisposed

Mast cell tumours
- Possible breed predisposition
- May be seen at any age (from 4 months onwards), but usually seen in older animals

Neurological conditions
Hemivertebrae
- Congenital
- Occasionally seen

Pug encephalitis
- Rare
- Age of onset: 6 months to 7 years

Ocular conditions
Entropion (usually medial lower lids)
- Breed predisposition; polygenic inheritance likely

Distichiasis
- Breed predisposition; mode of inheritance unclear

Caruncular trichiasis
- Breed predisposition

Keratoconjunctivitis sicca
- Breed predisposition

Congenital keratoconjunctivitis sicca (lacrimal gland hypoplasia)
- Affected breed

Proptosis
- Occurs more easily in this breed due to head shape

Pigmentary keratitis
- Breed predisposition

Refractory corneal ulceration
- Breed predisposition

Physiological conditions
Achondroplasia
- Genetic dwarfism
- Skull and limbs affected
- Accepted as a breed standard

Reproductive conditions
XX sex reversal
- Congenital condition reported in this breed

Dystocia
- Breed predisposition due to combination of narrow pelvis and large head/wide shoulders

Respiratory conditions
Brachycephalic upper airway syndrome
- Complex of anatomical deformities
- Common in this breed
- Probably a consequence of selective breeding for certain facial characteristics

DOGS

PYRENEAN MOUNTAIN DOG

Cardiovascular conditions
Tricuspid dysplasia
- Congenital
- Relative risk 43.6
- Males predisposed

Haematological conditions
Factor XI deficiency
- Autosomal inheritance, with homozygotes symptomatic

Musculoskeletal conditions
Chondrodysplasia
- Very short limbs
- Inherited as an autosomal recessive trait

Craniomandibular osteopathy
- Reported in two Pyreneans

Shoulder osteochondrosis
- Male:female ratio 2.24:1
- 50% bilateral
- Age of onset: usually 4–7 months, but can be older

Neurological conditions
Congenital deafness
- Signs seen from birth

Ocular conditions
Entropion (usually lateral lower lids; may be associated with 'diamond eye')
- Breed predisposition; polygenic inheritance likely

Ectropion (may be associated with 'diamond eye')
- Breed predisposition; polygenic inheritance likely

Combined entropion-ectropion ('diamond eye')
- Breed predisposition; polygenic inheritance likely

Medial canthal pocket syndrome
- Breed predisposition resulting from head shape

Micropapilla
- Congenital condition

Physiological conditions
Multiple hind-limb dew claws
- Inherited as an autosomal dominant trait

Additional prominence on medial aspect of central tarsal bone

RED KELPI

Dermatological conditions
Ehler-Danlos syndrome
- Also known as cutaneous asthenia
- Inherited group of diseases
- May be inherited as an autosomal dominant trait
- Probably lethal in homozygotes

RHODESIAN RIDGEBACK

Dermatological conditions
Zinc-responsive dermatosis
- Occurs in rapidly–growing dogs fed zinc-deficient diets

Coat-colour dilution and cerebellar degeneration in Rhodesian Ridgeback dogs
- Inherited as an autosomal recessive trait

Dermoid sinus/cyst
- May be inherited as a simple recessive gene
- Progeny testing necessary for eradication
- Not breeding from affected individuals should reduce disease incidence
- Rare
- Solitary or multiple
- Occur on dorsal midline
- See also under Neurological conditions

Onychodystrophy

Neurological conditions
Congenital deafness
- Signs seen from birth

Arachnoid cysts
- Breed predisposition
- Age of clinical onset: <1 year

Dermoid sinus
- Congenital defect
- Autosomal recessive inheritance
- Neurological signs can occur at any age
- See also under Dermatological conditions

Ocular conditions
Entropion (usually lateral lower lids)
- Breed predisposition; polygenic inheritance likely

Eversion of the cartilage of the nictitating membrane
- Breed predisposition
- Usually occurs in young dogs

Cataract
- Inheritance suspected
- Localisation: posterior subcapsular cortex
- Age of onset: 3 years; progress slowly; visual deficiencies uncommon

ROTTWEILER

Cardiovascular conditions
Aortic stenosis
- Congenital
- Relative risk 5.4
- No sex predilection
- Mode of inheritance is possibly autosomal dominant with modifying genes, or polygenic

Dermatological conditions
Follicular lipidosis of Rottweilers
- Suspected genetic predisposition
- Affects young dogs of either sex

Follicular parakeratosis
- Females predisposed
- Possible X-linked mode of inheritance

Muzzle folliculitis/furunculosis
- Also known as canine acne
- Local trauma, hormones and genetics may play a role in the pathogenesis

Mucocutaneous hypopigmentation
- Congenital in this breed; affects lips and nose

Ichthyosis
- Rare
- Congenital
- Possibly inherited as an autosomal recessive trait

Congenital hypotrichosis
- Present at birth or develops in the first month of life
- Predisposition for males suggests sex linkage

Hypopigmentary disorders
- Possibly inherited

Vitiligo
- Presumed to be hereditary

Onychodystrophy

Vasculitis
- Uncommon
- Usually type III hypersensitivity reaction

Skin tumours
- See under Neoplastic conditions

Gastrointestinal conditions
Parvovirus enteritis
- Breed predisposition
- Usually young dogs
- See also under Immunological conditions

Eosinophilic gastroenteritis, enteritis and enterocolitis
- Breed predisposition
- Most common in dogs 5 years and younger

Gastrointestinal eosinophilic granuloma
- Possible breed predisposition
- Most common in young to middle-aged dogs

Lobular dissecting hepatitis
- Possible breed predisposition
- Seen primarily in young dogs (7 months or younger)
- Females may be predisposed

Immunological conditions
Susceptibility to parvovirus
- This breed susceptible to severe and often fatal parvovirus infection
- Resistance to other diseases usually normal

DOGS

Immunodeficiency
- Several related Rottweilers showed multiple immunological defects
- Inheritance suspected

Infectious conditions
Parvovirus enteritis
- Breed predisposition
- See also under Immunological conditions

Infectious skin disease
- See under Dermatological conditions

Musculoskeletal conditions
Elbow dysplasia
- Also known as osteochondrosis
- Genetically determined in this breed
- Medial coronoid process disease is common in this breed

Polyarthritis/meningitis
- Idiopathic
- Affects dogs from 6–9 months old

Plasmacytic-lymphocytic gonitis
- Aetiology unknown
- Observed in less than 10% of dogs undergoing cruciate surgery

Chronic sesamoiditis
- Present in 44% of Rottweilers in one study
- Not necessarily associated with lameness

Juvenile onset distal myopathy
- Uncommon

Hock osteochondrosis
- Common disease
- Affects the proximal medial and lateral trochlear ridges in this breed

Cranial cruciate ligament rupture
- Common cause of hind-limb lameness
- Neutered individuals may be predisposed
- Young animals may be predisposed in this breed

Hip dysplasia
- A large 1989 study showed a prevalence of 24.6% in this breed

Osteosarcoma
- Reported to be familial in this breed
- See also under Neoplastic conditions

Neoplastic conditions
Squamous cell carcinoma of the digit
- Possible breed predisposition
- Older dogs
- Dogs with black coats seem to be more frequently affected

Canine cutaneous histiocytoma
- Possible breed predisposition
- More common in young dogs 1–2 years of age

Primary bone tumours (most commonly osteosarcoma)
- Breed predisposition
- Males may be predisposed

Neurological conditions
Congenital deafness
- Signs seen from birth

Spinal muscular atrophy
- Inheritance suspected
- Rare; has been reported in this breed
- Age of clinical onset: 4 weeks

Atlantoaxial subluxation
- Congenital
- Seen occasionally in this breed
- Age of clinical onset: <1 year

Meningitis and polyarteritis
- Reported in this breed
- Age of onset: <1 year

Neuroaxonal dystrophy
- Autosomal recessive inheritance suspected
- Rare
- Age of clinical onset: <1 year

Rottweiler distal sensorimotor polyneuropathy
- Reported in the USA
- Age of clinical onset: >1 year

Leukoencephalomyelopathy of Rottweilers
- Autosomal recessive inheritance suspected
- Occasionally seen in the USA, UK, Netherlands and Australia
- Age of clinical onset: 1.5–4 years

Ocular conditions
Entropion (usually lateral lower lids)
- Breed predisposition; polygenic inheritance likely

Distichiasis
- Breed predisposition; mode of inheritance unclear

Medial canthal pocket syndrome
- Breed predisposition resulting from head shape

Refractory corneal ulceration
- Breed predisposition
- Age of onset: 5–10 years

Persistent pupillary membranes
- Breed predisposition
- Schedule 3 of the BVA/KC/ISDS Eye Scheme

Iris cyst
- Breed predisposition

Iris coloboma
- Congenital; reported in this breed
- May be seen with other ocular defects

Cataract
- Inheritance suspected
- Localisation: posterior polar subcapsular cataract
- Age of onset: <2 years; slow progression

Multifocal retinal dysplasia
- Congenital condition autosomal recessive inheritance suspected
- Schedule 1 of the BVA/KC/ISDS Eye Scheme

Generalised progressive retinal atrophy (GPRA)
- Mode of inheritance unknown but presumed recessive
- Seen as an advanced condition at 3 years

Retinal detachment
- Inheritance suspected
- Seen at 2–3 years of age
- May be associated with vitreal abnormalities

Multiple ocular defects
- Inheritance suspected
- Defects may include microphthalmia, congenital cataract and retinal dysplasia
- Schedule 3 of the BVA/KC/ISDS Eye Scheme

Physiological conditions
Additional process on the medial aspect of the central tarsal bone

Lateral tarsal torsion and tarsal valgus deformity
- Unknown aetiology
- Cosmetic fault

Blood group
- Tend to be DEA 1.1 or 1.2 positive

Renal and urinary conditions
Familial renal disease
- Chronic renal failure has been reported in four related dogs aged 6–12 months
- Primary glomerular disease was diagnosed

Sphincter mechanism incompetence
- Possible breed predisposition in female dogs

Reproductive conditions
Variation in the interoestrus interval
- Fertile cycles may occur as often as every 4.5 months in this breed

ST BERNARD

Cardiovascular conditions
Dilated cardiomyopathy
- Prevalence of 2.6% in this breed compared to 0.16% in mixed breeds and 0.65% in pure breeds
- Increased prevalence with age
- Approximately twice as common in males as females
- Thought to be familial or genetic

Dermatological conditions
Pyotraumatic folliculitis
- Young dogs predisposed
- Also known as hot spot, wet eczema

DOGS

Ehler-Danlos syndrome
- Also known as cutaneous asthenia
- Inherited group of diseases
- May be inherited as an autosomal dominant trait
- Probably lethal in homozygotes

Callus dermatitis/pyoderma
- Most common over hock and elbow joints of this breed

Intertrigo
- This breed predisposed to lip fold pyoderma

Gastrointestinal conditions
Gastric dilatation-volvulus
- Breed predisposition

Haematological conditions
Haemophilia B
- Factor IX deficiency
- Also known as Christmas disease
- Inherited as a sex-linked trait
- Less common than haemophilia A

Musculoskeletal conditions
Increased anteversion of the femoral head and neck
- Conformational abnormality
- Component of hip dysplasia

Elbow dysplasia
- Also known as osteochondrosis
- Genetically determined in this breed
- Medial coronoid process disease is common in this breed

Hip dysplasia
- Seventh worst mean-scoring breed in the BVA/KC Hip Dysplasia Scheme as of October 2001
- Breed mean score 23

Cranial cruciate ligament rupture
- Common cause of hind-limb lameness
- Neutered individuals may be predisposed
- Young animals may be predisposed in this breed

Osteosarcoma
- Reported to be familial in this breed
- See also under Neoplastic conditions

Lateral patellar luxation
- Also known as genu valgum
- May be inherited

Neoplastic conditions
Non-epitheliotropic lymphoma
- Affects older dogs

Lymphosarcoma (malignant lymphoma)
- Higher incidence noted in this breed
- Most cases are seen in middle-aged dogs (mean 6–7 years)

Primary bone tumours (most commonly osteosarcoma)
- Breed predisposition
- Males may be predisposed

Neurological conditions
Congenital deafness
- Signs seen from birth

True epilepsy
- Inheritance suspected
- Age of onset: 6 months to 3 years

Narcolepsy-cataplexy
- Reported in this breed
- Age of clinical onset: <1 year

Distal polyneuropathy
- Reported in this breed
- Age of clinical onset: >1 year

Ocular conditions
Dermoid
- Breed predisposition

Entropion (usually lower lids; may be associated with macropalpebral fissure)
- Breed predisposition; polygenic inheritance likely

Ectropion (may be associated with macropalpebral fissure)
- Breed predisposition; polygenic inheritance likely

Macropalpebral fissure resulting in combined entropion-ectropion ('diamond eye')
- Breed predisposition; genetic basis incompletely understood

Eversion of the cartilage of the nictitating membrane
- Breed predisposition; possibly inherited as a recessive trait
- Usually occurs in young dogs

Prolapse of the gland of the nictitating membrane
- Breed predisposition; inheritance suspected

Cataract
- Inheritance suspected
- Posterior subcapsular cataracts occur at 6–18 months and are slowly progressive
- Posterior cortical cataracts are seen at 7–8 years and are slowly progressive

Optic nerve hypoplasia
- Congenital defect; not known if inherited

Multiple ocular defects
- Congenital condition; not known if inherited
- Defects include microphthalmia, collapsed anterior chamber and detached dysplastic retinas

Physiological conditions
Additional process on the medial aspect of the central tarsal bone

Lateral tarsal torsion and tarsal valgus deformity
- Unknown aetiology
- Cosmetic fault

Reproductive conditions
Vaginal hyperplasia
- Possible breed predisposition

SALUKI

Dermatological conditions
Black hair follicular dysplasia
- Rare
- Early onset
- Familial

Colour-dilution alopecia
- Coat-colour genes involved in the pathogenesis

Skin tumours
- See under Neoplastic conditions

Drug reactions
Thiopentone
- This breed has a greatly increased susceptibility to thiopentone
- Use of this drug is not recommended in this breed

Neoplastic conditions
Cutaneous haemangioma
- Possible breed predisposition
- Average age was 8.7 years in one study

Neurological conditions
Lysosomal storage disease – ceroid lipofuscinosis
- Inheritance suspected
- Rare
- Signs seen at 1–2 years

Ocular conditions
Neuronal ceroid lipofuscinosis
- Inheritance suspected

SAMOYED

Cardiovascular conditions
Pulmonic stenosis
- Third most frequent cause of canine congenital heart disease
- Polygenic inheritance likely
- Relative risk 2.7

Aortic stenosis
- Common congenital disease
- Not all studies confirm a predisposition

Atrial septal defect
- Uncommon congenital disease
- Not all studies confirm a predisposition

Dermatological conditions
Canine uveodermatological syndrome
- Also known as Vogt-Koyanagi-Harada-like syndrome
- See also under Ocular conditions

DOGS

DOGS

Adult-onset growth-hormone-responsive dermatosis
- See under Endocrine conditions

Nasal depigmentation
- Also known as Dudley nose
- Cause unknown

Granulomatous sebaceous adenitis
- No sex predisposition
- Affects face and ears, progressing to the neck and dorsal trunk

Endocrine conditions
Diabetes mellitus
- Possible breed predisposition
- Usual age range: 4–14 years; peak incidence: 7–9 years
- Old entire females are predisposed

Adult-onset growth-hormone-responsive dermatosis
- Breed predisposition
- Males may be predisposed
- Clinical signs usually seen at 1–5 years

Musculoskeletal conditions
Carpal ligament weakening
- Affects older obese dogs
- Tarsal ligaments may also be affected

Ocular-skeletal dysplasia
- Short forelegs; domed forehead
- Also associated with cataracts and eosinophilia
- Inherited as an autosomal recessive trait
- See also under Ocular conditions

Neoplastic conditions
Perianal (hepatoid) gland adenomas
- Breed predisposition suggested in one survey of 2700 cases
- Average age was 10.5 years
- Entire males were predisposed

Neurological conditions
Congenital deafness
- Signs seen from birth

Cerebellar degeneration
- Uncommon
- Age of clinical onset: 3–6 months

Hypomyelination of the central nervous system
- Inheritance suspected
- Signs seen at 2–8 weeks

Lissencephaly
- Rare developmental disease
- Age of onset: <1 year

Spongiform degeneration
- Rare; reported in this breed
- Age of clinical onset: 3 months

Ocular conditions
Distichiasis
- Breed predisposition

Lacrimal punctal aplasia
- Congenital condition, predisposed breed

Medial canthal pocket syndrome
- Breed predisposition resulting from head shape

Uveodermatological syndrome
- Also known as Vogt-Koyanagi-Harada-like syndrome
- Breed predisposition
- Young adults (1.5–4 years)

Refractory corneal ulceration
- Breed predisposition
- Usually middle-aged

Corneal dystrophy
- Mode of inheritance unknown
- Stromal lipid dystrophy
- Age of onset: 6 months to 2 years

Primary glaucoma
- Breed predisposition
- Age of onset: 2–3 years
- Most cases are associated with goniodysgenesis

Cataract
- Inheritance suspected
- Posterior polar subcapsular cortical cataracts seen <2 years
- Anterior subcapsular cortical cataracts seen at 4 years and older
- Visual deficits uncommon

Multifocal retinal dysplasia
- Congenital condition; inheritance as an autosomal recessive trait suspected
- May be seen with vitreal abnormalities

Generalised progressive retinal atrophy (GPRA)
- Autosomal recessive inheritance, possibly X-linked
- Visual problems are not usually seen until 5–7 years

Optic nerve colobomas
- Congenital defect; not known if inherited

Multiple ocular defects and dwarfism
- Possibly inherited in a similar way to the condition in Labrador Retrievers, i.e. the gene having recessive effects on the skeleton and incomplete dominant effects on the eye
- Ocular defects may include retinal dysplasia and detachments, cataracts, abnormal secondary vitreous and persistence of the hyaloid system

Renal and urinary conditions
Familial renal disease
- X-linked dominant inheritance suggested
- Glomerular basement membrane disorder
- In males there is progressive glomerular disease. Dogs present with proteinuria and isosthenuria at 2–3 months of age, renal failure at 6–9 months of age and usually die by 12–16 months of age
- In carrier females the condition is milder and non-progressive. Affected individuals may fail to attain normal adult body weight, but do not progress to terminal renal failure

SCHIPPERKE

Dermatological conditions
Black hair follicular dysplasia
- Rare
- Early onset
- Familial

Colour-dilution alopecia
- Coat-colour genes involved in the pathogenesis

Pemphigus foliaceous
- Uncommon disease
- No sex predisposition
- Mean age of onset: 4 years

Canine follicular dysplasia
- A genetic basis is suspected for this group of diseases

Endocrine conditions
Diabetes mellitus
- Possible breed predisposition
- Usual age range: 4–14 years; peak incidence: 7–9 years
- Old entire females are predisposed

Ocular conditions
Cataract
- Inheritance suspected
- Localisation: anterior subcapsular
- Age of onset: 7 years; slowly progressive

Generalised progressive retinal atrophy (GPRA)
- Simple autosomal recessive inheritance suspected
- Age of clinical onset: 2–7 years

SCHNAUZER

Cardiovascular conditions
Patent ductus arteriosus
- Common congenital abnormality
- Relative risk 2.2
- Females predisposed
- Miniature Schnauzers predisposed
- Mode of inheritance is polygenic

Pulmonic stenosis
- Third most frequent cause of canine congenital heart disease
- Polygenic inheritance possible
- Relative risk 4.7
- Miniature Schnauzers are predisposed

Endocardiosis
- Also known as chronic valvular disease
- Relative risk 4.4

- Increased prevalence with age
- Aetiology unknown but genetic basis likely
- Miniature Schnauzers predisposed

Sick sinus syndrome
- Middle-aged to old dogs
- Relative risk 126 in one small study and 6.9 in a larger study
- Females predisposed in this breed, at a ratio of 3:1
- Miniature Schnauzers predisposed

Dermatological conditions
Atopy (Miniature Schnauzers)
- Females probably predisposed
- Age of onset: from 6 months to 7 years
- May or may not be seasonal

Food hypersensitivity (Miniature Schnauzers)
- No age or sex predisposition reported

Superficial suppurative necrolytic dermatitis of Miniature Schnauzers
- Associated with the use of shampoos
- No sex predisposition

Seasonal flank alopecia
- Tends to occur in spring or autumn

Schnauzer comedo syndrome
- Affects Miniature Schnauzers
- May be inherited

Acquired aurotrichia in Miniature Schnauzers
- Uncommon
- Affects either sex
- Inheritance likely

Papilloma-virus-associated pigmented lesions
- May have a genetic basis
- Affects Miniature Schnauzers

Vitiligo
- Presumed to be hereditary

Canine subcorneal pustular dermatosis
- Miniature Schnauzers account for 40% of cases
- Very rare
- No age or sex predisposition

Follicular cyst
- No age or sex predisposition

Epidermal naevi
- Uncommon
- Affects young adult Miniature Schnauzers
- Probably inherited

Skin tumours
- See under Neoplastic conditions

Drug reactions
Sulphonamides
- Can cause cutaneous reactions

Gold
- Can cause cutaneous reactions

Shampoos
- Can cause superficial suppurative necrolytic dermatitis

Endocrine conditions
Central diabetes insipidus (CDI)
- One report of CDI diagnosed in three of a litter of five 7-week-old Schnauzers suggesting a possible familial basis

Hypothyroidism (Giant Schnauzers)
- One report of congenital secondary hypothyroidism due to thyroid stimulating hormone deficiency in a family of Giant Schnauzers
- Autosomal recessive mode of inheritance suggested

Hypothyroidism (Miniature Schnauzers)
- Possible breed predisposition
- Often middle-aged (2–6 years)

Diabetes mellitus (Miniature Schnauzers)
- Possible breed predisposition
- Usual age range: 4–14 years; peak incidence: 7–9 years
- Old entire females are predisposed

Primary hypoparathyroidism (Miniature Schnauzers)
- Uncommon condition
- Possible breed predisposition
- Occurs at any age

DOGS

Gastrointestinal conditions

Congenital idiopathic megaoesophagus
(Miniature Schnauzers)

- Inheritance compatible with simple autosomal dominance or autosomal recessive inheritance with 60% penetrance

Haemorrhagic gastroenteritis (Miniature Schnauzers)

- Breed predisposition
- Seen most commonly at 2–4 years of age

Vacuolar hepatopathy associated with hyperlipidaemia (Miniature Schnauzers)

- An inborn error of lipoprotein metabolism in this breed leads to hyperlipidaemia and liver disease

Congenital portosystemic shunt (Miniature Schnauzers)

- Breed predisposition
- Clinical signs usually seen <1 year

Cholelithiasis (Miniature Schnauzers)

- Breed predisposition
- Older female dogs may be predisposed

Pancreatitis (Miniature Schnauzers)

- Breed predisposition
- May be associated with hyperlipidaemia in this breed

Selective malabsorption of cobalamin
(vitamin B$_{12}$) (Giant Schnauzers)

- Autosomal recessive inheritance has been suggested
- Signs seen at 6–12 weeks
- See also under Haematological conditions

Haematological conditions

Selective malabsorption of cobalamin
(vitamin B$_{12}$) (Giant Schnauzers)

- Causes a non-regenerative anaemia with poikilocytosis and neutropaenia
- Inherited as an autosomal recessive trait

Primary idiopathic hyperlipidaemia
(Miniature Schnauzers)

- Familial; suspected to be due to an inherited defect

Musculoskeletal conditions

Myotonia

- Affects Miniature Schnauzers
- Congenital in this breed
- Inherited as an autosomal recessive trait

Neoplastic conditions

Trichoepithelioma (Miniature Schnauzers)

- Possible breed predisposition
- Average age reported as 9 years

Sebaceous gland tumours (Miniature Schnauzers)

- Possible breed predisposition to nodular sebaceous hyperplasia
- Seen in older dogs (average age 10 years)

Melanoma

- Breed predisposition
- Average age 8–9 years

Lipoma (Miniature Schnauzers)

- Possible breed predisposition
- Most common in middle-aged, obese female dogs

Canine cutaneous histiocytoma (Miniature Schnauzers)

- Breed predisposition
- More common in young dogs 1–2 years of age

Melanoma of the digit

- Possible breed predisposition
- Average age 10–11 years
- More common in dogs with heavily pigmented skin

Squamous cell carcinoma of the digit
(Giant Schnauzers)

- Possible breed predisposition
- Older dogs
- Dogs with black coats seem to be more frequently affected

Testicular neoplasia (Miniature Schnauzers)

- Believed to be a breed at increased risk

Limbal melanoma

- Possible breed predisposition

DOGS

Neurological conditions
Narcolepsy-cataplexy (Giant Schnauzers)
- Reported in this breed
- Age of clinical onset: <1 year

Hyperlipidaemia as a cause of seizures (Minature Schnauzers)
- Familial; possibly due to an inherited defect in lipoprotein metabolism

Partial seizures ('fly-biting' and 'star-gazing' seizures in Miniature Schnauzers)
- Reported in this breed

Ocular conditions
Keratoconjunctivitis sicca
- Breed predisposition

Limbal melanoma
- Possible breed predisposition

Glaucoma (Giant and Miniature Schnauzers)
- Possible breed predisposition
- Goniodysgenesis has been seen in Giant Schnauzers

Lens luxation (Miniature Schnauzers)
- Breed predisposition; autosomal recessive inheritance has been suggested
- Age of onset: 3–6 years
- Glaucoma is a common sequel

Congenital hereditary cataract (Miniature Schnauzers)
- Autosomal recessive inheritance
- Age of onset: <6 weeks
- Localisation: posterior nucleus/subcapsular cortex; may be associated with microphthalmia and rotary nystagmus
- Schedule 1 of the BVA/KC/ISDS Eye Scheme

Cataract 1 (Miniature Schnauzers)
- Autosomal recessive inheritance
- Age of onset: <2 years
- Localisation: nucleus and suture lines; progressive with visual deficiencies possible
- Schedule 1 of the BVA/KC/ISDS Eye Scheme

Cataract 2 (Miniature Schnauzers)
- Inheritance suspected
- Age of onset: 4–6 years
- Localisation: posterior subcapsular cortex; frequently progresses to completion

Cataract 3 (Standard Schnauzer)
- Inheritance suspected
- Posterior nuclear/cortical cataracts may be congenital and progress slowly; may be associated with microcornea
- Posterior subcapsular cataracts may be seen <1 year and progress to completion
- Posterior subcapsular cataracts may also be seen at 6 years

Cataract 4 (Giant Schnauzers)
- Inheritance suspected
- Localisation: posterior subcapsular cortex
- Age of onset: young puppy or 6–7 years; slowly progressive
- Schedule 3 of the BVA/KC/ISDS Eye Scheme

Multifocal retinal dysplasia (Giant Schnauzers)
- Congenital condition; inheritance as an autosomal recessive trait suspected
- Schedule 3 of the BVA/KC/ISDS Eye Scheme

Generalised progressive retinal atrophy (GPRA) (Giant Schnauzers)
- Autosomal recessive inheritance suspected
- Clinically apparent at 3–4 years

Generalised progressive retinal atrophy (GPRA) (photoreceptor dysplasia) (Miniature Schnauzers)
- Autosomal recessive inheritance
- Slow clinical progression; ophthalmoscopic signs not seen until 2–5 years
- Schedule 1 BVA/KC/ISDS Eye Scheme

Micropapilla (Miniature Schnauzers)
- Congenital condition
- Seen occasionally in this breed

Optic nerve hypoplasia (Miniature Schnauzers)
- Congenital condition; not known if inherited
- Seen occasionally in this breed

Renal and urinary conditions
Familial renal disease (renal dysplasia)
(Miniature Schnauzers)
- Chronic renal failure suggestive of renal dysplasia was reported in eight related dogs aged 4 months to 3 years

Urate urolithiasis (Miniature Schnauzers)
- Higher incidence has been noted in this breed in some surveys
- Average age at diagnosis is 3–6 years
- Males seem to be predisposed

Calcium oxalate urolithiasis (Miniature Schnauzers)
- Higher incidence has been noted in this breed in some surveys
- Average age at diagnosis is 5–12 years
- Males may be predisposed
- May be associated with absorptive hypercalciuria

Struvite (magnesium ammonium phosphate) urolithiasis (Miniature Schnauzers)
- Higher incidence has been noted in this breed in some surveys
- Average age at diagnosis is 2–8 years
- Females seem to be predisposed

Calcium phosphate urolithiasis (hydroxyapatite and carbonate apatite) (Miniature Schnauzers)
- Higher incidence has been noted in this breed in some surveys
- Average age at diagnosis is 7–11 years

Silica urolithiasis (Miniature Schnauzers)
- Higher incidence has been noted in this breed in some surveys
- Males seem to be predisposed

Reproductive conditions
Cryptorchidism (Miniature Schnauzers)
- Developmental defect believed to be inherited as a sex-limited, autosomal recessive trait
- Believed to be a breed at increased risk

Testicular neoplasia (Miniature Schnauzers)
- Believed to be a breed at increased risk

Male pseudohermaphroditism (Miniature Schnauzers)
- Congenital abnormality reported in this breed

SCOTTISH DEERHOUND

Cardiovascular conditions
Dilated cardiomyopathy
- Prevalence of 6.0% in this breed in a small population studied compared to 0.16% in mixed breeds and 0.65% in pure breeds
- Increased prevalence with age
- Approximately twice as common in males as females
- Thought to be familial or genetic

Musculoskeletal conditions
Pseudoachondrodysplasia
- Causes retarded growth
- Later in life osteopaenia leads to severe deformity

Renal and urinary conditions
Cystine urolithiasis
- Cystinuria results from an inherited defect in renal tubular transport of cystine and predisposes to cystine urolithiasis
- Increased incidence reported in this breed in some surveys
- Average age at diagnosis is 1–8 years
- Males seem predisposed

SCOTTISH TERRIER

Cardiovascular conditions
Pulmonic stenosis
- Third most frequent cause of canine congenital heart disease
- Polygenic inheritance possible
- Relative risk 12.6

Dermatological conditions
Generalised demodicosis
- Scottish Terriers are among the ten breeds at highest statistical risk of this disease in the Cornell, USA population

DOGS

Atopy
- Females probably predisposed
- Age of onset from 6 months to 7 years
- May or may not be seasonal

Seasonal flank alopecia
- Tends to occur in spring or autumn

Familial vasculopathy
- Reported in five Scottish Terrier puppies
- Probably autosomal dominant inheritance

Scrotal vascular nevus
- More common in older dogs

Skin tumours
- See under Neoplastic conditions

Haematological/immunological conditions
Immune-mediated thrombocytopaenia
- Common
- Familial in this breed; inheritance likely
- Females more commonly affected than males

Von Willebrand's disease
- This breed is affected by type III disease
- Inherited as an autosomal recessive trait

Haemophilia B
- Factor IX deficiency
- Also known as Christmas disease
- Inherited as a sex-linked trait
- Less common than haemophilia A

Infectious conditions
Coccidiomycosis
- Increased incidence in this breed possibly due to an increased likelihood of exposure
- Seen mainly in young male dogs
- Geographic distribution: California, Arizona, Texas, New Mexico, Nevada, Utah, Mexico, and parts of Central and South America; not reported in the UK

Infectious skin disease
- See under Dermatological conditions

Musculoskeletal conditions
Craniomandibular osteopathy
- May be inherited in this breed
- Usually affects dogs aged 3–8 months

Muscle cramping ('Scottie cramp')
- Recessive inheritance suspected
- Age of clinical onset: <6 months

Neoplastic conditions
Mast cell tumours
- Possible breed predisposition
- May be seen at any age (from 4 months onwards), but usually seen in older animals

Melanoma
- Breed predisposition
- Average age 8–9 years

Canine cutaneous histiocytoma
- Possible breed predisposition
- More common in young dogs 1–2 years of age

Squamous cell carcinoma of the skin
- Occurs at an average of 9 years of age

Non-epitheliotropic lymphoma
- Affects older dogs

Primary brain tumour
- See under Neurological conditions

Lymphosarcoma (malignant lymphoma)
- Higher incidence noted in this breed
- Most cases are seen in middle-aged dogs (mean 6–7 years)

Neurological conditions
Congenital deafness
- Signs seen from birth

Muscle cramping ('Scottie cramp')
- Recessive inheritance suspected
- Age of clinical onset: <6 months

Ocular conditions
Lens luxation
- Inheritance suspected
- Age of onset: 3–4 years

Cataract
- Inheritance suspected
- Age of onset: 5–7 years

Physiological conditions
Hypochondroplasia
- Accepted as breed standard
- Short bowed legs, but normal skulls seen

Reproductive conditions
Dystocia
- Breed predisposition due to the combination of a narrow pelvis and large head/wide shoulders

SEALYHAM TERRIER

Dermatological conditions
Waardenburg-Klein syndrome
- Inherited as an autosomal dominant trait with incomplete penetrance

Neurological conditions
Congenital deafness
- Signs seen from birth

Ocular conditions
Lacrimal punctal aplasia
- Congenital condition, predisposed breed

Glaucoma
- Possible breed predisposition
- Most cases are secondary and associated with lens luxation

Primary lens luxation
- Autosomal dominant inheritance suggested
- Age of onset: 4–6 years
- Often followed by glaucoma
- Schedule 1 of the BVA/KC/ISDS Eye Scheme

Cataract
- Inheritance suspected

Total retinal dysplasia with retinal detachment
- Congenital condition inherited as a simple autosomal recessive trait
- May be seen with a degree of microphthalmia

- Schedule 1 of the BVA/KC/ISDS Eye Scheme

Generalised progressive retinal atrophy (GPRA)
- Has been recognised in this breed in the UK

Reproductive conditions
Dystocia
- Breed predisposition due to the combination of a narrow pelvis and large head/wide shoulders

SHAR PEI

Dermatological conditions
Generalised demodicosis
- Shar Peis are in the ten breeds at highest statistical risk of this disease in the Cornell, USA population

Atopy
- Females probably predisposed
- Age of onset: 6 months to 7 years
- May or may not be seasonal

Food hypersensitivity
- No age or sex predisposition reported

Primary seborrhoea
- Probably inherited as an autosomal recessive trait
- Signs first appear at early age and get worse with age

Idiopathic cutaneous mucinosis
- Often a cosmetic problem only in this breed

Intertrigo
- May occur due to intentional breeding for excessive skin folding

Skin tumours
- See under Neoplastic conditions

Gastrointestinal conditions
Congenital idiopathic megaoesophagus
- Possible breed predisposition

DOGS

Congenital (sliding) hiatal hernia
- Breed predisposition

Lymphocytic-plasmacytic enteritis
- Possible breed predisposition
- Most common in middle-aged and older dogs

Amyloidosis
- Breed predisposition
- May affect many body systems including the liver and kidneys

Immunological conditions
Selective IgA deficiency
- Found in two colonies of Shar Peis
- Led to chronic skin disease and recurrent respiratory disease

Musculoskeletal conditions
Hip dysplasia
- Sixteenth worst mean-scoring breed in the BVA/KC Hip Dysplasia Scheme as of October 2001
- Breed mean score 18

Familial Mediterranean fever
- Renal amyloidosis and swollen joints seen
- See also under Renal and urinary conditions

Neoplastic conditions
Canine cutaneous histiocytoma
- Possible breed predisposition
- More common in young dogs 1–2 years of age

Mast cell tumours
- This breed is predisposed to developing this tumour at less than 2 years of age (5 out of 18 reported cases)
- Predilection sites are the inguinal and preputial regions

Ocular conditions
Entropion (often involves upper and lower lids)
- Breed predisposition; polygenic inheritance likely
- Very common and often very severe; may be secondary to excessive facial skin folds

Prolapse of the gland of the nictitating membrane
- Breed predisposition; possibly inherited

Glaucoma
- Possible breed predisposition

Cataract
- Inheritance suspected

Primary lens luxation
- Inheritance suspected
- Often followed by glaucoma

Fibrosing esotropia
- Breed predisposition
- Seen in young dogs
- Severe medial deviation of one or both globes

Renal and urinary conditions
Renal amyloidosis (as part of reactive systemic amyloidosis)
- Familial
- Age of clinical onset: 1.5–6 years
- In one report of 14 affected Shar Pei dogs, ten were female and four male
- Most dogs have medullary deposition of amyloid; only 66% have glomerular involvement. Amyloid deposits may be found in many other organs including liver, spleen, gastrointestinal tract and thyroid gland. The disease presents with chronic renal failure at a young age, recurrent fever and joint swelling or hepatomegaly, jaundice and, rarely, liver rupture

Respiratory conditions
Primary ciliary dyskinesia
- Signs usually seen early in life

SHETLAND SHEEPDOG

Cardiovascular conditions
Patent ductus arteriosus
- Common congenital abnormality
- Relative risk 3.9
- Mode of inheritance is polygenic

Dermatological conditions

Cutaneous histiocytosis
- No apparent age or sex predisposition

Superficial bacterial folliculitis
- Can resemble endocrine alopecia in this breed

Malassezia dermatitis
- Often seasonal
- Affects any age

Systemic lupus erythematosus
- Uncommon (incidence approximately 0.03% of general canine population)
- No age or sex predisposition

Discoid lupus erythematosus
- No age or sex predisposition
- Accounted for 0.3% of skin diseases at a referral institution

Familial canine dermatomyositis
- Inherited as an autosomal dominant trait with incomplete penetrance
- No predispositions for sex, coat colour or coat length

Idiopathic ulcerative dermatosis in Shetland Sheepdogs and Collies
- Unknown cause
- No sex predisposition
- Affects middle-aged to older dogs

Canine uveodermatological syndrome
- Also known as Vogt-Koyanagi-Harada-like syndrome
- See also under Ocular conditions

Colour-dilution alopecia
- Coat-colour genes are involved in the pathogenesis

Skin tumours
- See under Neoplastic conditions

Drug reactions

Ivermectin and milbemycin
- High doses can cause tremors, ataxia, coma and death

Endocrine conditions

Hypothyroidism
- Reported to be a breed at increased risk
- Often middle-aged (2–6 years)

Gastrointestinal conditions

Haemorrhagic gastroenteritis
- Possible breed predisposition
- Seen most commonly at 2–4 years of age

Haematological/immunological conditions

Von Willebrand's disease
- This breed is affected by type III disease
- Inheritance possibly determined by two mutations in this breed

Systemic lupus erythematosus
- Inherited, but not by a simple mechanism

Haemophilia B
- Factor IX deficiency
- Also known as Christmas disease
- Inherited as a sex-linked trait
- Less common than haemophilia A

Musculoskeletal conditions

Carpal ligament weakening
- Affects older obese dogs
- Tarsal ligaments may also be affected

Canine idiopathic polyarthritis
- Usually affects dogs aged 1–3 years, but any age can be affected
- Males predisposed

Congenital scapulohumeral luxation
- Rare condition
- Age of onset: usually 3–10 months

Congenital elbow luxation
- Uncommon; accounts for 15% of non-traumatic elbow lameness
- Severe disability in this breed (type I)
- Present at birth or in the first 3 months of life

Angular deformity of the tibia
- Uncommon
- Caused by injury to the distal tibial growth plate

DOGS

Calcaneoquartal subluxation due to plantar tarsal ligament rupture
- Common hock injury
- Affects athletic dogs during exercise

Hip dysplasia
- Eighteenth worst mean-scoring breed in the BVA/KC Hip Dysplasia Scheme as of October 2001
- Breed mean score 16
- Breed mean score improving

Superficial digital flexor tendon luxation
- Uncommon
- Usually lateral luxation

Neoplastic conditions
Canine cutaneous histiocytoma
- Possible breed predisposition
- More common in young dogs 1–2 years of age

Basal cell tumour
- Reported to be at increased risk

Liposarcoma
- Average age of onset: 10 years
- Males may be predisposed

Nasal cavity tumours
- Reported to be at increased risk
- Average age reported as 10.5–11 years
- Dogs in urban areas may be at increased risk

Testicular neoplasia
- Believed to be a breed at increased risk

Neurological conditions
Congenital deafness
- Signs seen from birth

Ocular conditions
Micropalpebral fissure
- Breed predisposition

Entropion (usually lower lids, may be associated with micropalpebral fissure)
- Breed predisposition; polygenic inheritance likely

Distichiasis
- Breed predisposition; mode of inheritance not defined

Nodular episclerokeratitis
- Seen occasionally in this breed
- Usually presents at 2–5 years

Congenital, sub-epithelial, geographic corneal dystrophy
- Congenital condition; predisposed breed
- Occurs in young puppies (<10 weeks); transient condition

Corneal (epithelial) dystrophy
- Inheritance suspected
- Superficial crystalline deposit
- Age of onset: 2–4 years

Persistent pupillary membranes
- Inheritance suspected

Uveodermatological syndrome
- Also known as Vogt-Koyanagi-Harada-like syndrome
- Breed predisposition
- Young adults (1.5–4 years)

Cataract
- Inheritance suspected
- Localisation: anterior and posterior cortex

Collie eye anomaly
- Congenital disorder originally thought to be inherited as a simple autosomal recessive trait; more recently polygenic inheritance has been suggested
- Higher incidence in this breed reported in the UK and parts of Europe than in the USA. In general, the condition is less severe than in Collies, with retinal detachment and haemorrhage uncommon
- Schedule 1 of the BVA/KC/ISDS Eye Scheme

Central progressive retinal atrophy (CPRA) or retinal pigment epithelial dystrophy (RPED)
- Breed predisposition; inheritance suspected

- More prevalent in the UK than in the USA; becoming less prevalent following the introduction of control schemes
- Age of clinical onset: 2–3 years
- Schedule 1 of the BVA/KC/ISDS Eye Scheme

Generalised progressive retinal atrophy (GPRA)

- Simple autosomal recessive inheritance suspected
- Clinically apparent at 5 years

Micropapilla

- Congenital condition

Optic nerve hypoplasia

- Congenital condition; not known if inherited

Optic nerve colobomas

- Congenital defect; not known if inherited
- Seen occasionally in this breed; unclear if this is a separate condition or a manifestation of Collie eye anomaly

Multiple ocular defects

- Congenital condition, seen in homozygous merles (the result of merle to merle breeding) with predominantly white coats
- Defects may include microphthalmia, microcornea, cataract, equatorial staphylomas and retinal defects. These dogs may also be deaf

Physiological conditions
Schirmer tear test

- This breed has a lower average Schirmer tear test than others
- Average was 15.8 +/− 1.8

Reproductive conditions
Cryptorchidism

- Developmental defect believed to be inherited as a sex-limited, autosomal recessive trait
- Believed to be a breed at increased risk

Testicular neoplasia

- Believed to be a breed at increased risk

Azoospermia with spermatogenic arrest

- Reported in this breed

SHIH TZU

Cardiovascular conditions
Ventricular septal defect

- Congenital
- Uncommon
- Relative risk 3.3

Endocardiosis

- Also known as chronic valvular disease
- Relative risk 3.0
- Increased prevalence with age
- Aetiology unknown but genetic basis likely

Dermatological conditions
Atopy

- Females probably predisposed
- Age of onset: from 6 months to 7 years
- May or may not be seasonal

Follicular cyst

- No age or sex predisposition

Skin tumours

- See under Neoplastic conditions

Drug reactions
Glucocorticoids

- Subcutaneous injections in this breed may cause local areas of alopecia

Gastrointestinal conditions
Cleft palate

- Congenital disorder with inheritance suspected in this breed

Pyloric stenosis (antral pyloric hypertrophy syndrome)

- Breed predisposition to adult-onset pyloric hypertrophy syndrome
- Males may be predisposed

Neoplastic conditions
Sebaceous gland tumours

- Possible breed predisposition to sebaceous epithelioma
- Seen in older dogs (average age 10 years)

DOGS

Perianal (hepatoid) gland adenomas
- Breed predisposition suggested in one survey of 2700 cases
- Average age was 10.5 years
- Entire males were predisposed

Neurological conditions
Intervertebral disc disease
- Breed predisposition
- Relatively common condition
- Age of clinical onset: 3–7 years

Ocular conditions
Entropion (usually medial lower lids)
- Breed predisposition; polygenic inheritance likely

Distichiasis
- Breed predisposition

Caruncular trichiasis
- Breed predisposition

Proptosis
- Occurs more easily in this breed, usually following trauma

Pigmentary keratitis
- Breed predisposition

Refractory corneal ulceration
- Breed predisposition

Keratoconjunctivitis sicca
- Breed predisposition

Vitreal syneresis
- Breed predisposition
- Age of onset: 2–4 years
- May be seen with retinal detachment and glaucoma

Micropapilla
- Congenital condition

Optic nerve hypoplasia
- Congenital condition; familial in this breed

Physiological conditions
Achondroplasia
- Genetic dwarfism
- Skull and limbs affected
- Accepted as a breed standard

Renal and urinary conditions
Familial renal disease (renal dysplasia)
- Mode of inheritance unknown
- Cases present with chronic renal failure at a few months to 5 years of age

Renal glucosuria
- May be seen with familial renal disease

Urate urolithiasis (see plate 13)
- Higher incidence has been noted in this breed in some surveys
- Average age at diagnosis is 3–6 years
- Males may be predisposed

Calcium oxalate urolithiasis
- Higher incidence has been noted in this breed in some surveys
- Average age at diagnosis is 5–12 years
- Males may be predisposed

Struvite (magnesium ammonium phosphate) urolithiasis
- Higher incidence has been noted in this breed in some surveys
- Average age at diagnosis is 2–8 years
- Females seem to be predisposed

Calcium phosphate urolithiasis (hydroxyapatite and carbonate apatite)
- Higher incidence has been noted in this breed in some surveys
- Average age at diagnosis is 7–11 years

Calcium phosphate urolithiasis (brushite)
- Higher incidence has been noted in this breed in some surveys
- Average age at diagnosis is 7–11 years
- Males may be predisposed

Silica urolithiasis
- Higher incidence has been noted in this breed in some surveys
- Males may be predisposed

Respiratory conditions
Tracheal collapse
- Aetiology unknown
- Usually affects middle-aged to old dogs

SIBERIAN HUSKY

Cardiovascular conditions
Essential hypertension
- Middle-aged to older dogs affected
- Males may be predisposed
- Hereditary essential hypertension has been reported in a line of Siberian Huskies

Dermatological conditions
Discoid lupus erythematosus
- No age or sex predisposition
- Accounted for 0.3% of skin diseases at one referral institution

Canine uveodermatological syndrome
- Also known as Vogt-Koyanagi-Harada-like syndrome
- See also under Ocular conditions

Follicular dysplasia
- May affect multiple dogs in a litter
- Clipped areas tend not to regrow

Post-clipping alopecia
- Relatively uncommon

Nasal depigmentation
- Also known as Dudley nose
- Cause unknown

Mucocutaneous hypopigmentation
- Nasal form common in this breed

Zinc-responsive dermatosis
- In this breed, skin lesions develop despite adequate levels of zinc in the diet

Canine eosinophilic granuloma
- Rare
- Idiopathic
- Young males predisposed
- Siberian Huskies account for 76% of cases

Onychodystrophy

Skin tumours
- See under Neoplastic conditions

Endocrine conditions
Congenital nephrogenic diabetes insipidus (NDI)
- One report of familial NDI in a litter of Husky puppies

Gastrointestinal conditions
Oral eosinophilic granuloma
- Breed predisposition
- Seen in young dogs

Neoplastic conditions
Basal cell tumour
- Reported to be at increased risk

Sebaceous gland tumours
- Possible breed predisposition to sebaceous epithelioma
- Seen in older dogs (average age 10 years)

Haemangiopericytoma
- Occurs at a mean age of 7–10 years

Perianal (hepatoid) gland adenomas
- Breed predisposition suggested in one survey of 2700 cases
- Average age was 10.5 years
- Entire males were predisposed

Testicular neoplasia
- Believed to be a breed at increased risk

Neurological conditions
True epilepsy
- Inheritance suspected
- Age of onset: 6 months to 3 years

Degenerative myelopathy
- Reported in this breed
- Adults affected

Ocular conditions
Entropion (usually lower lids)
- Breed predisposition; polygenic inheritance likely

DOGS

Chronic superficial keratitis (pannus)
- Breed predisposition
- Age of onset: 1–3 years

Corneal dystrophy
- Recessive inheritance with variable expression has been suggested
- Lipid stromal dystrophy
- Age of onset: 5 months to 8 years

Primary glaucoma/goniodysgenesis
- Inheritance suspected
- Age of onset: 1–2 years
- Schedule 1 of the BVA/KC/ISDS Eye Scheme

Persistent pupillary membranes
- Inheritance suspected
- Schedule 3 of the BVA/KC/ISDS Eye Scheme

Uveodermatological syndrome
- Also known as Vogt-Koyanagi-Harada-like syndrome
- Breed predisposition
- Young adults (1.5–4 years)

Cataract
- Autosomal recessive inheritance suspected
- Localisation: posterior sutures
- Age of onset: 6–18 months
- Schedule 1 of the BVA/KC/ISDS Eye Scheme

Generalised progressive retinal atrophy (GPRA)
- Autosomal recessive inheritance, possibly X-linked
- Clinically evident by 2–4 years
- Males more frequently affected

Optic nerve colobomas
- Congenital defect; not known if inherited

Microphthalmia
- Inheritance suspected
- Often associated with other ocular abnormalities, e.g. microcornea, cataract and retinal detachment

Physiological conditions
Hereditary cardiac hypertrophy
- May be an adaptation favouring endurance

Increased platelet aggregation
- May be an adaptation favouring endurance

Renal and urinary conditions
Ectopic ureters
- Congenital anomaly; higher incidence reported in this breed
- Usually presents <1 year of age
- More commonly diagnosed in females

Reproductive conditions
Testicular neoplasia
- Believed to be a breed at increased risk

Respiratory conditions
Laryngeal paralysis
- Idiopathic

SILKY TERRIER

Dermatological conditions
Malassezia dermatitis
- Affects adult dogs of any age or sex
- Often seasonal

Rabies-vaccine-associated vasculitis and alopecia
- Lesions appear at site of vaccine, 3–6 months after administration

Short hair syndrome of Silky breeds
- Usual onset: 1–5 years
- Unknown cause

Colour-dilution alopecia
- Coat-colour genes involved in the pathogenesis

Melanotrichia
- Often follows healing of deep inflammation

Drug reactions
Glucocorticoids
- Subcutaneous injections in this breed may cause local areas of alopecia

Neurological conditions
Lysosomal storage disease –
glucocerbrosidosis (Gaucher's disease)
- Inheritance suspected
- Rare
- Signs seen at 6–8 months

Spongiform degeneration
- Reported in this breed
- Age of clinical onset: 3 months

Ocular conditions
Refractory corneal ulceration
- Breed predisposition
- Usually middle-aged

Cataract
- Inheritance suspected
- Posterior polar subcapsular cataracts occur in 4–5 year olds and are slowly progressive leading to visual deficiencies at 7–11 years (possibly more rapidly progressive in Australia)
- Peripheral cortical cataracts occur in 4–5 year olds and are slowly progressive

Generalised progressive retinal atrophy (GPRA)
- Simple autosomal recessive inheritance suspected
- Clinically evident at 5–11 years of age
- Often associated with extensive cataract formation

Renal and urinary conditions
Cystine urolithiasis
- Cystinuria results from an inherited defect in renal tubular transport of cystine and predisposes to cystine urolithiasis
- Higher incidence reported in this breed in some American surveys
- Average age at diagnosis is 1–8 years
- Males seem predisposed

SKYE TERRIER

Gastrointestinal diseases
Chronic hepatitis
- Breed predisposition
- Chronic hepatitis may be seen with copper accumulation in this breed. Where it occurs, copper accumulation is perivenular and believed to be the result of intrahepatic canalicular cholestasis

Musculoskeletal conditions
Foramen magnum dysplasia
- Congenital

Ocular conditions
Glaucoma
- Possible breed predisposition

Lens luxation
- Possible breed predisposition

Physiological conditions
Hypochondroplasia
- Accepted as breed standard
- Short bowed legs but normal skulls seen

Renal and urinary conditions
Ectopic ureters
- Congenital anomaly; higher incidence reported in this breed
- Usually presents <1 year of age
- More commonly diagnosed in females

SOFT-COATED WHEATEN TERRIER

Dermatological conditions
Ehler-Danlos syndrome
- Also known as cutaneous asthenia
- Inherited group of diseases
- May be inherited as an autosomal dominant trait
- Probably lethal in homozygotes

Food hypersensitivity
- No age or sex predisposition reported

Gastrointestinal conditions
Lymphangiectasia and protein-losing enteropathy
- Possible breed predisposition
- May be accompanied by a protein-losing nephropathy in this breed

Ocular conditions
Cataract
- Inheritance suspected

DOGS

Persistence of the hyaloid apparatus
- Congenital condition; inheritance suspected
- May be associated with posterior capsular cataract

Micropapilla
- Congenital condition
- Seen commonly in this breed

Renal and urinary conditions
Familial renal disease (renal dysplasia)
- Mode of inheritance, if any, unknown
- Cases typically present with renal failure from 5–30 months
- Some cases may present with protein-losing nephropathy without uraemia due to membranoproliferative glomerulonephritis. These dogs range from 2–11 years

SPRINGER SPANIEL

Cardiovascular conditions
Patent ductus arteriosus
- Common congenital abnormality
- Relative risk 4.0
- Females predisposed
- Mode of inheritance is polygenic

Ventricular septal defect
- Marked risk in this breed (relative risk 5.0)
- No sex predilection
- Familial in this breed; inheritance suspected

Persistent atrial standstill
- Rare condition
- May be associated with scapulohumeral muscle wasting

Dermatological conditions
Acral mutilation syndrome
- Probably inherited as an autosomal recessive trait
- No sex predisposition
- Age of onset: 3–5 months

Malassezia dermatitis
- Affects adults of any age or sex
- May be seasonal

Grass awn migration
- Common in the summer months

Food hypersensitivity
- No age or sex predisposition reported

Primary seborrhoea
- Probably inherited as an autosomal recessive trait
- Signs first appear at an early age and get worse with age

Ichthyosis
- Rare
- Congenital
- Possibly inherited as an autosomal recessive trait

Psoriasiform-lichenoid dermatosis in English Springer Spaniels
- Rare
- Only affects English Springers
- Probably genetically determined

Ehler-Danlos syndrome
- Also known as cutaneous asthenia
- Inherited group of diseases
- May be inherited as an autosomal dominant trait
- Probably lethal in homozygotes

Intertrigo
- Lip fold pyoderma occurs in Spaniels

Idiopathic onychomadesis

Anal sac disease
- No sex or age predisposition noted

Skin tumours
- See under Neoplastic conditions

Gastrointestinal conditions
Secondary megaoesophagus
(English Springer Spaniels)
- Familial polymyopathy may predispose to megaoesophagus

Haematological/immunological conditions
Immune-mediated haemolytic anaemia
- Common disease
- Usually affects young adult and middle-aged animals
- May be more common in bitches
- May be seasonal variations

Factor XI deficiency
- Autosomal inheritance, with homozygotes symptomatic

Phosphofructokinase deficiency
- Inherited as an autosomal recessive trait
- DNA test available

Musculoskeletal conditions
Congenital myasthenia gravis
- See under Neurological conditions

Hip dysplasia
- Welsh Springers have the twelfth worst breed mean score in the BVA/KC Hip Dysplasia Scheme as of October 2001, with a breed average score of 19
- English Springers have a better mean score of 14

Neoplastic conditions
Trichoepithelioma (English Springer Spaniels)
- Possible breed predisposition
- Average age reported as 9 years
- This breed may be predisposed to multiple trichoepitheliomas

Canine cutaneous histiocytoma
- Possible breed predisposition
- More common in young dogs 1–2 years old

Haemangiopericytoma
- Occurs at a mean age of 7–10 years

Melanoma
- Breed predisposition
- Average age 8–9 years

Cutaneous haemangioma (English Springer Spaniels)
- Possible breed predisposition
- Average age was 8.7 years in one study

Anal sac adenocarcinoma (English Springer Spaniels)
- Breed predisposition suggested in one survey of 232 cases
- Average age was 10.5 years
- Some surveys suggest a predisposition for females

Neurological conditions
Hypomyelination of the central nervous system
- X-linked recessive inheritance suggested
- Signs seen at 2–4 weeks
- Males affected

Congenital myasthenia gravis
- Rare
- Autosomal recessive inheritance suspected
- Age of clinical onset: 6–8 weeks

Lysosomal storage disease – fucosidosis (English Springer Spaniels)
- Autosomal recessive inheritance
- Seen in Australia, New Zealand, the UK, North America
- Signs seen at 1–3 years

Lysosomal storage disease – GM_1 gangliosidosis (English Springer Spaniels)
- Autosomal recessive inheritance
- Rare
- Signs seen at 3–6 months

Springer Spaniel rage syndrome
- Seen in young to middle-aged dogs

Ocular conditions
Entropion (usually lower lids) (English Springer Spaniels)
- Breed predisposition, polygenic inheritance likely

Combined entropion-ectropion ('diamond eye') (English Springer Spaniels)
- Breed predisposition; polygenic inheritance likely

Distichiasis (Welsh Springer Spaniels)
- Breed predisposition

Plasma cell infiltration of the nictitating membrane (plasmoma) (English Springer Spaniels)
- Breed predisposition
- May be associated with pannus

Keratoconjunctivitis sicca (English Springer Spaniels)
- Breed predisposition

DOGS

DOGS

Chronic superficial keratitis (pannus)
(English Springer Spaniels)
- Breed predisposition
- Age of onset: 1–3 years

Refractory corneal ulceration
(English Springer Spaniels)
- Breed predisposition
- Usually middle-aged

Congenital, sub-epithelial, geographic
corneal dystrophy (English Springer
Spaniels)
- Congenital condition; predisposed breed
- Occurs in young puppies (<10 weeks); transient condition

Corneal dystrophy
- Breed predisposition
- Endothelial dystrophy with progressive corneal oedema

Primary glaucoma/goniodysgenesis
(English Springer Spaniels)
- Inheritance suspected
- Schedule 3 of the BVA/KC/ISDS Eye Scheme

Primary glaucoma/goniodysgenesis (Welsh
Springer Spaniels)
- Autosomal dominant inheritance has been suggested
- Age of onset: 10 weeks to 10 years; females seem predisposed
- Schedule 1 of the BVA/KC/ISDS Eye Scheme

Cataract (English Springer Spaniels)
- Inheritance suspected
- Posterior polar subcapsular cataracts occur at 1–3 years
- Nuclear cataracts occur at 5 years and older

Cataract (Welsh Springer Spaniels)
- Autosomal recessive inheritance
- Localisation: posterior cortex
- Age of onset: 8–12 weeks; rapidly progressive to blindness at 1–2 years
- Schedule 1 of the BVA/KC/ISDS Eye Scheme

Multifocal retinal dysplasia (English Springer
Spaniels)
- Congenital condition, inheritance as an autosomal recessive trait suspected
- Schedule 1 of the BVA/KC/ISDS Eye Scheme

Geographic retinal dysplasia (English Springer
Spaniels)
- Congenital condition; inheritance suspected
- Reported in the UK

Total retinal dysplasia (English Springer
Spaniels)
- Congenital condition; inheritance suspected
- Reported in the UK

Generalised progressive retinal atrophy
(GPRA) (English Springer Spaniels)
- Autosomal recessive inheritance
- Clinically apparent within the first 2 years, progressing to blindness at 3–5 years
- A second form is clinically apparent at 7 years and progresses more slowly
- Schedule 1 BVA/KC/ISDS Eye Scheme

Generalised progressive retinal atrophy
(GPRA) (Welsh Springer Spaniels)
- Autosomal recessive inheritance suspected
- Clinical onset at 5–7 years

Central progressive retinal atrophy (CPRA) or
retinal pigment epithelial dystrophy (RPED)
(English Springer Spaniels)
- Breed predisposition; inheritance suspected
- Schedule 1 of the BVA/KC/ISDS Eye Scheme

Microphthalmia (with multiple ocular defects)
(English Springer Spaniels)
- Recessive inheritance suggested

Renal and urinary conditions
Sphincter mechanism incompetence
- Suggested breed predisposition in female dogs

Calcium phosphate urolithiasis
(hydroxyapatite and carbonate apatite)
- Higher incidence has been noted in this breed in some surveys
- Average age at diagnosis is 7–11 years

Reproductive conditions
Vaginal hyperplasia
- Possible breed predisposition

Azoospermia with spermatogenic arrest (Welsh Springer Spaniels)
- Reported in this breed

Respiratory conditions
Primary ciliary dyskinesia
- Inherited defect
- Usually signs seen within first few weeks of life

STAFFORDSHIRE BULL TERRIER

Dermatological conditions
Canine follicular dysplasia
- A marked predilection in this breed implies a genetic basis for this group of diseases
- Hair loss begins at 2–4 years of age and occurs mainly on the flank

Skin tumours
- See under Neoplastic conditions

Endocrine conditions
Hyperadrenocorticism: pituitary-dependent (PDH)
- Possible breed predisposition
- Middle-aged / older
- 55–60% female

Gastrointestinal conditions
Gastric neoplasia
- Higher risk for this breed noted in one study
- Male dogs more commonly affected
- Age of occurrence: 8–10 years

Musculoskeletal conditions
Myotonia
- Condition described in this breed in the USA
- First seen in young puppies
- Familial, mode of inheritance not known

Sub-patellar pain
- Uncommon
- May or may not be associated with patellar luxation

Neoplastic conditions
Mast cell tumours
- Possible breed predisposition
- May be seen at any age (from 4 months onwards), but usually seen in older animals

Pituitary tumour resulting in hyperadrenocorticism
- See under Endocrine conditions

Ocular conditions
Cataract
- Autosomal recessive inheritance
- Localisation: nucleus and sutures
- Age of onset: < 1 year; progresses to blindness
- Schedule 1 of the BVA/KC/ISDS Eye Scheme

Persistent hyperpalstic tunica vasculosa lentis/persistent hyperplastic primary vitreous (PHTVL/PHPV)
- Developmental disorder
- Inheritance suspected
- Schedule 1 of the BVA/KC/ISDS Eye Scheme (PHPV)

Renal and urinary conditions
Cystine urolithiasis
- Cystinuria results from an inherited defect in renal tubular transport of cystine and predisposes to cystine urolithiasis
- Higher incidence reported in this breed in some surveys
- Average age at diagnosis is 1–8 years
- Males seem to be predisposed

SUSSEX SPANIEL

Musculoskeletal conditions
Mitochondrial myopathy
- Rare
- Primary defect is in mitochondrial function
- Can cause sudden death

Hip dysplasia
- Sixteenth worst mean-scoring breed in the BVA/KC Hip Dysplasia Scheme as of October 2001
- Breed mean score 37

DOGS

Ocular conditions
Distichiasis
- Breed predisposition

Persistent hyaloid artery
- Inheritance suspected

Multifocal retinal dysplasia
- Mode of inheritance not defined
- Schedule 3 of the BVA/KC/ISDS Eye Scheme

SWEDISH LAPLAND

Neurological conditions
Spinal muscular atrophy
- Autosomal recessive inheritance suggested
- Rare
- Age of clinical onset: 5–6 weeks

Glycogenosis (glycogen storage disease type 2)
- Autosomal recessive inheritance suggested
- Rare
- Age of clinical onset: <1 year

TIBETAN MASTIFF

Neurological conditions
Hypertrophic neuropathy
- Inherited as an autosomal recessive trait
- Age of clinical onset: 7–10 weeks

TIBETAN SPANIEL

Ocular conditions
Entropion (usually medial lower lids)
- Breed predisposition; polygenic inheritance likely

Cataract
- Inheritance suspected

Generalised progressive retinal atrophy (GPRA)
- Mode of inheritance unknown, but presumed to be recessive
- Ophthalmoscopic signs seen from 3–5 years
- Schedule 1 BVA/KC/ISDS Eye Scheme

Micropapilla
- Congenital condition

Optic nerve colobomas
- Congenital defect; not known if inherited

Multiple ocular defects with microphthalmia
- Congenital condition; inheritance suspected

TIBETAN TERRIER

Endocrine conditions
Diabetes mellitus
- Possible breed predisposition
- Usual age range: 4–14 years; peak incidence: 7–9 years
- Old entire females are predisposed

Neurological conditions
Lysosomal storage disease – ceroid lipofuscinosis
- Autosomal recessive inheritance
- Rare
- Signs seen at 1–2 years

Congenital vestibular disease
- Signs seen <3 months

Ocular conditions
Glaucoma
- Possible breed predisposition

Primary lens luxation
- Simple autosomal recessive inheritance suggested
- Age of onset: 3–6 years
- Often followed by glaucoma
- Schedule 1 of the BVA/KC/ISDS Eye Scheme

Cataract
- Inheritance suspected
- Posterior cortical cataracts are seen <1 year and progress to cause visual deficiencies at 4–5 years
- Schedule 3 of the BVA/KC/ISDS Eye Scheme

Multifocal retinal dysplasia
- Congenital condition; autosomal recessive inheritance suggested

Generalised progressive retinal atrophy (GPRA)

- Autosomal recessive inheritance suspected
- Night blindness is present at 1 year, complete blindness as early as 2 years; secondary cataracts occur
- A second type of PRA may exist with night blindness at 2 months but no ophthalmoscopic changes until 3–4 years of age
- Schedule 1 BVA/KC/ISDS Eye Scheme

Neuronal ceroid lipofuscinosis

- Inheritance suspected

WEIMARANER

Cardiovascular conditions

Tricuspid dysplasia

- Congenital
- Males predisposed

Peritoneopericardial diaphragmatic hernia

- Accounts for 0.5% of congenital heart disease but may be under-reported

Dermatological conditions

Muzzle folliculitis/furunculosis

- Also known as canine acne
- Local trauma, hormones and genetics may play a role in the pathogenesis

Pododermatitis

- Can affect any age or sex
- Males predisposed
- Front feet more commonly affected

Blastomycosis

- See under Infectious conditions

Histoplasmosis

- See under Infectious conditions

Generalised demodicosis

- Weimaraners are in the ten breeds at highest statistical risk of this disease in the Cornell, USA population

Idiopathic sterile granuloma and pyogranuloma

- Uncommon
- No age or sex predisposition

Skin tumours

- See under Neoplastic conditions

Gastrointestinal conditions

Oropharyngeal neoplasia

- Possible breed predisposition

Gastric dilatation-volvulus

- Possible breed predisposition

Haematological/immunological conditions

Neutrophil function defect of Weimaraners

- Primary defect in neutrophil function
- Males predisposed
- Reduced concentration of IgG, which may be primary or secondary
- Leads to recurrent infection with left shift neutrophilia

T-cell dysfunction

- Described in a colony of Weimaraners in 1980
- Causes a wasting syndrome and increased susceptibility to infection

Vaccine-associated vasculitis with hypertrophic osteodystrophy

- Gastrointestinal signs also seen

Infectious conditions

Blastomycosis

- Increased incidence in this breed possibly due to an increased likelihood of exposure
- Seen mainly in young male dogs living near water
- Geographic distribution: around the Mississippi, Ohio, Missouri, Tennessee and St Lawrence Rivers, the southern Great Lakes and the southern mid-Atlantic states; Not reported in the UK

Histoplasmosis

- Uncommon
- Mainly restricted to the central United States
- Usually affects dogs less than 4 years old

Infectious skin disease

- See under Dermatological conditions

DOGS

Musculoskeletal conditions
Vaccine-associated vasculitis with hypertrophic dystrophy
- Gastrointestinal signs also seen

Polyarthritis/meningitis
- Idiopathic
- This breed prone to a more severe form of the disease

Umbilical hernia

Neoplastic conditions
Mast cell tumours
- Possible breed predisposition
- May be seen at any age (from 4 months onwards), but usually seen in older animals

Lipoma
- Possible breed predisposition
- Most common in middle-aged, obese female dogs

Neurological conditions
Hypomyelination of the central nervous system
- Reported in this breed
- Signs seen at 2–8 weeks

Meningitis and polyarteritis
- Reported in this breed
- Age of onset: <1 year

Spinal dysraphism
- Congenital; inherited
- Seen most commonly in this breed
- Signs seen at 3–4 weeks

Ocular conditions
Entropion
- Breed predisposition; polygenic inheritance likely

Distichiasis
- Breed predisposition

Eversion of the cartilage of the nictitating membrane
- Breed predisposition; possibly inherited as a recessive trait
- Usually occurs in young dogs

Conjunctival melanoma
- Possible breed predisposition

Medial canthal pocket syndrome
- Breed predisposition resulting from head shape

Refractory corneal ulceration
- Breed predisposition
- Age of onset: 4–8 years

Corneal dystrophy
- Breed predisposition
- Subepithelial, paracentral, lipid dystrophy
- Age of onset: 1–8 years

Renal and urinary conditions
Sphincter mechanism incompetence
- Possible breed predisposition in female dogs

Reproductive conditions
Vaginal hyperplasia
- Possible breed predisposition

XX sex reversal
- Congenital condition reported in this breed

WELSH CORGI

Dermatological conditions
Ehler-Danlos syndrome
- Also known as cutaneous asthenia
- Inherited group of diseases
- May be inherited as an autosomal dominant trait
- Probably lethal in homozygotes

Haematological/immunological conditions
Severe combined immunodeficiency
- Inherited as an X-linked recessive trait
- Thymic hypoplasia and lymphopaenia seen

Von Willebrand's disease (Pembroke Welsh Corgis)
- Possibly inherited as an autosomal recessive trait
- Mainly type I disease seen in this breed

Ocular conditions
Refractory corneal ulceration (Pembroke and Cardigan Welsh Corgis)
- Breed predisposition
- Usually middle-aged

Corneal dystrophy (Pembroke Welsh Corgis)
- Not known if inherited
- Bilateral corneal vascularisation and pigmentation in young dogs

Lens luxation (Pembroke and Cardigan Welsh Corgis)
- Inheritance suspected
- Reported mainly in the UK

Persistent pupillary membranes (Pembroke and Cardigan Welsh Corgis)
- Familial condition; recessive inheritance has been suggested
- Severity varies

Cataract (Pembroke Welsh Corgis)
- Inheritance suspected
- Congenital cataracts have been reported
- Posterior cortical cataracts are seen at 1 year and are slowly progressive

Multifocal retinal dysplasia (Pembroke and Cardigan Welsh Corgis)
- Autosomal recessive inheritance suggested
- A second severe form exists, with abnormality (liquefaction) of the vitreous

Generalised progressive retinal atrophy (GPRA) (Pembroke and Cardigan Welsh Corgis)
- Mode of inheritance unknown, but presumed to be recessive
- Rod-cone dysplasia type 3 (Cardigan Welsh Corgis)
- May be clinically apparent as early as 3 months of age in Cardigan Welsh Corgis
- Schedule 1 of the BVA/KC/ISDS Eye Scheme (Cardigan Welsh Corgis only)

Central progressive retinal atrophy (CPRA) or retinal pigment epithelial dystrophy (RPED) (Cardigan Welsh Corgis)
- Breed predisposition; inheritance suspected
- Reported mainly in the UK

- Schedule 1 of the BVA/KC/ISDS Eye Scheme

Physiological conditions
Hypochondroplasia
- Accepted as breed standard
- Short, bowed legs but normal skulls seen

Renal and urinary conditions
Renal telangiectasia (Pembroke Welsh Corgis)
- Possible breed predisposition
- Affected dogs are 5–13 years of age
- Anomalous development of the blood vessels leads to marked haematuria

Ectopic ureters
- Congenital anomaly; higher incidence reported in this breed
- Usually presents <1 year of age

Cystine urolithiasis
- Cystinuria results from an inherited defect in renal tubular transport of cystine and predisposes to cystine urolithiasis
- Higher incidence reported in this breed in some surveys
- Average age at diagnosis is 1–8 years
- Males seem to be predisposed

WELSH TERRIER

Ocular conditions
Primary glaucoma/goniodysgenesis
- Inheritance suspected
- Age of onset: 5–6 years
- Schedule 3 of the BVA/KC/ISDS Eye Scheme

Lens luxation
- Breed predisposition
- Age of onset: 5–6 years

WEST HIGHLAND WHITE TERRIER

Cardiovascular conditions
Ventricular septal defect
- Congenital
- Uncommon
- Relative risk 13.4

DOGS

DOGS

Tetralogy of Fallot
- Congenital
- Rare
- Relative risk 14.1

Pulmonic stenosis
- Third most frequent cause of canine congenital heart disease
- May be polygenic mode of inheritance
- Relative risk 4.2

Dermatological conditions
Malassezia dermatitis
- Affects adult dogs of any age or sex
- Often seasonal

Generalised demodicosis
- West Highland Whites are in the ten breeds at highest statistical risk of this disease in the Cornell, USA population

Atopy
- Females probably predisposed
- Age of onset: from 6 months to 7 years
- May or may not be seasonal

Food hypersensitivity
- No age or sex predisposition reported

Primary seborrhoea
- Probably inherited as an autosomal recessive trait
- Signs first appear at early age and get worse with age

Ichthyosis
- Rare
- Congenital
- Possibly inherited as an autosomal recessive trait

Epidermal dysplasia in West Highland White Terriers
- Also known as Armadillo Westie syndrome
- Uncommon
- Familial
- Probably inherited as an autosomal recessive trait
- Usually affects dogs aged 6–12 months

Skin tumours
- See under Neoplastic conditions

Gastrointestinal conditions
Chronic hepatitis
- Breed predisposition in the USA
- Seen in young to middle-aged dogs
- Chronic hepatitis may be seen with or without copper accumulation. Copper levels do not appear to increase with age as seen in the Bedlington. The relationship between copper accumulation and chronic hepatitis is not clear in this breed

Haematological conditions
Pyruvate kinase deficiency
- Affected dogs have abnormal red blood cells with a lifespan of about 20 days
- DNA test available in this breed

Musculoskeletal conditions
Aseptic necrosis of the femoral head
- Also known as Legg-Calve-Perthe's disease
- Mean age of onset: 7 months
- Aetiology unknown

Craniomandibular osteopathy (see figure 15)
- Inherited as an autosomal recessive trait in this breed
- Usually affects dogs aged 3–8 months

Pyruvate kinase deficiency
- Causes intramedullary osteosclerosis
- Inherited disease

Inguinal hernia

Neoplastic conditions
Canine cutaneous histiocytoma
- Possible breed predisposition
- More common in young dogs 1–2 years of age

Neurological conditions
Congenital deafness
- Signs seen from birth

Lysosomal storage disease – globoid cell Leukodystrophy (Krabbe's disease)
- Autosomal recessive inheritance
- Rare
- Signs seen at 3–6 months

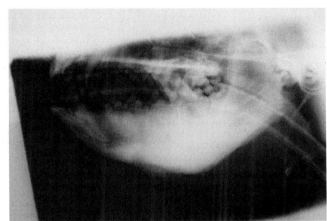

DOGS

Figure 15
Lateral skull radiograph of an eighteen-month-old neutered male West Highland White Terrier with craniomandibular osteopathy. There is extensive new bone formation along the ventral aspect of the mandible.

Shaker dog disease
- Breed predisposition
- Age of clinical onset: 9 months to 2 years

Hemivertebrae
- Congenital
- Occasionally seen

Ocular conditions
Keratoconjunctivitis sicca
- Breed predisposition; high incidence in this breed
- Age of onset: 4–7 years
- Females predisposed (70%)

Refractory corneal ulceration
- Breed predisposition
- Usually middle-aged

Persistent pupillary membranes
- Congenital defect; inheritance not defined in this breed
- Schedule 3 of the BVA/KC/ISDS Eye Scheme

Lens luxation
- Autosomal dominant inheritance suggested
- Age of onset: 3–4 years, later in the USA
- Often followed by glaucoma

Congenital cataract
- Inheritance suspected

- Localisation: posterior sutures
- Schedule 3 of the BVA/KC/ISDS Eye Scheme

Multiple ocular defects
- Autosomal recessive inheritance has been suggested
- Defects may include congenital cataract, retinal dysplasia, persistent pupillary membranes and microphthalmia
- Schedule 3 of the BVA/KC/ISDS Eye Scheme

Physiological conditions
Gestation
- Mean gestation reported as 62.8 days

Renal and urinary conditions
Polycystic kidney disease
- Autosomal recessive inheritance suspected
- Reported in young (5 week-old) dogs

Ectopic ureters
- Congenital anomaly; higher incidence reported in this breed
- Usually presents <1 year of age
- More commonly diagnosed in females

Respiratory conditions
Pulmonary interstitial fibrosis
- Aetiology unknown
- Affects older dogs

DOGS

WHIPPET

Dermatological conditions
Pinnal alopecia
- Age of onset: usually >1 year

Congenital hypotrichosis
- Present at birth or develops in the first month of life
- Predisposition for males

Pattern baldness
- Affects almost exclusively females
- Ventral neck and ventrum affected

Colour-dilution alopecia
- Coat-colour genes involved in the pathogenesis

Canine solar dermatitis
- Sunnier climates predispose

Idiopathic onychomadesis

Skin tumours
- See under Neoplastic conditions

Drug reactions
Thiopentone
- This breed has a greatly increased susceptibility to thiopentone
- Use of this drug is not recommended in this breed

Musculoskeletal conditions
Accessory carpal bone fracture
- Sprain/avulsion-type fractures due to carpal hyperextension during exercise

Neoplastic conditions
Cutaneous haemangioma
- Reported breed predisposition
- Average age was 8.7 years in one study

Ocular conditions
Corneal dystrophy
- Breed predisposition
- Stromal lipid dystrophy
- Age of onset: 3–5 years

Cataract
- Inheritance suspected
- Several types

Lens luxation
- Possible breed predisposition
- Age of onset: 8 years

Vitreal syneresis
- Breed predisposition
- Age of onset: 6 years

Generalised progressive retinal atrophy
- Mode of inheritance not known but presumed recessive
- Clinical onset at 5 years

Micropapilla
- Congenital condition, familial in this breed

YORKSHIRE TERRIER

Cardiovascular conditions
Patent ductus arteriosus
- Common congenital abnormality
- Relative risk 4.2
- Mode of inheritance is polygenic

Endocardiosis
- Also known as chronic valvular disease
- Relative risk 2.6
- Increased prevalence with age
- Aetiology unknown but genetic basis likely

Dermatological conditions
Rabies-vaccine-associated vasculitis and alopecia
- Lesions appear at site of vaccine 3–6 months after administration

Short-hair syndrome of Silky breeds
- Usual onset: 1–5 years
- Cause unknown

Cyclic follicular dysplasia
- Seems to be a particular problem in Alaska, suggesting duration of daylight exposure may be a factor

Ichthyosis
- Rare
- Congenital
- Possibly inherited as an autosomal recessive trait

Congenital hypotrichosis
- Present at birth or develops in first month of life
- Predisposition for males suggests sex linkage

Colour-dilution alopecia
- Coat-colour genes involved in the pathogenesis

Melanotrichia
- Often follows healing of deep inflammation

Melanoderma and alopecia in Yorkshire Terriers
- Probably genetic
- Usually affects dogs aged 6 months to 3 years

Skin tumours
- See under Neoplastic conditions

Drug reactions
Glucocorticoids
- Subcutaneous injections in this breed may cause local areas of alopecia

Endocrine conditions
Hyperadrenocorticism: pituitary-dependent (PDH)
- Possible breed predisposition
- Middle-aged / older
- 55–60% female

Gastrointestinal conditions
Lymphangiectasia and protein-losing enteropathy
- Possible breed predisposition

Hepatic lipidosis
- Breed predisposition
- Seen in puppies

Congenital portosystemic shunt
- Breed predisposition
- Onset of clinical signs <1 year

Microvascular portal dysplasia
- Breed predisposition

Musculoskeletal conditions
Aseptic necrosis of the femoral head
- Also known as Legg-Calve-Perthe's disease
- Mean age of onset: 7 months
- Aetiology unknown

Cartilaginous exostosis

Congenital elbow luxation
- Type I and type II luxation seen in this breed
- Type I (90° rotation of proximal ulna) causes severe disability in this breed from birth or in first 3 months of life
- Type II (proximal radius displaced caudolaterally) usually presents at 4–5 months of age

Medial patellar luxation
- Significant hereditary component suspected

Odontoid process dysplasia
- Congenital

Delayed/non-union of fractures of the distal third of the radius and ulna in miniature and toy breeds
- May be associated with inadequate immobilisation

Neoplastic conditions
Keratoacanthoma
- Uncommon
- Possibly inherited
- Affects dogs of 5 years or younger

Pituitary tumour resulting in hyperadrenocorticism
- See under Endocrine conditions

Testicular neoplasia
- Believed to be a breed at increased risk

Neurological conditions
Hydrocephalus
- Congenital
- Relatively common
- Onset of signs: usually 4–5 months

DOGS

Atlantoaxial subluxation
- Congenital
- Relatively common in this breed
- Age of clinical onset: <1 year

Hemivertebrae
- Congenital
- Occasionally seen in this breed

Ocular conditions
Distichiasis
- Breed predisposition

Keratoconjunctivitis sicca
- Breed predisposition

Congenital keratoconjunctivitis sicca
(lacrimal gland hypoplasia)
- Affected breed

Congenital, sub-epithelial, geographic
corneal dystrophy
- Congenital condition; predisposed breed
- Occurs in young puppies (<10 weeks); transient condition

Cataract
- Inheritance suspected
- Progressive cortical cataracts; may result in vision loss by 5 years
- Schedule 3 of the BVA/KC/ISDS Eye Scheme

Generalised progressive retinal atrophy
- Autosomal recessive inheritance suggested
- There may be two types: one presenting with night blindness at 4–8 months, the other at 6 years or later
- Schedule 3 of the BVA/KC/ISDS Eye Scheme

Renal and urinary conditions
Urate urolithiasis
- Higher incidence has been noted in this breed in some surveys

- Average age at diagnosis is 3–6 years
- Males may be predisposed

Calcium oxalate urolithiasis
- Higher incidence has been noted in this breed in some surveys
- Average age at diagnosis is 5–12 years
- Males may be predisposed

Struvite (magnesium ammonium phosphate) urolithiasis
- Higher incidence has been noted in this breed in some surveys
- Average age at diagnosis is 2–8 years
- Females seem to be predisposed

Calcium phosphate urolithiasis
(hydroxyapatite and carbonate apatite)
- Higher incidence has been noted in this breed in some surveys
- Average age at diagnosis is 7–11 years

Calcium phosphate urolithiasis (brushite)
- Higher incidence has been noted in this breed in some surveys
- Average age at diagnosis is 7–11 years
- Males may be predisposed

Silica urolithiasis
- Higher incidence has been noted in this breed in some surveys
- Males seem to be predisposed

Reproductive conditions
Cryptorchidism
- Developmental defect believed to be inherited as a sex-limited, autosomal recessive trait
- Believed to be a breed at increased risk

Testicular neoplasia
- Believed to be a breed at increased risk

Respiratory conditions
Tracheal collapse
- Aetiology unknown
- Usually affects middle-aged to old dogs

PART II
CATS

ABYSSINIAN

Cardiovascular conditions
Dilated cardiomyopathy
- Less common than in the past
- Genetic factors may influence susceptibility to disease
- Males predisposed

Dermatological conditions
Shaft disorder of Abyssinian cats
- Uncommon
- Probably inherited

Psychogenic alopecia
- Thought to be a result of anxiety

Blastomycosis
- See under Infectious conditions

Cryptococcosis
- See under Infectious conditions

Drug reactions
Griseofulvin
- Anecdotal reports suggest a predisposition to side effects with this drug in this breed

Endocrine conditions
Congenital hypothyroidism
- One report of congenital hypothyroidism in a family of Abyssinian cats due to a defect in iodine organification
- Autosomal recessive inheritance was suspected

Gastrointestinal conditions
Amyloidosis
- Breed predisposition
- May affect many body systems including the liver and kidneys

Haematological conditions
Increased osmotic fragility of erythrocytes
- Initial presentation in first few years of life
- Mode of inheritance unknown

Pyruvate kinase deficiency
- Inherited as an autosomal recessive trait
- Carriers are asymptomatic
- Causes severe anaemia

Infectious conditions
Blastomycosis
- Very rare
- Seen in areas with sandy soil close to water

163

Cryptococcosis
- Uncommon

Musculoskeletal conditions
Mysasthenia gravis
- See under Neurological conditions

Neurological conditions
Hyperaesthesia syndrome
- Breed predisposition

Myasthenia gravis
- Rare in cats
- Usually adult-onset

Ocular conditions
Progressive retinal atrophy: rod-cone retinal dysplasia
- Autosomal dominant inheritance
- Presents with retinal changes at 8–12 weeks and progresses rapidly

Progressive retinal atrophy: rod-cone retinal degeneration
- Autosomal recessive inheritance
- Clinical onset at 1.5–2 years, progressing to complete degeneration over 2–4 years

Physiological conditions
Blood group
- In the USA, 80% are group A and 20% group B
- Group B Abyssinians are rare in the UK

Renal and urinary conditions
Renal amyloidosis (usually as part of reactive systemic amyloidosis)
- Familial
- Age of clinical onset: <5 years
- In one report of 119 affected Abyssinian cats, 73 were female and 46 male
- Renal amyloid deposits are found principally in the medulla, but there may be variable (usually mild) glomerular involvement. Amyloid deposits may also be found in adrenal and thyroid glands, spleen, stomach, small intestine, heart, liver, pancreas and colon. These deposits often do not contribute to the clinical signs which are principally due to chronic renal failure.

Respiratory conditions
Nasopharyngeal polyps
- Usually diagnosed in young cats
- No sex predisposition

AMERICAN SHORT HAIR

Cardiovascular conditions
Hypertrophic cardiomyopathy
- Common disease
- Middle-aged to older cats predisposed
- Males predisposed
- May be inherited as an autosomal dominant trait in this breed

Physiological conditions
Blood group
- In the USA, 100% of reported types are group A

BALINESE

Dermatological conditions
Feline acromelanism
- Temperature-dependent enzyme involved in pathogenesis

BIRMAN

Dermatological conditions
Congenital hypotrichosis
- Inherited as an autosomal recessive trait in this breed

Tail-tip necrosis
- See under Haematological/immunological conditions

Haematological/immunological conditions
Haemophilia B
- Factor IX deficiency
- Also known as Christmas disease
- Inherited as a sex-linked trait
- Less common than haemophilia A

Tail-tip necrosis
- Thought to be due to neonatal isoerythrolysis

Thymic aplasia
- Signs usually seen at 1–3 months of age

Ocular conditions
Corneal dermoid
- Rare condition; reported in this breed

Corneal sequestration
- Breed predisposition

Congenital cataract
- Reported in this breed

Neurological conditions
Spongiform degeneration
- Reported in this breed
- Age of clinical onset: 7 weeks

Birman cat distal polyneuropathy
- Recessive inheritance suspected
- Age of clinical onset: 8–10 weeks

Physiological conditions
Blood group
- In the USA, 82% are group A and 18% group B
- In the UK, 71% are group A and 29% are group B

Atypical granulation of neutrophils in Birman cats
- Inherited as an autosomal recessive trait
- Common, with 46% of cats studied affected
- Neutrophils have prominent eosinophilic granules
- No clinical abnormalities of neutrophil function defects detected

BRITISH SHORT HAIR

Cardiovascular conditions
Hypertrophic cardiomyopathy
- Common disease
- Middle-aged to older cats predisposed
- Males predisposed
- May be inherited in this breed

Haematological conditions
Haemophilia B
- Factor IX deficiency
- Also known as Christmas disease
- Inherited as a sex-linked trait
- Less common than haemophilia A

Physiological conditions
Blood group
- In the USA and UK, 41% were group A, 59% group B

BURMESE

Cardiovascular conditions
Dilated cardiomyopathy
- Less common than in the past
- Genetic factors may influence susceptibility to disease
- Males predisposed

Endocardial fibroelastosis
- Age of onset: <6 months
- Thought to be inherited in this breed

Dermatological conditions
Generalised demodicosis
- Rare in cats
- Usually less severe in cats than in dogs

Congenital hypotrichosis
- Familial

Feline acromelanism
- Temperature-dependent enzyme involved in pathogenesis

Psychogenic alopecia
- Thought to be a result of anxiety

Musculoskeletal conditions
Hypokalaemic polymyopathy
- Possibly inherited
- Signs occur from 4–12 months of age

Burmese head defect
- Inherited as autosomal recessive
- Cats with shorter faces may be carriers

Neurological conditions
Congenital vestibular disease
- Signs seen <3 months

Congenital deafness
- Signs seen from birth

Hyperaesthesia syndrome
- Breed predisposition

CATS

Meningoencephalocoele
- Autosomal recessive inheritance
- Lethal malformation with a reported high rate of carriers in this breed

Ocular conditions
Corneal and lateral limbal dermoid
- Rare condition; reported in this breed

Prolapse of the gland of the nictitating membrane
- Reported in this breed

Eversion of the cartilage of the nictitating membrane
- Reported in this breed

Corneal sequestration
- Breed predisposition

Physiological conditions
Blood group
- In the USA, 100% reported were group A

Renal and urinary conditions
Calcium oxalate urolithiasis
- Higher incidence reported in this breed

Respiratory conditions
Agenesis of the nares
- Congenital

CORNISH AND DEVON REX

Dermatological conditions
Congenital hypotrichosis
- Familial

Malassezia dermatitis
- No age or sex predisposition

Haematological conditions
Vitamin-K-dependent coagulopathy
- Prevalence unknown but may be uncommon
- Possibly inherited as an autosomal recessive trait

Musculoskeletal conditions
Hereditary myopathy of Devon Rex cats
- Inherited as an autosomal recessive trait

Patellar luxation
- Usually apparent at an early age

Umbilical hernia
- Polygenic inheritance likely

Physiological conditions
Coat
- Rex cats have short, curly or absent whiskers
- May moult during oestrus or pregnancy

Blood group
- In the USA 57% were group A, 59% group B
- Similar figures reported in the UK

DOMESTIC LONG HAIR

Cardiovascular conditions
Hypertrophic cardiomyopathy
- Common disease
- Middle-aged to older cats predisposed
- Males predisposed

Dermatological conditions
Ehler-Danlos syndrome
- Also known as cutaneous asthenia
- Inherited group of diseases
- May be inherited as an autosomal dominant trait
- Probably lethal in homozygotes

Gastrointestinal conditions
Congenital portosystemic shunt
- Usually extrahepatic shunts

Neoplastic conditions
Basal cell tumour
- Reported to be at increased risk
- Average age is 7–10 years

Neurological conditions
Lysosomal storage disease – alpha mannosidosis
- Inheritance suspected
- Rare
- Signs seen at 6–12 months

Renal and urinary conditions
Polycystic kidney disease
- Breed predisposition

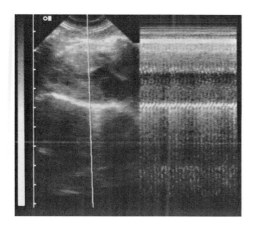

Figure 16a
B-mode and M-mode echocardiogram (left ventricular short axis) of a fourteen-year-old neutered male Domestic Short Hair cat with hypertrophic cardiomyopathy.

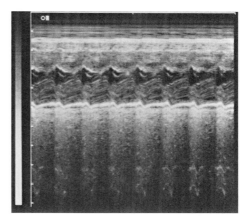

Figure 16b
M-mode echocardiogram (left ventricular short axis) of a fourteen-year-old neutered male Domestic Short Hair cat with hypertrophic cardiomyopathy.

DOMESTIC SHORT HAIR

Cardiovascular conditions
Hypertrophic cardiomyopathy
(see figures 16a and 16b)
- Common disease
- Middle–aged to older cats predisposed
- Males predisposed

Dermatological conditions
Ehler-Danlos syndrome
- Also known as cutaneous asthenia
- Inherited group of diseases
- May be inherited as an autosomal dominant trait
- Probably lethal in homozygotes

Lentigo simplex
- Cause unknown
- Usually affects cats less than 1 year old

Solar dermatitis
- Blue–eyed white cats predisposed

Psychogenic alopecia
- Thought to be a result of anxiety

Skin tumours
- See under Neoplastic conditions

Gastrointestinal conditions
Congenital portosystemic shunt
- Usually extrahepatic shunts

Haematological conditions
Pelger-Huet anomaly
- Inherited as an autosomal dominant trait
- Homozygous form is lethal
- Heterozygotes do not appear predisposed to infectious diseases

Methaemoglobin reductase deficiency
- Inherited as an autosomal recessive trait
- Heterozygotes are asymptomatic

Pyruvate kinase deficiency
- Inherited as an autosomal recessive trait
- Carriers are asymptomatic
- Causes severe anaemia

Haemophilia A
- Incidence of sponataneous haemorrhages lower in cats than dogs

CATS

Musculoskeletal conditions
Mucopolysaccharidosis I
- Uncommon
- Skeletal, cardiac and ocular lesions seen
- See lysosomal storage diseases under Ocular conditions and Neurological conditions

Congenital myasthenia gravis
- See under Neurological conditions

Neoplastic conditions
Sebaceous gland tumours
- Possible breed predisposition
- Seen in older cats (average age 10 years)

Neurological conditions
Neuroaxonal dystrophy (Domestic Tricolour cat)
- Autosomal recessive inheritance suspected
- Rare
- Age of clinical onset: 5–6 weeks

Lysosomal storage disease – sphingomyelinosis (Niemann-Pick disease)
- Inheritance suspected
- Rare
- Signs seen at 3–6 months

Lysosomal storage disease – mucopolysaccharidosis
- Inheritance suspected
- Rare
- Signs seen at 3–6 months

Lysosomal storage disease – GM_1 gangliosidosis
- Autosomal recessive inheritance
- Rare
- Signs seen at 3–6 months

Lysosomal storage disease – globoid cell leukodystrophy (Krabbe's disease)
- Inheritance suspected
- Rare
- Signs seen at 6–12 months

Lysosomal storage disease – alpha mannosidosis
- Inheritance suspected
- Rare
- Signs seen at 6–12 months

Hyperoxaluria
- Autosomal recessive inheritance suggested
- Age of clinical onset: 5–9 months
- Results in renal failure and neurological damage

Congenital myasthenia gravis
- Has been reported
- Age of clinical onset: 4 months

Ocular conditions
Coloboma
- Congenital condition; breed predisposition
- May occur in one or more ocular tissues including eyelid, iris, optic nerve and sclera

Corneal dermoid
- Rare condition; reported in this breed

Congenital cataract
- Rare condition; reported in this breed

Microphakia
- Rare condition; reported in this breed

Lysosomal storage diseases
- Rare conditions; inheritance suspected
- Types affecting ocular tissues: GM_1 gangliosidosis, GM_2 gangliosidosis, α-mannosidosis, mucopolysaccharidosis 1

Physiological conditions
Hereditary porphyria
- Not usually associated with anaemia in this breed

Renal and urinary conditions
Hyperoxaluria
- Autosomal recessive inheritance suggested
- Age of clinical onset: 5–9 months
- Results in renal failure and neurological damage

EGYPTIAN MAU

Neurological conditions
Spongiform degeneration
- Inheritance suspected
- Age of clinical onset: 7 weeks

CATS

HAVANA BROWN

Dermatological conditions
Blastomycosis
- See under Infectious conditions

Infectious conditions
Blastomycosis
- Very rare
- Seen in areas with sandy soil close to water

HIMALAYAN

Dermatological conditions
Dermatophytosis
- Common

Multiple epitrichial cysts
- Affect eyelids

Systemic lupus erythematosus
- Rare in cats
- No age or sex predisposition

Ehler-Danlos syndrome
- Also known as cutaneous asthenia
- Inherited group of diseases
- May be inherited as an autosomal dominant trait
- Probably lethal in homozygotes

Feline acromelanism
- Temperature-dependent enzyme involved in pathogenesis

Idiopathic facial dermatitis in Persians and Himalayans
- Uncommon
- Unknown cause; possibly genetic basis

Skin tumours
- See under Neoplastic conditions

Drug reactions
Griseofulvin
- Anecdotal reports suggest a predisposition to side effects with this drug in this breed

Gastrointestinal conditions
Congenital portosystemic shunt
- Usually extrahepatic shunts

Neoplastic conditions
Basal cell tumour
- Reported to be at increased risk
- Average age is 7–10 years

Neurological conditions
Hyperaesthesia syndrome
- Breed predisposition

Ocular conditions
Corneal sequestration
- Breed predisposition

Congenital cataract
- Rare condition; reported in this breed

Physiological conditions
Blood group
- Colourpoint Himalayans reported as 80% group A, 20% group B in the USA

Renal and urinary conditions
Calcium oxalate urolithiasis
- Higher incidence reported in this breed
- Males have been found to be more commonly affected in one survey

KORAT

Neurological conditions
Lysosomal storage disease – GM_1 gangliosidosis
- Autosomal recessive inheritance
- Rare
- Signs seen at 3–6 months

Lysosomal storage disease – GM_2 gangliosidosis
- Autosomal recessive inheritance
- Rare
- Signs seen at 3–6 months

Ocular conditions
Lysosomal storage diseases
- Autosomal recessive inheritance
- Rare
- Types affecting ocular tissues: GM_1 gangliosidosis, GM_2 gangliosidosis

CATS

MAINE COON

Cardiovascular conditions
Hypertrophic cardiomyopathy
- Common disease
- Middle-aged to older cats predisposed
- Males predisposed
- Inherited as an autosomal dominant trait in this breed

Musculoskeletal conditions
Hip dysplasia
- One study showed 51% of Maine Coon cats examined had radiographic evidence of hip dysplasia
- Heritability not known in cats

MANX

Dermatological conditions
Intertrigo
- Predisposed to rump fold intertrigo

Gastrointestinal conditions
Megacolon and constipation
- Breed predisposition
- Seen in older cats

Rectal prolapse
- Breed predisposition

Musculoskeletal conditions
Sacrocaudal dysgenesis
- Congenital
- See also under Neurological conditions

Neurological conditions
Spina bifida
- Congenital

Sacrocaudal dysgenesis
- Congenital, autosomal dominant inheritance
- Relatively common in this breed

Ocular conditions
Corneal dystrophy
- Breed predisposition; possibly inherited as a simple autosomal recessive trait
- Progressive condition, presenting at 4 months with corneal oedema

Renal and urinary conditions
Sacrocaudal dysgenesis (causing urinary incontinence)
- Congenital, autosomal dominant inheritance
- See also under Neurological conditions

NORWEGIAN FOREST

Neurological conditions
Glycogenosis (glycogen storage disease type 4)
- Autosomal recessive inheritance suspected
- Rare
- Age of clinical onset: <6 months

Physiological conditions
Blood group
- Reported as being 100% group A in the USA

ORIENTAL

Dermatological conditions
Psychogenic alopecia
- Common in nervous cats

PERSIAN

Cardiovascular conditions
Hypertrophic cardiomyopathy
- Common disease
- Middle-aged to older cats predisposed
- Males predisposed
- May be inherited in this breed

Peritoneopericardial diaphragmatic hernia
- Accounts for 0.5% of congenital heart disease but may be under-reported
- Females may be predisposed
- May be inherited as an autosomal recessive trait in cats

Dermatological conditions
Dermatophytosis
- Common
- This breed may develop dermatophytic pseudomycetoma, characterised by one or more ulcerated and discharging nodules over the dorsal trunk or tail base

CATS

Systemic lupus erythematosus
- Rare in cats
- No age or sex predisposition

Primary seborrhoea
- Rare in cats
- Autosomal recessive mode of inheritance

Chédiak-Higashi syndrome (blue smoke Persians only)
- Autosomal recessive inheritance
- See under Haematological conditions

Idiopathic periocular crusting
- May be associated with *Malassezia* or feline acne

Facial fold pyoderma

Idiopathic facial dermatitis in Persians and Himalayans
- Uncommon
- Unknown cause; possibly genetic basis

Multiple epitrichial cysts
- Affect eyelids

Skin tumours
- See under Neoplastic conditions

Drug reactions
Griseofulvin
- Anecdotal reports suggest a predisposition to side effects with this drug in this breed

Gastrointestinal conditions
Congenital portosystemic shunt
- Usually extrahepatic shunts

Congenital polycystic liver disease
- Breed predisposition
- May be associated with polycystic kidney disease

Haematological/immunological conditions
Chédiak-Higashi syndrome (blue smoke Persians only)
- Autosomal recessive inheritance
- Abnormal lysosomes and neutrophil granules seen

Susceptibility to dermatophytosis
- Can lead to severe and long-term infections

Systemic lupus erythematosus
- Rare in cats
- No age or sex predisposition

Neoplastic conditions
Basal cell tumour
- Reported to be at increased risk
- Average age is 7–10 years

Sebaceous gland tumours
- Possible breed predisposition
- Seen in older cats (average age 10 years)

Neurological conditions
Lysosomal storage disease – alpha mannosidosis
- Inheritance suspected
- Rare
- Signs seen at 2–4 months

Ocular conditions
Coloboma
- Congenital condition; breed predisposition
- May occur in one or more ocular tissues including eyelid, iris, optic nerve and sclera

Entropion
- Breed predisposition

Lacrimal punctal aplasia
- Congenital condition; predisposed breed

Idiopathic epiphora
- Breed predisposition; may relate to head and eyelid shape

Corneal sequestration
- Breed predisposition

Congenital cataract
- Rare condition; reported in this breed

Chédiak-Higashi syndrome (blue smoke Persians only)
- Autosomal recessive inheritance
- See under Haematological conditions

CATS

Retinal degeneration
- Autosomal recessive inheritance suspected

Lysosomal storage diseases
- Inheritance suspected
- Rare
- Types affecting ocular tissues: α-mannosidosis

Physiological conditions
Blood group
- In the USA 76% reported as group A and 24% as group B
- In the UK 12% were reported as group B

Prognathism
- A longer lower jaw than upper jaw is accepted as a breed standard

Renal and urinary conditions
Polycystic kidney disease
- Autosomal dominant inheritance
- Cysts arise in both the medulla and cortex and enlarge over time. They may be detected by ultrasound as early as 6–8 weeks of age. Most cases do not develop renal failure until later in life (average age 7 years).

Calcium oxalate urolithiasis
- Higher incidence reported in this breed

Reproductive conditions
Cryptorchidism
- Suspected inherited defect with a simple autosomal recessive, sex-linked mode of inheritance
- Possible breed predisposition

RAGDOLL

Cardiovascular conditions
Hypertrophic cardiomyopathy
- Common disease
- Middle-aged to older cats predisposed
- Males predisposed
- May be inherited in this breed

SCOTTISH FOLD

Musculoskeletal conditions
Arthropathy associated with Scottish Fold cats
- Homozygotes develop cartilage abnormalities and a progressive arthropathy
- Occasionally heterozygotes develop a milder form of the disease

Physiological conditions
Blood group
- In the USA 85% reported as group A, 15% as group B

SIAMESE

Cardiovascular conditions
Dilated cardiomyopathy
- Less common than in the past
- Genetic factors may influence susceptibility to disease
- Males predisposed

Endocardial fibroelastosis
- Age of onset: <6 months
- May be familial in this breed

Patent ductus arteriosus
- A possible slightly increased predisposition for this condition in this breed has been suggested
- Familial
- No sex predisposition in cats

Persistent atrial standstill
- Uncommon disease
- Marked predisposition in this breed

Dermatological conditions
Cutaneous tuberculosis
- Rare unless there is a high degree of exposure

Blastomycosis
- See under Infectious conditions

Cryptococcosis
- See under Infectious conditions

CATS

Histoplasmosis
- Rare

Generalised demodicosis
- Rare in cats
- Usually less severe in cats than in dogs

Food hypersensitivity
- Siameses and Siamese crosses accounted for 30% of cases in two studies
- Odds ratio 5.0

Systemic lupus erythematosus
- Rare in cats
- No age or sex predisposition

Feline pinnal alopecia
- Cause unknown

Junctional epidermolysis bullosa
- Claw shedding noted
- Autosomal recessive inheritance likely

Congenital hypotrichosis
- Familial

Feline acromelanism
- Temperature-dependent enzyme involved in pathogenesis

Vitiligo
- Presumed to be hereditary

Periocular leukotrichia
- Bilateral
- No age predilection

Aguirre syndrome
- Unilateral periocular depigmentation
- May be associated with Horner's syndrome, corneal necrosis and upper respiratory tract infection

Psychogenic alopecia
- Thought to be a result of anxiety

Tail sucking
- Psychogenic disorder

Sporotrichosis
- Uncommon
- Entire males predisposed
- Mainly affects cats <4 years old

Eyelid coloboma
- Congenital

Skin tumours
- See under Neoplastic conditions

Drug reactions
Griseofulvin
- Anecdotal reports suggest a predisposition to side effects with this drug in this breed

Endocrine conditions
Parathyroid tumours (resulting in primary hyperparathyroidism)
- Rare
- In a report of seven feline cases, five were Siamese
- Older cats affected

Insulinoma
- Rare disease
- In three reported cases where signalment was included, all were male Siamese and the average age was 14 years

Gastrointestinal conditions
Cleft palate
- Congenital disorder; familial occurrence in this breed

Congenital idiopathic megaoesophagus
- Breed predisposition

Pyloric dysfunction
- Breed predisposition

Small intestinal adenocarcinoma
- Possible breed predisposition
- Seen in older cats

Congenital portosystemic shunt
- Usually extrahepatic shunts

CATS

Amyloidosis
- Familial
- Age of onset: 1–4 years
- Amyloid deposits are found mainly in the liver and thyroid glands, resulting in clinical signs of cachexia, jaundice and occasionally liver rupture. This may be another example of systemic amyloidosis.

Haematological conditions
Haemophilia B
- Factor IX deficiency
- Also known as Christmas disease
- Inherited as a sex-linked trait
- Less common than haemophilia A

Hereditary porphyria
- May be anaemia with renal failure in this breed

Infectious conditions
Mycobacterium avium
- Rare condition
- Possible breed predisposition

Blastomycosis
- Rare condition in cats. Most reported cases have been in this breed
- Geographic distribution: around the Mississippi, Ohio, Missouri, Tennessee, and St Lawrence Rivers, the southern Great Lakes, and the southern mid–Atlantic states. Not reported in the UK

Cryptococcosis
- Uncommon

Histoplasmosis
- Rare

Infectious skin disease
- See under Dermatological conditions

Musculoskeletal conditions
Cleft palate/lip
- See under Gastrointestinal conditions

Hip dysplasia
- Case reports suggest an over-representation of Siamese with hip dysplasia
- Heritability in cats poorly understood

Congenital myasthenia gravis
- See under Neurological conditions

Mucopolysaccharidosis VI
- Lysosomal storage disease
- Inherited as an autosomal recessive trait
- Causes dwarfism and multiple skeletal, neurological and retinal deficits

Neoplastic conditions
Mast cell tumours
- Possible breed predisposition
- Usually seen in cats >4 years
- There are reports of two litters of Siamese kittens with cutaneous mast cell tumours. One litter was 6 weeks and the other 8 weeks at diagnosis. In all kittens the lesions had disappeared at 4 months

Lipoma
- Usually occurs in animals older than 8 years

Basal cell tumour
- Reported to be at increased risk
- Average age is 7–10 years

Sweat gland tumour
- Reported to be at increased risk
- Average age reported as 11.6 years

Nasal cavity tumours
- Reported to be at increased risk
- Average age reported as 8–10 years
- A predisposition for neutered males has been suggested

Parathyroid tumours (resulting in primary hyperparathyroidism)
- See under Endocrine conditions

Insulinoma
- See under Endocrine conditions

Small intestinal adenocarcinoma
- See under Gastrointestinal conditions

Mammary tumours
- Possible breed predisposition
- Seen in older cats (mean age 10–12 years)

CATS

Neurological conditions
Congenital vestibular disease
- Signs seen <3 months

Congenital deafness
- Signs seen from birth

Hydrocephalus
- Congenital; inherited as an autosomal recessive trait

Lysosomal storage disease – GM_1 gangliosidosis
- Autosomal recessive inheritance
- Rare
- Signs seen at 3–6 months

Lysosomal storage disease – ceroid lipofuscinosis
- Inheritance suspected
- Rare
- Signs seen at 6–12 months

Lysosomal storage disease – sphingomyelinosis (Niemann-Pick disease)
- Autosomal recessive inheritance
- Rare
- Signs seen at 3–6 months

Lysosomal storage disease – mucopolysaccharidosis type VI
- Autosomal recessive inheritance
- Rare
- Signs seen at 2–3 months

Hyperaesthesia syndrome
- Breed predisposition

Congenital myasthenia gravis
- Has been reported
- Age of clinical onset: 5 months

Ocular conditions
Convergent strabismus and nystagmus
- Congenital condition found in this breed
- Results from abnormal visual pathway development

Corneal sequestration
- Breed predisposition

Glaucoma
- Breed predisposition

Congenital cataract
- Has been reported in this breed

Microphakia
- Rare condition; reported in this breed

Retinal degeneration
- Inheritance suspected
- Seen in older cats (10 years) in the UK

Lysosomal storage diseases
- Autosomal recessive inheritance
- Rare
- Types affecting ocular tissues: GM_1 gangliosidosis, mucopolysaccharidosis VI
- See under Neurological conditions

Physiological conditions
Blood group
- In the USA 100% of Siamese reported to be group A

Respiratory conditions
Feline asthma
- Common
- Affects all ages

Chylothorax
- No sex predisposition
- This breed over-represented in one study

SOMALI

Haematological conditions
Increased osmotic fragility of erythrocytes
- Initial presentation in first few years of life
- Mode of inheritance unknown

Pyruvate kinase deficiency
- Inherited as an autosomal recessive trait
- Carriers are asymptomatic
- Causes severe anaemia

Musculoskeletal conditions
Mysasthenia gravis
- See under Neurological conditions

CATS

Neurological conditions
Mysasthenia gravis
- Rare in cats
- Usually adult–onset

Physiological conditions
Blood group
- In the USA 78% reported as group A, 22% as group B

TONKINESE

Neurological conditions
Congenital vestibular disease
- Signs seen <3 months

Physiological conditions
Blood group
- In the USA 100% reported as group A

CATS

PART III
DISEASE SUMMARIES

CARDIOVASCULAR CONDITIONS

Aortic stenosis (see figure 17)

This important condition accounts for up to a third of reported cases of congenital canine heart disease. It appears to be inherited, but not in a simple way, with more than one gene thought to be involved. The lesion develops in the first three to eight weeks of life, and may be first detected as a heart murmur at this age. If the condition is mild, clinical signs are minimal, but more severely affected animals may suffer from weakness, collapse and sudden death. Dogs with aortic stenosis should not be used for breeding.

Atrial fibrillation

This arrhythmia is usually seen in conjunction with severe heart disease such as dilated cardiomyopathy. However, some large-breed dogs can show an asymptomatic atrial fibrillation.

Atrial septal defect

This congenital condition, involving a defect in the septum between the atria, is uncommon, accounting for 14 out of 1000 cases in a survey of dogs with congenital heart disease. Small defects may be asymptomatic, but larger lesions can lead to congestive heart failure.

Boxer cardiomyopathy

An arryhthmogenic cardiomyopathy is seen in this breed. Affected animals can present with syncope, weakness or congestive heart failure (CHF).

Bypass tract macrore-entrant tachycardia of Labrador Retrievers

This rare condition involves tachycardia caused by abnormal conduction within the heart. The high heart rate can induce acute pulmonary oedema.

Canine juvenile polyarteritis syndrome

Young Beagles from various laboratories have been reported to suffer from a pain syndrome caused by systemic vasculitis.

Coronary artery vasculitis

Spontaneous, asymptomatic coronary artery vasculitis has been documented in up to 34% of young Beagles studied.

179

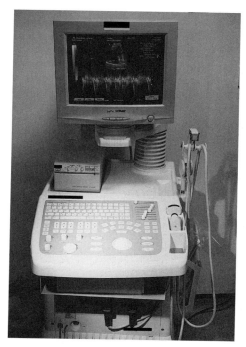

Figure 17
An ultrasound machine capable of Doppler echocardiography is useful in the diagnosis of congenital cardiac abnormalities.

Dilated cardiomyopathy (see figures 18a and 18b)

This condition involves a dilation of the heart involving larger chamber size, thinner heart walls and reduced power of the heartbeat. Pure-bred dogs suffer from this condition at a prevalance rate of about 0.65% compared to 0.16% for mixed breed dogs. It is thought that the majority of cases are genetic or familial, but it is not certain that all cases are genetic in origin. Nutritional abnormalities may also contribute, and it is possible that viral and immune-mediated causes may be involved in some cases.

Duchenne's X-linked muscular dystrophy cardiomyopathy

Also known as Golden Retriever muscular dys-trophy. In this rare, inherited condition, skeletal muscle signs predominate, starting at about eight weeks of age, but severe cardiac involve-ment may develop later. Few dogs affected with this condition survive past five years of age. See also section on Musculoskeletal conditions.

Endocardial fibroelastosis

Severe thickening of the endocardium is seen in this condition, sometimes involving the mitral valve leaflets. Heart murmur, failure to thrive and congestive heart failure are seen.

Endocardiosis

Also known as chronic degenerative valvular disease. This is the most common cause of heart disease in the dog, with up to 75% of dogs with congestive heart failure suffering from this con-dition. The heart valves become deformed by a myxomatous degeneration, leading to regurgita-tion and congestive heart failure. This condition is likely to be inherited, although other proposed causes include stress, hypertension, hypoxia, infection and endocrine abnormalities.

Essential hypertension

Increased blood pressure may be secondary or primary. In Greyhounds, a higher blood pres-sure compared to other breeds is a physiological condition, and the same may be true of Siberian Huskies, where a hereditary essential hyperten-sion was reported in Husky crosses.

Familial cardiomyopathy

This is a form of dilated cardiomyopathy seen in English Cockers and other breeds.

Hereditary stenosis of bundle of His

This condition leads to an atrioventricular con-duction block.

Hypertrophic cardiomyopathy

In this condition a hypertrophied ventricle causes congestive heart failure and dysrhythmias. The incidence is reported as being 1.6–5.2%. It is likely that the condition is inherited, although modifying factors may cause variable expression of the condition.

Mitral valve dysplasia

This is the commonest congenital heart disease of cats, and is thought to be inherited in some

DISEASE SUMMARIES

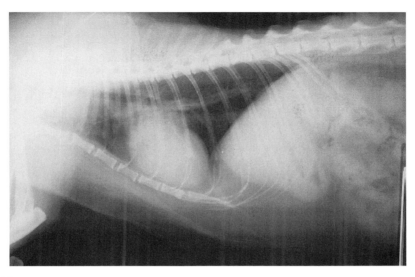

Figure 18a
Lateral thoracic radiograph of a ten-year-old female Domestic Short Hair cat with idiopathic dilated cardiomyopathy.

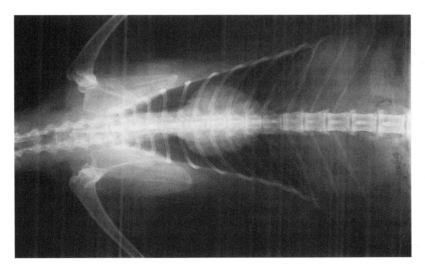

Figure 18b
Dorsoventral thoracic radiograph of a ten-year-old female Domestic Short Hair cat with idiopathic dilated cardiomyopathy.

DISEASE SUMMARIES

breeds of dog, although this is not yet proven. The lesion consists of a malformation of the mitral valve, the normal function of which is to prevent blood flowing back from the left ventricle to the left atrium. Many animals with this condition do not show symptoms, and those that do usually demonstrate exercise intolerance and congestive heart failure.

Patent ductus arteriosus

The ductus arteriosus carries blood from the pulmonary artery to the aorta in the foetus to bypass the lung, which is not in use. It normally closes within the first week after birth. It is probably the commonest congenital heart condition of dogs, but is less common in cats. Females are at a higher risk of developing the condition than males. Symptoms range from none, to congestive heart failure and poor body condition, to weakness, collapse and seizures.

Pericardial effusion

This condition involves a build up of fluid between the heart wall and the pericardium. It can be caused by tumours of the heart, but often has no apparent cause ('benign' or 'idiopathic' pericardial effusion). The idiopathic form is poorly understood, and it is not known whether it is inherited. However, it does tend to affect large-breed and giant dogs. Symptoms are precipitated by the inability of the heart to fill properly because of restriction caused by the fluid-filled pericardial sac. Chronic cases exhibit weight loss, ascites and dyspnoea resulting from pleural effusion. Acute cases may show rapidly progressing weakness, collapse and death.

Peritoneopericardial hernia

This uncommon congenital disease is seen in only about 0.5% of cases of congenital heart disease. It involves a continuation of the pericardium with the peritoneum, and often abdominal viscera are found within the pericadial sac. It may be asymptomatic, or may cause signs of respiratory distress, vomiting and colic.

Persistent atrial standstill

This is a rare condition caused by an enlargement and thinning of the atria. It is often

associated with scapulohumeral wasting in English Springers.

Persistent left cranial vena cava

The left cranial vena cava is normally present in the foetus, but may persist abnormally after birth. This abnormality is relatively common, but is of no significance to the animal unless it is undergoing thoracic surgery.

Persistent right aortic arch

This is a malformation in the foetal development of the vascular system, which leads to the oesophagus being partially occluded. This leads to regurgitation once the animal starts weaning. See also *Vascular ring anomaly* under Gastrointestinal conditions.

Pulmonic stenosis

This is a common congenital condition, affecting 20% of dogs diagnosed with congenital heart disease. The condition may be asymptomatic, or may cause signs of syncope and right-sided congestive heart failure.

Sick sinus syndrome

This dysrhythmia often involves periods of bradycardia and tachycardia, leading to syncope.

Tetralogy of Fallot

This condition accounts for approximately 4% of congenital heart disease. Pulmonic stenosis, ventricular septal defect, a dextrapositioned or overriding aorta and a secondary right ventricular hypertrophy comprise the four parts of this abnormality.

Tricuspid dysplasia

This is a malformation of the tricuspid valve, the consequence of which is to allow blood to flow back from the right ventricle into the right atrium. Affected dogs may have other congenital heart lesions. In some cases the animals are asymptomatic for many years, while others show progressive heart failure leading to death.

Ventricular ectopy

Ventricular ectopic beats are abnormal beats of the heart arising within the ventricles instead of the normal pacemaker in the atria. They can

DISEASE SUMMARIES

have a number of causes, such as heart disease, kidney disease and sepsis. They are also inherited in German Shepherd Dogs. If they occur frequently they can cause symptoms of collapse, and the rhythm can degenerate into fatal ventricular fibrillation.

Ventricular septal defect

This condition accounts for approximately 7% of canine congenital heart disease. Defects vary in size but can be very large. Small defects may be asymptomatic, but larger defects can cause congestive heart failure, pulmonary vascular disease and pulmonary hypertension.

DERMATOLOGICAL CONDITIONS

Acanthosis nigricans

This is an uncommon condition which can be primary or secondary to intertrigo, endocrine disorders or hypersensitivities. It is characterised by bilateral axillary hyperpigmentation which progresses to alopecia and seborrhoea.

Acquired aurotrichia

Silver or black hairs turn gold, especially on the dorsal thorax and abdomen.

Acquired depigmentation

Affects dogs from about 18 months of age. There is loss of pigment around the face and sometimes the coat.

Acral lick dermatitis

Also known as lick granuloma. This condition may be psychogenic in origin, but underlying causes should be considered.

Acral mutilation syndrome

This is an unusual neurological condition which results in mutilation of the distal extremities. Pups are affected between three and five months of age. Temperature and pain sensation of the toes is lost. The prognosis is poor.

Acrodermatitis

Inherited condition of Bull Terriers, causing coat, skin and footpad lesions. There may be

respiratory and gastrointestinal signs, and the prognosis is poor. A defect in zinc metabolism may be involved in the pathogenesis.

Aguirre syndrome

Unilateral periocular depigmentation. It may be associated with Horner's syndrome, ocular and respiratory problems.

Alopecia areata

This condition is uncommon, leading to an asymptomatic, non-inflammatory alopecia.

Anal sac disease

Infections and impactions of the anal sacs are common, causing self-trauma to the perineal area and other parts of the body.

Atopy (see plate 14)

This is a common condition involving hypersensitivity reactions to environmental allergens. It is thought to be inherited but the exact mode of inheritance has not yet been determined. Symptoms consist of pruritus, erythema and self-trauma with secondary bacterial infection.

Black hair follicular dysplasia

A rare disorder causing alopecia in areas of black hair.

Blastomycosis

See under Infectious conditions.

Bullous pemphigoid

A rare autoimmune condition leading to ulceration of the mucocutaneous junctions, skin and oral cavity.

Calcinosis circumscripta

An uncommon condition, usually of unknown cause, although it may be associated with hyperadrenocorticism. Most affected dogs are of large breeds, and pressure points are commonly involved.

Callus dermatitis/pyoderma

Calluses form in response to trauma. Secondary infection occurs in chronic cases, leading to ulceration.

DISEASE SUMMARIES

Canine benign familial chronic pemphigus

In this condition lesions develop in response to trauma or infection due to a genetic weakness in desmosomes.

Canine linear IgA dermatosis

A very rare condition characterised by a generalised pustular dermatitis. It appears to affect adult Dachshunds exclusively.

Canine ear margin dermatosis

This condition begins as a mild seborrheoa which can progress to severe crusting and painful fissuring.

Canine eosinophilic granuloma

This condition is rare in dogs. It consists of nodules, plaques, ulcers or vegetative masses of the skin or, more commonly, the oral cavity. See also under Gastrointestinal conditions.

Canine juvenile cellulitis

This condition is also known as juvenile pyoderma, puppy strangles or juvenile sterile granulomatous dermatitis and lymphadenitis. It is an uncommon disorder, causing pustules on the face and pinnae of puppies. The submandibular lymph nodes are often greatly enlarged.

Chédiak-Higashi syndrome

See under Ocular and Haematological/immunological conditions.

Coat-colour dilution and cerebellar degeneration in Rhodesian Ridgeback dogs

This condition has been reported in a family of Rhodesian Ridgebacks. Pups were born with a bluish coat, and developed ataxia at two weeks of age. Most were euthanased at four to six weeks of age.

Collagenous naevus

A naevus is a developmental skin defect leading to skin hyperplasia. Collagenous naevi can be solitary or multiple. They may be associated with bilateral renal cystadenocarcinomas and multiple uterine leiomyomas.

Colour-dilution alopecia

Hypotrichosis and recurrent bacterial folliculitis occur in colour dilute areas.

Congenital hypotrichosis

Animals affected with this condition are born wihout their normal coats or lose them in the first few months of life.

Contact hypersensitivity

Also called allergic contact dermatitis, this condition is rare, as opposed to irritant contact dermatitis which is quite common. The paws and sparsely haired areas of skin are usually affected. Plants, medications and home furnishings are reported as sources of allergens.

Cryptococcosis

See under Infectious conditions.

Cutaneous histiocytosis

This benign proliferative condition is thought to be a reactive histiocytosis. There may be generalised or localised clusters of plaques or nodules.

Cutaneous tuberculosis

It is uncommon for dogs and cats to be affected. Dermatological signs include ulcers, plaques, nodules and abscesses.

Cyclic follicular dysplasia

A temporary pattern alopecia which usually affects the trunk and especially the flank. It seems to be a problem in Alaska, suggesting that duration of daylight may be important.

Dermatophytosis

Also known as ringworm. This common condition is particularly prevalent in long-haired cats.

Demodicosis, generalised (see figure 19)

Generalised demodicosis is a severe skin disease caused by the *Demodex* mite. It can lead to pyoderma and deep folliculitis.

Dermoid cyst

A rare developmental abnormality. It can be solitary or multiple, and occurs along the dorsal midline.

DISEASE SUMMARIES

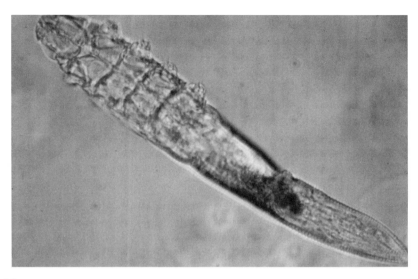

Figure 19
Demodex mite. Courtesy of A. Foster, University of Bristol.

Dermoid sinus
See under Neurological conditions.

Discoid lupus erythematosus
Uncommon in dogs and very rare in cats, this condition is an immune-mediated dermatosis with no systemic involvement. Clinical signs include depigmentation, scaling, erosion and ulceration. The nose is primarily affected, but the pinnae, limbs and genitalia can be involved.

Disorder of the footpads in German Shepherd Dogs
Affected dogs show soft pads, depigmentation and ulceration.

Ehlers-Danlos syndrome
Also known as cutaneous asthenia, dermato-praxis. This group of diseases is characterised by fragile, hyperextensible, easily torn skin.

Eosinophilic dermatitis and oedema
This rare condition presents as acute-onset erythematous macules which progress to form plaques. Variable oedema is seen.

Epidermal dysplasia in West Highland Whites
Also known as armadillo Westie syndrome. *Malassezia* is involved in the pathogenesis. The skin becomes inflamed, greasy, itchy and, in advanced cases, lichenified.

Epidermolysis bullosa, junctional and dystrophic
These are a group of inherited bullous diseases, involving abnormal keratin production. Junctional epidermolysis bullosa causes bullae, vesicles and erosions in various locations. Dystrophic epidermolysis bullosa shows erosions in the mucocutaneous junctions.

Eyelid coloboma
This is a congenital discontinuity in the eyelid.

Facial fold pyoderma/intertrigo
This condition arises due to friction in a facial skin fold. Surface bacteria and *Malassezia* contribute to inflammation.

Familial canine dermatomyositis
This is a hereditary disease causing skin lesions around the face, ear tips and digits.

DISEASE SUMMARIES

Familial vasculopathy

This is a rare group of conditions which can cause dermatological and systemic signs. In some breeds the disease is inherited.

Feline acromelanism

Coat-colour changes in some Oriental cat breeds with environmental and physiologically-induced temperature variations. If the temperature change is addressed, the colour changes may be reversible.

Feline pinnal alopecia

Bilateral spontaneous pinnal alopecia occurs in some Siamese cats. There is usually spontaneous recovery after a period of months.

Feline solar dermatitis

This is a chronic dermatitis involving white ears and occasionally the eyelids, nose and lips. UVB in sunlight is implicated in the pathogenesis.

Fibropruritic nodule

Multiple alopecic, firm or pedunculated lesions occur in this condition. Chronic self-trauma or flea-bite hypersensitivity are usually involved.

Flank sucking

This may be a form of psychomotor epilepsy, but primary skin diseases should be eliminated by biopsy.

Flea-bite hypersensitivity

Severe inflammatory reactions may occur due to hypersensitivity reactions to allergens in flea saliva.

Follicular cyst

These cysts occur in the dermis or subcutaneous region. They are usually solitary and well-circumscribed. Often they do not cause problems, but if they rupture they can cause foreign body reactions.

Follicular dysplasia

These are a group of conditions having alopecia and coat changes in common. They are suspected to be inherited in many breeds.

Follicular lipidosis of Rottweilers

This condition has been recently described, and affects young Rottweilers of either sex. A variable degree of alopecia of the red-coloured points is seen. The condition appears to be largely self-limiting.

Follicular parakeratosis

This disorder of cornification is congenital and hereditary. All cases so far reported have been in females and it is postulated that there is an X-linked mode of inheritance. Clinical signs include generalised seborrhoea that worsens with age.

Food hypersensitivity

This is a pruritic skin disease associated with the ingestion of one or more allergens present in food. Type I hypersensitivity reactions are usually involved, although type III and IV reactions are suspected.

Footpad hyperkeratosis

This condition is familial in some breeds. Signs of severe hyperkeratosis are usually seen by six months of age.

German Shepherd Dog folliculitis, furunculosis and cellulitis

This is an idiopathic deep pyoderma affecting German Shepherd Dogs. Probably an inherited immunodeficiency causes susceptibility to infection.

Granulomatous sebaceous adenitis

This condition is uncommon in dogs and rare in cats. Different breeds show different manifestations, including scaling, alopecia, hyperkeratosis and occasional systemic signs. Generally the disease is non-pruritic unless there is secondary bacterial infection.

Grass awn migration

Grass awns are reported to comprise 61% of foreign bodies. Predilection sites include ears, eyes, interdigital web and nose.

Hereditary lupoid dermatosis

This is a familial disease of unknown cause. Scaling begins on the head and progresses to become generalised. There may be systemic signs. No consistently successful treatment has been described.

DISEASE SUMMARIES

Histoplasmosis

See under Infectious conditions.

Hyperoestrogenism

This condition associated with polycystic ovaries in middle-aged intact females can cause bilateral endocrine alopecia.

Hypopigmentary disorders

There are a variety of causes for loss of hair or skin pigment. There may be a hereditary involvement in some breeds.

Ichthyosis

Also known as fish scale disease. Extreme hyperkeratosis is seen, and affected dogs are abnormal at birth. Scaling, erythema and severe seborrhoea are seen.

Idiopathic cutaneous and renal glomerular vasculopathy

Lesions consist of purpura and ulceration. They are slow to heal. Some dogs develop renal failure with accompanying clinical signs.

Idiopathic cutaneous mucinosis

Clinical signs of mucinosis include a puffy skin, vesicles and bullae. Shar Peis have large amounts of mucin in the skin, leading to excessive skin folding.

Idiopathic facial dermatitis in Persians and Himalayans

This an uncommon disease demonstrating crusting, erythema and self-trauma to the head and neck. Secondary bacteria and yeasts are common.

Idiopathic onychomadesis

Onychomadesis is a sloughing of the nail, usually involving multiple nails. Abnormal mineral composition of the affected nails has been documented, but the cause is unknown.

Idiopathic sterile granuloma and pyogranuloma

Clinical signs of this disorder include papules, plaques and nodules on the head, pinnae and paws.

Idiopathic sterile nodular panniculitis

This condition can look like deep pyoderma. There are often multiple skin lesions in predisposed breeds, and systemic signs, such as lethargy and pyrexia, are often present.

Idiopathic ulcerative dermatosis of Collies and Shetland Sheepdogs

This condition may be related to dermatomyositis. Vesicles and bullae progress to ulcers, especially in the inguinal and axillar regions and mucocutaneous junctions.

Intertrigo

Inflammation and bacterial infection caused by the trauma of friction between two apposing surfaces.

Lentigo simplex

In this condition, lesions start as small black spots that gradually enlarge and become more numerous over time. They are non-pruritic and are not pre-malignant.

Lentiginosa profusa

This is reported as a hereditary form of lentigo, but may actually be a pigmented epidermal naevus.

Malassezia dermatitis

This yeast commonly causes pruritus and a greasy, scaly skin disease.

Melanoderma and alopecia

In this condition, a symmetrical alopecia and hyperpigmentation is seen on the nasal planum and pinnae.

Melanotrichia

May occur after deep areas of inflammation heal. The hairs darken in focal areas.

Mucocutaneous hypopigmentation

The cause of this condition is unknown, but it is generally a cosmetic problem only.

Multiple epitrochial cysts

These lesions occur around the eyelids. The cysts are soft and fluid-filled and can be quite large. Both eyelids are usually involved.

DISEASE SUMMARIES

Muzzle folliculitis/furunculosis

Also known as canine acne. This is a chronic inflammation of the chin and lips, affecting young dogs. The underlying cause is unknown and bacterial infections are secondary. Treatment options include shampoos, and, in advanced cases, long courses of antibiotics. Scarring commonly occurs.

Nasal depigmentation

Affected dogs are normal at birth, but over time the black nasal planum slowly fades to a paler colour. The cause is not known.

Nasal folliculitis/furunculosis

This is a painful but uncommon condition of the nose whose cause is unknown. Clinical signs consist of papules and pustules progressing to folliculitis and furunculosis.

Nasal hyperkeratosis

The nasal planum becomes dry, rough and brown in this presumed inherited condition.

Nasal solar dermatitis

This photodermatitis is seen more commonly in sunny regions. Lesions, consisting of crusting and ulceration, are mainly seen at the junction between haired and hairless areas on the nose.

Oestrogen-responsive dermatosis

This is a rare condition of spayed female dogs causing a bilaterally symmetric alopecia. There may be accompanying juvenile genitalia.

Onychodystrophy

In this condition multiple claws are affected and no underlying cause can be ascertained.

Papilloma-virus-associated pigmented lesions

This condition causes rough black pigmented plaques to appear in the groin, on the abdomen, ventral thorax and neck. They do not regress and may transform into squamous cell carcinomas.

Pattern baldness

This acquired baldness is probably genetic in origin. Different syndromes of this condition affect different breeds.

Pemphigus erythematosus

This autoimmune condition is probably a less aggressive form of pemphigus foliaceous. Pustules and erythema are seen on the face and ears, which progress to erosions, scales and crusts.

Pemphigus foliaceous

This is probably the most common autoimmune skin condition of dogs and cats. Clinical signs of crusting and pustules usually start on the face and ears and progress to become multifocal or generalised. Secondary bacterial infection is common.

Periocular leukotrichia

Goggles can appear around the eyes of Siamese cats after various precipitating factors such as pregnancy and systemic illness.

Persistent scratching in Cavalier King Charles Spaniels

This condition is neurogenic, and is thought to be familial.

Pinnal alopecia

In this condition, the hair around the ears thins with age. Occasionally it may progress to complete alopecia of the pinnae. Diagnosis is by exclusion of other diseases. There is no known treatment.

Pododemodicosis

In this condition infection with the *Demodex* mite is confined to the feet.

Pododermatitis

Various factors, such as foreign bodies or trauma, can trigger folliculitis and furunculosis in the feet. Fungal, parasitic and psychogenic dermatitis can also cause pododermatitis.

Post-clipping alopecia

In this condition, hair fails to regrow for up to 24 months after clipping. This has been variously described as uncommon and relatively common. It may be caused by vascular changes in the skin resulting from cutaneous temperature changes.

DISEASE SUMMARIES

Primary lymphoedema

Lymphoedema is an abnormal lymph flow causing swelling. Primary lymphoedema results from defects in the lymphatic system. The hind-limbs are most commonly affected.

Primary seborrhoea

This is an inherited disorder of keratinisation and cornification which has an early age of onset. Clinical signs include flaking, scaling, crusting and greasy, smelly skin. The claws may also be affected. Secondary bacterial and fungal infections are common.

Protothecosis

The causal organisms of this condition, *Prototheca*, are ubiquitous algae. Infection is rare. Gastrointestinal, ocular and nervous signs are more common than dermatological signs.

Psoriasiform-lichenoid dermatosis in English Springer Spaniels

This is a rare condition causing plaques and papules on the pinnae and inguinal region. In time, the disease can become more generalised.

Psychogenic alopecia

Anxiety and stress can lead to overgrooming and alopecia. Elimination of underlying causes and examination of hair shafts aids in diagnosis.

Pyotraumatic folliculitis

This infection may be a complication of pyotraumatic dermatitis (wet eczema) and involves a deeper infection which may progress to furunculosis.

Pythiosis

The causal organism of this condition, *Pythium*, is an aquatic fungus which attacks damaged animal tissue. Lesions can be solitary or multiple and consist of ulcerated nodules which progress to discharging tracts.

Rabies-vaccine-associated vasculitis

Alopecia and hyperpigmentation are occasionally seen at the sites of rabies vaccination.

Schnauzer comedo syndrome

In this condition, mutiple comedos are seen along the dorsum.

Seasonal flank alopecia

This is a localised cyclic follicular dysplasia causing a symmetrical alopecia. Some dogs lose their hair in spring and regrow it spontaneously in autumn, for others the reverse occurs.

Seasonal nasal hypopigmentation

Also known as snow nose, this condition causes a decrease in nasal pigment in the winter months.

Shaft disorder of Abyssinian cats

This is a rare disorder affecting the whiskers and primary hairs. The coat is rough and lacking lustre, and hair fracture occurs.

Short-hair syndrome of silky breeds

Some Yorkshire and Silky Terriers lose their long coat, which is replaced by a much shorter one. No other skin lesions occur, and this is of cosmetic significance only.

Skin tumours

See under Neoplastic conditions.

Spiculosis

In this condition, mutiple bone spicules are found, particularly over the lateral hock.

Sporotrichosis

This is a rare fungal condition which can cause cutaneous signs such as ulcerated nodules and skin necrosis, regional lymphadenopathy and systemic signs such as depression, anorexia and pyrexia.

Subcorneal pustular dermatosis

This is a very rare idiopathic condition which leads to a generalised pustular or seborrhoea-like dermatitis. The head and trunk are particularly affected. Pruritus is variable.

Superficial bacterial folliculitis

In Collies and Shetland Sheepdogs, superficial bacterial folliculitis can have a bilaterally symmetrical distribution, mimicking endocrine alopecia.

Superficial suppurative necrolytic dermatitis of Miniature Schnauzer

This is a drug reaction to certain shampoos. Cutaneous and systemic signs usually occur within three days. Cutaneous signs include papules, plaques and pustules, and systemic signs include pyrexia and depression.

Symmetric lupoid onychodystrophy
Multiple claws slough, and when they regrow are misshapen and brittle.

Systemic lupus erythematosus
This is an uncommon autoimmune disorder affecting multiple body systems. Various cutaneous signs are seen including seborrhoea, vesicobullous disorders and alopecia. Systemic manifestations include cardiorespiratory, neurological and musculoskeletal signs. See also Haematological/immunological conditions.

Tail dock neuroma
This occurs rarely, following docking of tails. Transected nerves occasionally proliferate in a disorganised manner. Self-trauma to the lesion can cause a painful dermatosis.

Testosterone-responsive dermatosis
This is a rare dermatosis of castrated males, leading to a bilaterally symmetric alopecia.

Truncal solar dermatitis
Sparse hair and poorly-pigmented skin predispose to sun damage to the skin in sunny climates. The area affected can vary with the animal's sunbathing habits.

Tyrosinase deficiency
This extremely rare disease of Chow Chows causes colour changes of the tongue and hair shafts.

Uveodermatological syndrome
See under Ocular conditions.

Vasculitis
This uncommon condition causes various skin lesions such as wheals, papules, oedema, ulceration and scarring. Various cell types may be involved histologically, but the classification is usually of a type III hypersensitivity reaction. Various triggering factors may be involved, such as vaccinations, arthropod bites and mast cell tumours.

Vascular naevus, scrotal
Single or multiple plaques are seen, usually on the scrotum. Occasionally, the lesions bleed.

Ventral comedo syndrome
In this condition, comedos form because of pressure and friction on the sternum. Secondary bacterial infection, which may respond to topical antibiotic preparations, is common.

Vitamin-A-responsive dermatosis
This condition is characterised by a relatively refractory seborrhoea. There is often a waxy otitis externa. Vitamin A supplementation can lead to complete resolution, but therapy may need to be lifelong.

Vitiligo
This is thought to be an autoimmune disease causing depigmentation of the face. The condition is usually seen in young adults.

Waardenburg-Klein syndrome
This condition arises due to a lack of melanocytes in the affected skin. Affected animals are also deaf.

Waterline disease of black Labradors
Severe pruritus, seborrhoea and alopecia of the legs and ventrum are seen in this condition.

Zinc-responsive dermatosis
Two syndromes of this condition are recognised. Syndrome I occurs in diets with sufficient zinc. Erythema, alopecia, crusting, scaling and suppuration are seen around the mouth, chin, eyes and ears. In syndrome II, zinc-deficient diets can lead to hyperkeratotic plaques on the footpads and nasal planum.

ENDOCRINE CONDITIONS

Adult-onset growth-hormone-responsive dermatosis
A poorly-understood syndrome of unknown cause. Basal growth hormone levels are low and unresponsive to stimulation. Other pituitary functions seem normal. The condition is characterised by bilaterally symmetrical areas of

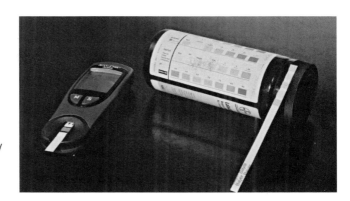

Figure 20
A portable glucometer and
urine dipsticks are commonly
used in the diagnosis and
monitoring of diabetes
mellitus.

alopecia and hyperpigmentation initially in the areas of friction, e.g. the neck.

Central diabetes insipidus (CDI)

A polyuric state caused by a complete or partial lack of antidiuretic hormone (vasopressin) which is normally produced in the neuro-hypophysis of the pituitary. Urine specific gravity is usually hyposthenuric. In the dog, most cases are idiopathic, but the condition may be acquired secondary to trauma, neoplasia or cystic malformations of the neurohypophysis. Although rare, there are a few reports of suspected hereditary CDI.

Congenital nephrogenic diabetes insipidus (congenital NDI)

NDI is a polyuric state caused by the reduced responsiveness of the renal tubules to anti-diuretic hormone. Acquired NDI occurs sec-ondarily to a wide variety of disorders. Congenital NDI is an extremely rare condition of which there are only a few reports in the dog.

Congenital hypothyroidism

Congenital hypothyroidism occurs where there is a congenital defect in thyroid hormone pro-duction or transport and results in dispro-portionate dwarfism. It is suspected it may also be a cause of neonatal death or fading puppy syndrome.

Cushing's syndrome

See *Hyperadrenocorticism*.

Diabetes mellitus (see figure 20)

Diabetes mellitus occurs where there is hyper-glycaemia resulting from an absolute or rel-ative lack of insulin. Where the blood glucose level exceeds the renal threshold, glycosuria results.

Hyperadrenocorticism (Cushing's syndrome)

One of the most commonly diagnosed endocrinopathies in the dog, but rare in the cat. Hyperadrenocorticism occurs where there is a sustained and inappropriately elevated secretion of cortisol from the adrenal cortex. Hyperadrenocorticism may be pituitary dependent, where there is excessive adrenocor-ticotrophic hormone (ACTH) secretion leading to bilateral adrenal cortical hyperplasia and increased cortisol secretion, or it may be adrenal dependent where there is a unilateral or bilat-eral functional adrenocortical tumour.

Hypoadrenocorticism

Hypoadrenocorticism is a condition wherein there is inadequate adrenocortical hormone production leading to a deficiency in miner-alocorticoids and/or glucocorticoids. Primary hypoadrenocorticism (Addison's disease) results most commonly from immune-mediated destruc-tion of the adrenal cortices leading to defici-encies of all adrenocortical hormones. Whilst there is no apparent breed predilection, a hered-itary factor has been suggested in some breeds. It is very rare in the cat.

DISEASE SUMMARIES

Hypothyroidism

Hypothyroidism is a common endocrine disease in the dog. There is a deficiency in the secretion of thyroid hormone either as a result of thyroid gland destruction (primary hypothyroidism), inadequate pituitary production of thyroid stimulating hormone (TSH) (secondary hypothyroidism) or inadequate hypothalamic secretion of thyrotropin releasing hormone (TRH) (tertiary hypothyroidism). Many breeds seem predisposed to hypothyroidism, most notably Dobermann Pinschers and Golden Retrievers.

Immune-mediated destruction of the thyroid gland (*Lymphocytic thyroiditis*) is a common cause of primary hypothyroidism and has been demonstrated to be hereditary in laboratory Beagles and a family of Borzois.

Insulinoma

Insulinomas are functional insulin-secreting tumours of the pancreatic beta cells. Insulin secretion is independent of the normal negative feedback control, resulting in hypoglycaemia. These tumours are generally malignant with a high metastatic potential.

Lymphocytic thyroiditis

See *Hypothyroidism*.

Phaeochromocytoma

Uncommon in dogs and rare in cats, phaeochromocytomas are catecholamine-secreting tumours of the adrenal medulla. Most are slow-growing and benign, but some are malignant and may invade locally, and/or metastasise. The high level of circulating catecholamines produced results in hypertension and tachycardia.

Pituitary dwarfism

Pituitary dwarfism results from a failure of growth hormone secretion in an immature animal. The most striking abnormality is a failure to grow, animals remaining of small stature, but with normal proportional shape (proportionate dwarfism). There may be concurrent failure of other pituitary hormones (panhypopituitarism). The condition is most commonly seen in the German Shepherd Dog but has been identified in several other breeds.

Primary hypoparathyroidism

This is an uncommon condition, wherein lymphocytic plasmacytic destruction of the parathyroid glands results in a deficiency of parathyroid hormone and hypocalcaemia.

Primary hyperparathyroidism
(see plate 15)

Primary hyperparathyroidism is usually the result of a functional parathyroid adenoma (see also *Parathyroid tumours* under Neoplastic conditions). The excess of parathyroid hormone results in hypercalcaemia. The Keeshond seems particularly susceptible to the condition.

Thyroid neoplasia in dogs

Most thyroid tumours in the dog are invasive and malignant carcinomas presenting as readily detectable masses in the neck. Adenomas do occur but are usually small and rarely detected during life. Thyroid tumours in the dog are generally non-functional, only 5–20% being functional, producing clinical signs of hyperthyroidism. Up to 30% of cases become hypothyroid as normal thyroid tissue is destroyed by the tumour. The remainder are euthyroid.

GASTROINTESTINAL CONDITIONS

Alpha-1-antitrypsin related hepatitis

A form of chronic progressive hepatitis associated with the accumulation of the acute-phase protein alpha-1-antitrypsin.

Amyloidosis

Amyloidosis results from the deposition of an insoluble fibrillar protein (amyloid) in a variety of organs, resulting in organ dysfunction. It may occur as an abnormal response to inflammatory or lymphoproliferative disease.

Antral pyloric hypertrophy syndrome (pyloric stenosis)

In this syndrome, gastric-outlet obstruction is caused by hypertrophy of the pyloric muscle, hyperplasia of the antral mucosa or both, and results in persistent vomiting. Congenital

DISEASE SUMMARIES

hypertrophy of the pyloric muscle is seen in young Boxers and Boston Terriers and may be referred to as congenital pyloric stenosis.

Adult-onset antral pyloric hypertrophy syndrome is seen in older (>6 years) small Oriental canine breeds. In these cases there may be antropyloric mucosal hyperplasia only or a combination of mucosal and muscular hypertrophy.

Cholelithiasis

The development of gallstones. Gallstones are uncommon in the dog and where found are usually asymptomatic.

Chronic hepatitis

Inflammatory liver disease which usually progresses to cirrhosis. There are many types of hepatitis, and classification remains controversial, however certain breeds of dog may be predisposed, and individual breeds may demonstrate particular patterns of inflammation.

Chronic idiopathic (lymphocytic-plasmacytic) colitis

Colonic inflammation characterised by the presence of large numbers of lymphocytes and plasma cells in the mucosa. Patients have chronic, intermittent large-bowel-type diarrhoea.

Cleft palate

A congenital defect in the hard or soft palate allowing abnormal communication between the oral cavity and the nasal cavity/nasopharynx.

Congenital bronchoesophageal fistula

This is an abnormal communication between the oesophagus and a bronchus resulting from incomplete separation of these structures in the developing embryo. Symptoms of regurgitation and coughing (especially after eating and drinking) are seen.

Congenital polycystic liver disease

Multiple hepatic cysts usually derived from the bile duct epithelium. They may be associated with cysts in other organs (especially the kidneys). Cysts may also be seen as an acquired lesion.

Congenital portosystemic shunts

Failure of foetal venous shunts to close after birth leads to persistent shunting of blood from the gastrointestinal tract to the systemic circulation without hepatic metabolism. Shunts may be single or multiple, intrahepatic or extrahepatic. Large breeds of dog are more likely to have intrahepatic shunts than small breeds.

Copper storage hepatopathy

Copper accumulation in the liver may be the result of a primary defect in copper excretion resulting in hepatic necrosis, as seen in the Bedlington. Alternatively, copper may accumulate as a result of chronic hepatitis and reduced biliary excretion.

Cricopharyngeal achalasia

Difficulty in swallowing due to failure of the cricopharyngeal sphincter (the upper oesophageal sphincter) to relax.

Diarroheal syndrome of Lundehunds

A chronic progressive form of lymphocytic-plasmacytic enteritis specific to this breed.

Dysphagia

Difficulty swallowing.

Eosinophilic gastroenteritis, enteritis and enterocolitis

Chronic inflammatory disease of the stomach and small intestine, small intestine only, or small intestine and colon. Eosinophilic infiltration is a predominant feature of the inflammation and peripheral eosinophilia may also be present.

Exocrine pancreatic insufficiency

Inadequate production of digestive enzymes leading to malabsorption and chronic diarrhoea. This is most commonly due to *Pancreatic acinar atrophy*, or occasionally due to chronic pancreatitis or pancreatic neoplasia.

Gastric carcinoma (see plate 16)

A primary, malignant stomach tumour derived from epithelial cells.

Gastric dilatation/volvulus

Gastric distension due to the rapid accumulation of food, fluid or gas resulting in torsion of

DISEASE SUMMARIES

the stomach. Usually an acute and severe condition which is rapidly fatal without treatment. Large deep-chested dogs are predisposed.

Gastric neoplasia

Primary stomach tumours include gastric carcinomas, lymphosarcoma, leiomyoma/sarcoma, adenomatous polyps, fibroma/fibrosarcoma, plasmacytoma and squamous cell carcinoma.

Gastro-oesophageal intussusception

Invagination of the stomach into the thoracic oesophagus. A rare condition with high mortality.

Gastrointestinal eosinophilic granuloma

Chronic inflammatory masses which may be found anywhere in the gastrointestinal tract. Histologically, the predominant cell type is the eosinophil.

Gluten-sensitive enteropathy

An intolerance to gluten-containing foods, most commonly seen in Irish Setters. Weight loss and chronic diarrhoea due to malabsorption are seen.

Haemangiosarcoma

See under Neoplastic conditions.

Haemorrhagic gastroenteritis

A haemorrhagic diarrhoea syndrome of unknown cause.

Hepatic lipidosis

A potentially severe liver disease wherein hepatocyte function is compromised by extensive lipid accumulation. Seen most commonly in anorexic, obese female cats, but occasionally seen in puppies of toy breeds.

Hiatal hernia

Displacement of part of the stomach or other abdominal organs cranially through the oseophageal hiatus in the diaphragm. The condition may be congenital or acquired.

Histiocytic colitis

Chronic inflammatory disease of the colon characterised histologically by an inflammatory infiltrate with large numbers of histiocytes. Ulceration of the mucosa may be a prominent feature and the disease tends to be refractory to treatment.

Hypertrophic gastritis

A chronic condition of the stomach characterised by hypertrophy of the mucosa. A diffuse form is seen in the Basenji, whereas a focal form affecting primarily the antrum (part of the *Antral pyloric hypertrophy syndrome*) is seen in small breeds of dog.

Idiopathic hepatic fibrosis

Fibrosis of the liver of unknown cause which is seen without preceeding active inflammation. Various patterns of fibrosis are described. The condition is mostly seen in young dogs. Fibrosis results in portal hypertension, vascular shunting, ascites and hepatic encephalopathy.

Immunoproliferative enteropathy of Basenjis

A specific disease of Basenjis, of unknown cause. Several forms of pathology may be identified in the gastrointestinal tract including hypertrophic gastritis and lymphocytic-plasmacytic enteritis resulting in chronic diarrhoea and protein-losing enteropathy.

Intestinal adenocarcinoma

A malignant tumour found most frequently in the colon of dogs and the jejunum and ileum of cats. Most are locally invasive and metastasise early to the lymph nodes and liver.

Lobular dissecting hepatitis

A form of progressive hepatitis where there is a random pattern of inflammation and fibrosis leading to weight loss and ascites. Seen mostly in young dogs.

Lymphangiectasia

Distension of the lymphatic vessels in the intestinal mucosa. It may be a primary congenital disease, or it may be secondary to other disorders including right-sided heart failure or lipogranulomatous inflammation.

Lymphocytic-plasmacytic enteritis

A form of inflammatory bowel disease in which the cellular infiltrate of the intestinal mucosa is mainly composed of lymphocytes and plasma cells.

DISEASE SUMMARIES

Megacolon

Dilation of the colon which results in constipation.

Megaoesophagus

Oesophageal dilation and reduced motility resulting in regurgitation. Megaoesophagus can be classified as congenital idiopathic megaoesophagus, which presents shortly after weaning, adult-onset idiopathic megaoesophagus which occurs later in life or secondary megaoesophagus where an underlying primary cause can be found.

Microvascular portal dysplasia

Congenital malformation of the intrahepatic portal circulation resulting in vascular shunting and hepatic dysfunction.

Oral eosinophilic granuloma of the Siberian Husky

Raised, ulcerative lesions usually seen on the lateral and ventral areas of the tongue.

Oropharyngeal neoplasia (see plate 17)

The most common canine oropharyngeal tumours are squamous cell carcinomas, malignant melanomas, epulides and fibrosarcomas. The most common feline oropharyngeal tumours are squamous cell carcinomas and fibrosarcomas.

Pancreatic acinar atrophy

A condition where there is spontaneous and progressive loss of pancreatic acinar cells, responsible for the production of digestive enzymes, leading to *Exocrine pancreatic insufficiency*.

Pancreatic carcinoma

A tumour of the duct cells of the pancreas. Uncommon, but usually highly malignant.

Pancreatitis

Inflammation of the pancreas.

Parvovirus enteritis

An infectious viral disease which most commonly causes a severe gastroenteritis, however may also manifest as acute myocarditis or neonatal mortality.

Perianal fistula (anal furunculosis)

Chronically infected and often deep tracts in the soft tissues around the anus.

Portosystemic shunts

See *Congenital portosystemic shunts*.

Protein-losing enteropathy

Excessive loss of plasma proteins via the gastrointestinal tract. It is seen with a number of gastrointestinal and systemic disorders, but particularly with inflammatory enteropathies and lymphangiectasia.

Pyloric dysfunction

Delayed gastric emptying with no evidence of pyloric stenosis. Seen in Siamese cats.

Pyloric stenosis

See *Antral pyloric hypertrophy syndrome*.

Rectal Prolapse

Eversion of the rectum through the anus. Generally seen in young animals.

Salivary mucocoele

An accumulation of saliva in the subcutaneous tissues.

Selective malabsorption of cobalamin (vitamin B$_{12}$)

Malabsorption of vitamin B$_{12}$ (cobalamin) may occur as a result of an absence of the appropriate receptors in the ileum. The condition is inherited in the Giant Schnauzer and symptoms include inappetance, failure to grow and anaemia.

Small intestinal bacterial overgrowth (SIBO)

Increased numbers of bacteria in the upper small intestine associated with chronic diarrhoea. SIBO is often a secondary condition, however in some cases it may be primary with no evidence of other underlying gastrointestinal disease.

Small-intestinal volvulus

A rare condition where the small intestine rotates about its mesenteric axis resulting in

DISEASE SUMMARIES

intestinal obstruction and ischaemia. The condition is rapidly fatal.

Tuberculosis (See also *Mycobacterial infections* under Infectious conditions)
Infection with a species of *Mycobacterium*. Infection may be gained by the oral, respiratory or percutaneous routes and usually gives rise to granulomas in the affected organs. Infected animals are a public health risk.

Vacuolar hepatopathy
A type of liver disease (seen primarily in Miniature Schnauzers with hyperlipidaemia) wherein the hepatocytes appear severely vacuolated on biopsy.

Vascular ring anomaly
Congenital abnormalities of the major thoracic arteries leading to entrapment of the oesophagus and clinical signs of regurgitation at or after weaning. Persistent right aortic arch is the most common vascular ring anomaly.

HAEMATOLOGICAL/ IMMUNOLOGICAL CONDITIONS

Basset Hound thrombopathia
This condition is seen only in Bassets. Clinical signs include prolonged haemorrhage, particularly at surgery and oestrus. Aural haematomas and petechiae are also seen. The platelets demonstrate defective aggregation and retention. The underlying cause is unknown.

Blood groups
Canine blood groups are classified according to the dog erythrocyte antigen (DEA). There are six main groups, DEA 1.1, 1.2, 3, 4, 5 and 7. DEA 1.1 and 1.2 are alleles so it is not possible to be positive for both. Since there are no naturally-occurring autoantibodies to these two groups, an initial blood transfusion doesn't usually cause an acute transfusion reaction. However, if the donor and recipient are incompatible, an immune response will be mounted after the first transfusion, so subsequent incompatible transfusions are likely to cause a

reaction. DEA 1.1 is inherited as an autosomal dominant. A DEA 1.1 negative female bred with a DEA 1.1 positive male may therefore have DEA 1.1 postive pups, and this can lead to neonatal isoerythrolysis.

Feline blood groups are classified into A, B and AB. A is dominant over B, but the inheritance of the rare AB blood group is determined by a different gene. There are high levels of naturally-occurring antibodies against the other groups, so there are no universal donors, and cross-matching or typing is vital before transfusing.

C3 complement deficiency
The complement system is important in neutrophil function and in fighting bacterial infection. There are two pathways, however, so a defect in one does not always lead to immunodeficiency.

Canine leucocyte adhesion deficiency
An inherited defect in the ability of neutrophils to bind to endothelial cells causes severe and recurrent bacterial infections. A molecular diagnostic test is available to diagnose this condition.

Chédiak-Higashi syndrome
In this condition, abnormal lysosomes and neutrophil granules lead to neutrophil dysfunction. Platelet function is also impaired, leading to bleeding. See also under Ocular conditions.

Combined B- and T-cell immunodeficiency
This condition causes severe bacterial infections in young dogs once maternal immunity wanes, from 8–16 weeks of age.

Cyclic haematopoiesis
In this condition, neutrophil numbers decrease every 12 days. There may also be cyclic decreases in platelet, monocyte and reticulocyte numbers.

Factor VII deficiency
This condition leads to a mild clotting disorder. Prothrombin time (PT) is usually prolonged, but activated partial thromboplastin time (APTT) is usually normal, as is consistent with a disorder of the extrinisic pathway.

DISEASE SUMMARIES

Factor X deficiency

Factor X is part of the common pathway, so PT and APTT are both prolonged. A specific factor X assay is used to confirm the diagnosis. The severity of bleeding is variable, and some affected dogs may survive into adulthood.

Factor XI deficiency

Heterozygotes for this condition have about 25–50% of the normal activity of factor XI and are asymptomatic. Homozygotes have about 10% activity and suffer from severe and often lethal bleeding.

Glanzmann's thrombasthenia

This condition affects platelets, leading to decreased platelet retention and absent platelet aggregation. This causes severe mucosal bleeding. Platelet count is usually normal or possibly slightly decreased. The buccal mucosal bleeding time is increased and clot retraction is abnormal. It is inherited as an autosomal recessive trait.

Haemolytic uraemic syndrome

This condition involves hyperaggregability of platelets, leading to platelet thrombi and tissue ischaemia. Clinical signs include neurological symptoms, renal failure, microangiopathic haemolytic anaemia, thrombocytopaenia and pyrexia.

Haemophilia A

This deficiency of factor VIII can cause moderate to severe bleeding. APTT is prolonged, but PT is normal. Many cases may arise from new mutations. The condition is inherited as a sex-linked recessive.

Haemophilia B

Also known as Christmas disease, this clotting deficiency is caused by a deficiency in factor IX. This is a sex-linked condition, but because the size of the gene for factor IX is smaller than for factor VIII, spontaneous mutations are less common for haemophilia B than haemophilia A. APTT is prolonged, but PT is normal.

Hereditary porphyria

This condition leads to anaemia in Siamese cats, but is also seen in non-anaemic domestic short hairs. Affected animals have a defect in haem synthesis. There may also be photosensitisation and red cell haemolysis.

Hereditary stomatocytosis

This condition may lead to a mild anaemia but is usually clinically insignificant.

Immune-mediated haemolytic anaemia
(see plate 18)

Mild to severe anaemia, chronic or acute, can be seen with this condition. Haematology shows anaemia (with a regenerative response if the anaemia is not too acute) and spherocytosis. Although many cases respond well to treatment, the potential for serious complications means the prognosis for this condition is guarded.

Immune-mediated thrombocytopaenia

This is a common disorder, characterised by immune-mediated destruction of platelets. Epistaxis, haematochezia and mucosal haemorrhage are often seen.

Immunodeficiency syndrome of Irish Wolfhounds

Respiratory conditions in related Irish Wolfhounds have been attributed to an underlying immunodeficiency, possibly in cell-mediated immunity or in IgA.

Increased osmotic fragility of erythrocytes

Extreme fragility of the erythrocytes can lead to recurrent and severe anaemia, with splenomegaly and weight loss. Prednisolone and blood transfusions may be helpful.

Lethal acrodermatitis

Clinical signs of this condition include dermatological and respiratory problems and stunted growth. Plasma zinc levels are low and tissue T-lymphocytes are depleted.

Methaemoglobin reductase deficiency

This condition causes dark brown mucous membranes and cyanotic blood vessels. Severe methaemoglobinaemia is seen which may be life-threatening. Management is by avoidance of oxidative agents such as onion, drugs and certain food components.

DISEASE SUMMARIES

Non-spherocytic haemolytic anaemia

This condition is due to a defect in the calcium pump system. Chronic haemolysis may lead to myelofibrosis.

Neutrophil function defect

Defects in neutrophil function lead to recurrent and/or severe bacterial infections. A pronounced left shift neutrophilia may be present.

Pelger-Huet anomaly

This anomaly involves a decreased segmentation of granulocyte nuclei. There doesn't seem to be an increased predisposition to infection in these cases.

Phosphofructokinase deficiency

Haemolytic crises and exertional myopathy are seen with this relatively common enzyme deficiency. Exercise intolerance is often seen. A PCR-based DNA test is available for affected dogs and carriers.

Platelet storage-pool deficiency

This condition leads to moderate to severe haemorrhage. Platelet counts are normal, but buccal mucosal bleeding time is prolonged.

Predisposition to tuberculosis

A report has shown five Bassets that developed systemic tuberculosis. It is thought that an immune deficiency, possibly in cell-mediated immunity, was responsible.

Primary idiopathic hyperlipidaemia

This poorly understood familial condition can cause multisystemic signs such as abdominal pain, seizures and pancreatitis.

Pyruvate kinase deficiency

In this condition of erythrocytes, the affected cells lose the ability to retain their normal shape and have a reduced affinity for oxygen and a shortened lifespan.

Selective IgA deficiency

This condition causes different clinical signs in different breeds, including dermatological disease, respiratory disease such as rhinitis, and gastrointestinal disease such as small intestinal bacterial overgrowth and anal furunculosis.

Selective malabsorption of cobalamin (vitamin B$_{12}$)

See under Gastrointestinal conditions.

Spitz Dog thrombopathia

This condition is similar to Basset Hound thrombopathia. Intermittent mucosal bleeding is seen.

Systemic lupus erythematosus

Diagnosis of this uncommon disease is made on the basis of the presence of at least two signs of autoimmune disease, together with high levels of antinuclear antibodies (ANA) (although 10% of cases are ANA negative). Clinical manifestations include polyarthritis, mucocutaneous lesions, glomerular disease, autoimmune haemolytic anaema, autoimmune thrombocytopaenia and neurological signs.

T-cell dysfunction

This condition of Weimaraners is associated with growth hormone deficiency, thymic aplasia and dysfunction of T-cells.

Tail tip necrosis

This condition has been reported in Birman kittens and is thought to be due to neonatal isoerythrolysis involving cold agglutins.

Thymic aplasia

This congenital condition causes signs of stunted growth, wasting and suppurative pneumonia.

Transient hypogammaglobulinaemia

This condition can lead to a delay in developing active immunity, leading to recurrent respiratory infections. However, most affected puppies are normal by eight months of age.

Undefined immunodeficiency syndrome (susceptibility to *Pneumocystis carinii*)

A predisposition to respiratory disease caused by this organism is suspected to be caused by an underlying immunodeficiency, but the exact nature of this is not known.

Vaccine-associated vasculitis

Routine vaccinations in Weimaraners occasionally cause an acute systemic vasculitis, with gastrointestinal signs, hypertrophic osteodystrophy and lameness.

Vitamin-K-dependent coagulopathy

Clinical signs of this condition include prolonged bleeding post surgery or trauma. It is thought that an autosomal recessive defect in hepatic vitamin K metabolism leads to reduced levels of factors II, VII, IX and X. Affected animals can be detected by demonstrating a prolonged PT and APTT.

Von Willebrand's disease

This is the commonest inherited disorder of haemostasis in dogs, and is caused by a deficiency in von Willebrand's factor (vWF), which is vital for platelet function. There are three recognised types: type I involves a quantitative reduction in vWF, and the severity of the disease varies with breed. Some individuals respond to desmopressin (DDAVP) treatment; type II disease also involves a quantitative reduction in vWF, but the condition is more severe than type I, and there is no response to DDAVP; type III disease is characterised by a complete absence of vWF leading to the most severe clinical disease, again with no response to DDAVP. Genetic tests are also available to identify carriers of the gene to allow appropriate selection of breeding stock.

INFECTIOUS CONDITIONS

Aspergillosis (see figure 21)

Aspergillosis is an opportunist fungal infection. In the dog it generally presents as a nasal and frontal sinus infection and dolichocephalic breeds seem predisposed. In cats the condition is much less common and presents as a systemic disease with variable organ involvement.

Blastomycosis

Blastomycosis is systemic fungal infection, caused by *Blastomyces dermatitidis* seen primarily in North America. The lungs are the site of initial infection and from there it may spread to the lymphatics, skin, eyes and bones. Dogs are more commonly infected than cats, young, male, large sporting-breed dogs living close to water being at greatest risk.

Coccidiomycosis

Coccidiomycosis is a systemic fungal infection, caused by *Coccidioides immitis*, seen primarily in

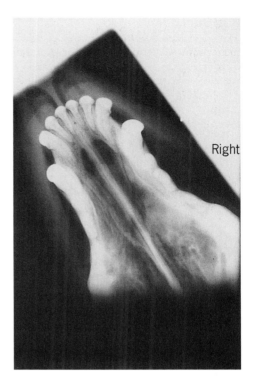

Right

Figure 21
Nasal aspergillosis in a two-year-old female Jack Russell Terrier. The right side of the nose shows loss of the turbinate pattern, increased radiodensity due to exudate and some punctate lucencies caudally.

the desert regions of North America. Infection originates in the lungs but may disseminate. Young, male, large-breed dogs kept outside seem predisposed, possibly due to increased chance of contact with the pathogen.

Cryptococcosis

Cryptococcosis is a systemic fungal infection, caused by *Cryptococcus neoformans*, which is found worldwide and may be spread by pigeons. It infects a wide range of mammalian species but is most commonly seen in the cat. Clinical signs may reflect nasal, respiratory, central nervous system, ocular or cutaneous involvement.

DISEASE SUMMARIES

Histoplasmosis

The causal organism, *Histoplasma capsulatum*, is a saprophytic soil fungus. It is uncommon and occurs mainly in the central USA. Clinical signs include fever, anorexia, weight loss, cough, dyspnoea and ocular and skin lesions.

Mycobacterial infections

Mycobacteria are aerobic, acid-fast bacteria with each species having a variation in host affinity and disease potential. Tuberculosis is caused by *M. tuberculosis*, *M. bovis*, *M. microti* or *M. avium*. The organisms cause granulomas and the site of formation determines the symptoms. Respiratory disease is more common in the dog, cutaneous or alimentary disease in the cat. Treatment is not always recommended as the disease has zoonotic potential.

Parvovirus enteritis

See under Gastrointestinal conditions.

Pneumocystis carinii infection

A protozoal infection which may result in pneumonia in the presence of immunosuppression (see also Haematological/immunological conditions).

Infectious conditions of the skin

See under Dermatological conditions.

MUSCULOSKELETAL CONDITIONS

Accessory carpal bone fracture

These fractures are sprain-avulsion type injuries caused by carpal hyperextension during racing. Carpal pain may be present.

Achondroplasia

Achondroplastic breeds are specifically bred for this condition. They have short maxillae, flared metaphyses and short, bowed limbs. This is accepted as part of the breed standard.

Alaskan Malamute chondrodysplasia

This condition leads to short limbs with bowed front legs and laterally deviated paws. Haemolytic anaemia is often also seen.

Angular deformity of tibia

In this condition, distal tibial growth plate injury or premature closure of the lateral aspect results in tarsal valgus.

Arthropathy associated with Scottish Fold cats

This condition has recently been characterised as an osteochondrodysplasia associated with inadequate cartilage maturation. A radiographic survey showed that all Scottish Fold cats examined were affected, whether or not they were symptomatic.

Avulsion of the tibial tuberosity

(see figure 22)

This is a fracture of the growth plate, which is seen more commonly in dogs with large quadriceps muscles.

Bilateral radial agenesis

In this inherited condition, the radius is partially or completely absent, and the ulna is shorter and thicker.

Bone cysts

These are benign, uncommon cystic lesions. Intramedullary metaphyseal haemorrhage may be involved. They are often asymptomatic, but may enlarge to cause pain or even pathological fracture.

Brachyury

Dogs of breeds with normally long tails occasionally develop with short tails. This is known as brachyury.

Bull Terrier osteochondrodysplasia

This condition leads to an abnormal gait with possible femoral neck fractures. Some long bones are distorted.

Burmese head defect

This congenital defect is inherited and has been described as autosomal recessive or autosomal dominant with incomplete penetrance. Heterozygotes have a range of facial dimensions. The condition is fatal to homozygotes. It is seen in the eastern, 'new look' or contemporary strain

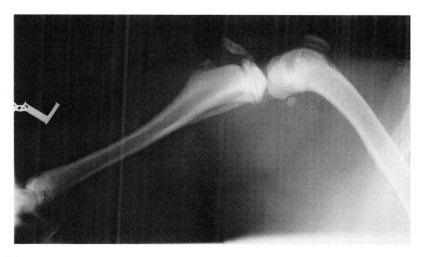

Figure 22
Lateral radiograph of the left stifle of an eight-month-old male Staffordshire Bull Terrier with avulsion of the tibial crest.

of Burmese. The upper maxillary region is duplicated.

Calcaneoquartal subluxation due to plantar tarsal ligament rupture

This is a common condition in athletic dogs, usually occurring in racing, but can also occur without a history of trauma in middle-aged pet dogs. The condition may be bilateral.

Calcaneus fracture

Extreme tension on the plantar side of the calcaneus or central tarsal bone fracture lead to calcaneal fractures, particularly in racing dogs. The right is usually affected due to the stresses generated while cornering left.

Carpal ligament weakening

Gradual degeneration and subsequent weakening of the carpal ligaments leads to subluxation and luxation of the carpus. The tarsus is also sometimes involved. Obesity predisposes, so weight loss is recommended.

Carpal soft-tissue injury

Soft-tissue injuries of the carpus are common in working dogs. Collateral ligament injuries,

hyperextension injuries and luxations can be involved.

Cartilaginous exostosis

Osteochondromatous outgrowths from the long bones, scapula, ilium, vertebrae and phalanges can be seen radiographically in this condition.

Central core myopathy

This very rare condition leads to signs of muscle weakness which becomes progressively more severe. The reported cases were euthanased before two years of age.

Central tarsal bone fracture

This fracture is very uncommon in non-athletic dogs, but is common in racing Greyhounds. The fracture usually involves an avulsion of the plantar process. There are usually other tarsal bone fractures associated.

Chronic sesamoid disease

Chronic sesamoiditis may be an incidental finding on radiographs or a cause of lameness. Clinical signs include a gradual onset of lameness in one or both forelimbs.

DISEASE SUMMARIES

Cleft palate/lip

This congenital condition involves a variety of possible defects including a unilateral cleft lip, incomplete fusion of the soft palate or an oronasal fistula.

Congenital elbow luxation

This condition is uncommon. There are two recognised types: type I is more severe and results in a 90° outward rotation of the proximal ulna. Lateral deviation of the antebrachium is seen, with marked reduction in elbow extension. The cause is unknown. Diagnosis is by radiography. Closed reduction is the treatment of choice, but some cases require open reduction. In type II luxation, the proximal radius is displaced caudolaterally. This type is less severe than type I. Some animals require no treatment, while others may require surgery, such as osteotomy of the radius or ulna.

Congenital scapulohumeral luxation

This is a rare condition, usually occurring at an early age, but may be a sequel to minor trauma in an adult. The deviation is usually medial, and craniocaudal radiographs will confirm this.

Cranial cruciate ligament rupture
(see figure 23)

This common injury often presents as a severe, acute onset lameness. Diagnosis is by ascertaining the presence of a 'cranial drawer' motion in the stifle, by radiography and by arthroscopy or arthrotomy.

Craniomandibular osteopathy

This condition is inherited in some breeds, but other factors may be important in others. Clinical signs include mandibular swelling, drooling and pain on opening the mouth. Irregular bone proliferation is seen on radiographs. The disorder is usually self-limiting, although in some cases hemimandibulectomy may be necessary.

Delayed/non-union of fractures of the distal third of the radius and ulna in Miniature and Toy breeds

There is a disproportionately high incidence of malunion following repair of fractures of the

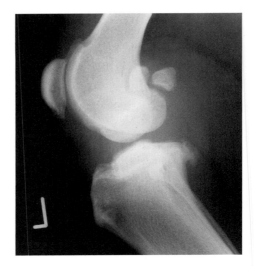

Figure 23
Lateral radiograph of a stifle, demonstrating cranial cruciate ligament disease. Courtesy of Andy Moores.

distal third of the radial and ulnar diaphyses. Inadequate immobilisation, infection and an easily disrupted blood supply to the bones may be responsible. Rigid fixation with plates or external fixators help reduce the risk.

Elbow dysplasia

Genetics and rapid growth predispose to this complex of diseases which include an ununited anconeal process, medial coronoid process disease and osteochondritis dissecans of the medial humeral condyle. It may be that elbow dysplasia is caused by osteochondrosis, possibly relating to incongruities of the trochlear notch. In the UK and USA there are screening schemes for elbow dysplasia in operation.

English Pointer enchondrodystrophy

This condition leads to short limbs and bowed front legs, with an abnormal gait.

Enostosis

Also known as panosteitis or eosinophilic panosteitis. This condition is fairly common, affecting young dogs aged 6–18 months. Acute intermittent lameness affecting one or more

DISEASE SUMMARIES

limbs is seen, often associated with pyrexia. A viral aetiology is suspected. The condition is usually self-limiting.

Exertional myopathy

Precipitated by over-exertion in unfit dogs or in hot and humid conditions, this condition has a variable severity. Hyperacute cases show severe pain leading to myoglobinuria, acute renal failure and death, whereas acute cases have a lower mortality. A non-fatal subacute form is also seen.

Familial Mediterranean fever (See also *Renal amyloidosis* under Renal conditions)

Renal failure, associated with amyloidosis and swollen joints, is found in this condition. Hypergammaglobulinaemia and raised serum levels of interleukin-6 are seen.

Fibrotic myopathy of semitendinosus muscle

This condition is seen in young to middle-aged dogs. A fibrous band of tissue develops in the semitendinosus muscle, leading to a reduced ability to extend the affected limb. This condition may be part of a complex with *Gracilis contracture*.

Foramen magnum dysplasia

This condition involves a malformation of the occipital bone and enlargement of the foramen magnum. There may be concurrent hydrocephalus and exposure of the brain stem and cerebellum. See also *Hydrocephalus* under Neurological conditions.

Gastrocnemius tendon avulsion

The gastrocnemius tendon becomes avulsed from the calcaneus, leading to an acute lameness or a chronic lameness with thickened tendons.

Glycogen storage diseases types II and III

Type II glycogen storage disease (Pompe's disease) causes weakness and exercise intolerance. Vomiting and cardiovascular abnormalities are seen. The prognosis is poor. Type III glycogen storage disease (Cori's disease) leads to poor growth, weakness and liver disease. This disease is rare and also has a poor prognosis.

Gracilis contracture

This is usually seen in athletic dogs and leads to a gait alteration. This condition may be part of a complex with *Fibrotic myopathy of semitendinosus*. Surgery can help but the condition can recur.

Hemivertebrae

These abnormal vertebrae are wedge-shaped and are often associated with angulation of the spine. See also under Neurological conditions.

Hereditary canine spinal muscular atrophy

This condition is a motor neurone disease. Homozygotes for the condition have an accelerated form of the disease, whereas heterozygotes have an intermediate or chronic form. Dogs are usually affected at less than one year of age.

Hereditary myopathy of Devon Rex

This hereditary disease leads to clinical signs of generalised muscle weakness, collapse on exercise, ventroflexion of the neck and sometimes death from laryngospasm, possibly due to oropharyngeal weakness.

Hip dysplasia (HD)

This very common condition occurs in a wide range of breeds. Various deformities in the hip lead to joint instability with the development of degenerative joint disease. Genetics undoubtedly play a role, but environmental factors, such as nutrition and exercise, are also important. Various screening programmes are used around the world to attempt to reduce the incidence of this condition. Estimates of heritability vary from 20–60%, depending on breed, population examined and methods applied. Note that, for the purposes of this text, only the top 20 breeds for HD, as scored by the British Veterinary Association/Kennel Club Hip Dysplasia Scheme, have been included. However, this is potentially misleading, as variable numbers have been scored, and there is some inherent bias in the scheme in that some vets do not send the worst X-rays for scoring. More information can be obtained from the British Veterinary Association.

DISEASE SUMMARIES

Hypokalaemic myopathy

Clinical signs of this condition include ventroflexion of the neck and transient weakness. There may also be a tremor. Serum potassium levels of less than 3 mmol/l are seen.

Idiopathic polyarthritis

Pain in more than one joint often suggests an immune-mediated polyarthritis. Canine idiopathic polyarthritis is the most common form of immune-mediated arthropathy. Approximately 25% of cases are associated with chronic infection remote from the joint, 15% are associated with gastrointestinal disease and another subset is associated with neoplasia remote from the joints. In the other cases, which account for about 50%, there is no other pathology or underlying aetiology detected.

Incomplete ossification of the humeral condyle

This condition may present with a history of mild intermittent lameness which is unresponsive to anti-inflammatory drugs. Acute severe lameness may follow exercise or mild trauma, corresponding with a humeral condylar fracture.

Increased anteversion of the femoral head and neck

This is associated with gait abnormalities, joint laxity and pain. It is a component of hip dysplasia.

Inguinal/scrotal herniation

Females are over-represented in this common condition. An inguinal mass or swelling is usually seen, although occasionally gastrointestinal signs are present.

Irish Setter hypochondroplasia

The limbs are slightly shortened in this condition. The ulna and radius may be bowed and carpal valgus is seen.

Juvenile onset distal myopathy

This recently recognised condition has been reported in several pups and has been described as a muscular dystrophy. Clinical signs include decreased activity and various postural abnormalities.

Labrador Retriever myopathy

This is an uncommon condition, but is widespread throughout the UK. Clinical signs include generalised muscle weakness, exercise intolerance and muscle wasting. Black- and yellow-coated Labradors are affected, and the condition is more common in working lines.

Lateral patellar luxation

Also known as genu valgum. This condition is often seen in the same breeds that are affected by hip dysplasia. There may be a genetic pattern of occurrence. Both stifles are often affected, causing a knock-kneed stance from five to six months of age.

Lateral torsion and tarsal valgus deformity

This condition is untreatable but rarely causes a clinical problem, being mainly a cosmetic fault.

Legg-Calve-Perthe's disease
(see figure 24)

This condition involves an aseptic, avascular necrosis of the femoral head. Signs are usually seen from five months of age. Ischaemia of the femoral head leads to degeneration of the bone which presents as a progressive uni- or bilateral hind-limb lameness.

Lumbosacral disease

Inefficient facet geometry at the lumbosacral junction leads to an increase in osteophyte formation. This can be associated with a risk of lumbosacral stenosis.

Masticatory myopathy

Also known as eosinophilic myositis, masticatory myositis. This is a common condition and demonstrates acute and chronic forms. The acute disease presents with swelling of the masticatory muscles and trismus. The chronic form demonstrates atrophy of the masticatory muscles, with histology showing marked muscle fibrosis. The condition is immune mediated.

Medial coronoid process disease

This common condition is part of the osteochondrosis complex which affects the elbow. Fragmentation of the medial coronoid process

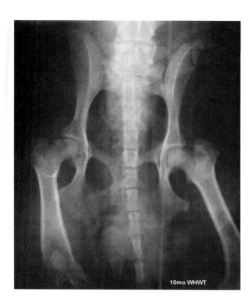

10mo WHWT

Figure 24
Ventrodorsal radiograph of a ten-month-old
West Highland White with aseptic necrosis
of the femoral head and neck – Legg-Calve-
Perthes – disease. Courtesy of Andy
Moores.

occurs, with the fragments usually remaining
attached to the annular ligament. Degenerative
joint disease usually ensues. Signs of lameness
are seen from four to five months of age.

Medial displacement of biceps brachii tendon

A gradual onset in lameness which is exacer-
bated by exercise is seen with this unusual
condition. Palpation and manipulation of the
shoulder can reveal pain, crepitus and sometimes a palpable popping of the tendon out of
the intertubercular groove.

Medial patellar luxation

This condition usually presents as an intermittent lameness, although in bilateral cases it may
present as a hind-limb gait abnormality. It is
usually seen from six months of age, although in
some cases may not cause clinical signs until the
animal is older.

Mitochondrial myopathy

A defect in mitochondrial function leads to
decreased exercise tolerance with tachycardia
and tachypnoea resulting from severe acidosis.
This condition can occasionally cause sudden
death.

Mucopolysaccharidosis

This group of conditions results from inherited
chromosomal abnormalities and leads to a
metabolic bone disease. Type I disease causes a
large broad head which may be associated with
ocular and cardiac abnormalities. Pectus excava-
tum, fusion of the cervical vertebrae and hip
subluxations also occur. Type VI disease causes
dwarfism and skeletal, neurological and retinal
abnormalities. There is no treatment, although
some affected animals may have an acceptable
quality of life.

Multiple enchondromatosis

This inherited condition leads to short bowed
limbs with distorted diaphyses. Femoral neck
fractures are seen, and the sternum lacks bone.

Multiple epiphyseal dysplasia

This inherited condition leads to short limbs,
enlarged joints, hip dysplasia and osteoar-
thropathy in adults.

Muscular dystrophy

A sex-linked muscular dystrophy of Golden
Retriever's found in the USA has been found to
be similar to Duchenne's muscular dystrophy of
humans. Clinical signs include exercise intolerance, gait abnormalities, trismus and occasionally
cardiac involvement. Creatinine kinase (CK)
is massively elevated on biochemistry. Other
muscular dystrophies in dogs include the
facioscapulohumeral type in Springers, which is
associated with persistent atrial standstill. A
condition resembling oculopharyngeal muscular
dystrophy of humans has been reported in
Bouviers.

Myasthenia gravis

See under Neurological conditions.

DISEASE SUMMARIES

Myopathy associated with falling Cavalier King Charles Spaniels

Episodic collapse, often associated with exercise or excitement may be due to ultrastructural changes in the affected dog's myocytes, but the exact cause is currently unclear. See also *Episodic collapse* under Neurological conditions.

Myotonia

Clinical signs of this condition include excess muscle mass, stiff gait after rest and collapse. Dyspnoea may be seen if the respiratory muscles are involved.

Ocular-skeletal dysplasia

This condition is inherited as an autosomal recessive, and causes clinical signs of shortened limbs and deviated joints, associated with ocular signs such as cataracts and retinal detachment. See also *Retinal dysplasia with skeletal defects* under Ocular conditions.

Odontoid process dysplasia

This condition results in atlantoaxial subluxation causing signs ranging from neck pain to quadraplegia. See also *Atlantoaxial subluxation* under Neurological conditions.

Osteochondrosis

Osteochondrosis is characterised by abnormal development of the cartilage in the physeal and epiphyseal sites. Common regions for osteochondrosis are the caudal humeral head, the medial condyle of the humerus, the medial coronoid process of the ulna, the anconeal process of the elbow, the lateral and medial condyles of the stifle and the medial ridge of the talus.

Osteogenesis imperfecta

This group of inherited diseases causes osteopaenia and increased bone fragility. The underlying defect is probably in collagen formation. The condition is rare, and the exact mode of inheritance is unknown. Cases may present with a history of multiple fractures with little or no trauma.

Osteosarcoma

This malignant tumour tends to affect the metaphyses of long bones, although they may also be seen in the axial skeleton. Rapid bone growth during early development, particularly in large- and giant-breed dogs may be involved in the aetiology, but a genetic predisposition is also suspected in some breeds. See also Neoplastic conditions.

Patellar luxation

Luxation of the patella can be due to abnormalities of the patellar groove or of the position of the tibial crest. It can cause chronic or intermittent lameness.

Patellar pain

This condition may be associated with patellar luxation, even after surgery, or may occur in the absence of luxation. Pain is seen on pressing the patella into the trochlear groove.

Perineal hernia

This relatively common condition presents as a swelling in the perineal region or as a defect palpable per rectum. Urinary bladder retroflexion with associated metabolic complications is seen in 20% of dogs.

Pes varus

This is seen at five to six months of age, and is probably related to an underlying tibial dysplasia.

Plasmacytic-lymphocytic gonitis

This condition of unknown aetiology leads to joint laxity and instability and is seen in up to 10% of dogs undergoing surgery of the cranial cruciate ligament.

Polyarthritis/meningitis

The underlying disorder in this condition is an idiopathic polyarteritis, which may be becoming more common. The main clinical signs are related to meningitis, such as neck pain and fever, but joint inflammation is not unusual. The severity of the disease varies with breed. Milder forms are often self-limiting, but the more severe forms may not be.

Polydactyly/syndactyly

Several breeds show a tendency to more than the normal number of digits (polydactyly) or

DISEASE SUMMARIES

fused digits (syndactyly). Often these abnormalities do not cause a clinical problem.

Prognathia
Overshot jaw.

Pseudoachondrodysplasia
This condition leads to short, bent limb bones and short vertebrae. Osteopaenia may be seen.

Pyruvate kinase deficiency
As well as haematological abnormalities, this inherited condition can lead to intramedullary osteosclerosis.

Retrognathia
Undershot jaw.

Sacrocaudal dysgenesis
See under Neurological conditions.

Scottish Fold arthropathy
Scottish Fold cats have abnormally shaped ears, due to an abnormality in the ear cartilage (inherited as a simple autosomal dominant). Homozygotes for this defect can develop generalised cartilage defects causing a shortening and thickening of the bones of the limbs, tail and spine and a progressive arthropathy.

Shoulder luxation
This condition usually occurs at three to four months. Flexed and rotated views of the shoulders can reveal the abnormality on radiography.

Spondylosis deformans
Also known as ankylosing spondylitis. Bony spurs (osteophytes) form around the margins of the vertebral endplates. They become more common with age, and are often apparent radiographically, but are rarely of clinical significance.

Spontaneous tibial fracture
Spontaneous fractures of the caudal distal articular margin of the tibia have been reported in racing Greyhounds, often associated with malleolar fractures. Degenerative joint disease is a common sequel, so prognosis after internal fixation is guarded.

Superficial digital flexor tendon luxation
This uncommon condition causes acute but moderate lameness. A calcaneal bursal effusion is seen. The luxation is usually lateral.

Temporomandibular dysplasia/luxation
Abnormal development of the articular surfaces leads to temporomandibular dysplasia with laxity of the joint. The condition can be seen from six months of age. Clinical signs include open mouth locking, often associated with yawning, and luxation which may be chronic. Degenerative joint disease and masticatory muscle wastage may be seen in chronic cases.

Transitional lumbosacral vertebra
This anomaly is characterised by separation of the first sacral segment identified on the lateral view of a radiograph by the presence of a radiolucent disc space between what are normally the first and second sacral segments. On the ventrodorsal view, there is separation of the spinous processes between what are normally the first and second sacral segments. The sacroiliac attachment is often weakened, leading to premature disc degeneration. Together with spinal canal stenosis, this can lead to cauda equina syndrome.

Umbilical hernia
In this condition, the umbilical ring fails to close at birth, and as abdominal pressure increases with age, abdominal fat and even intestines can be forced through. Many of these cases require surgical repair.

Ununited anconeal process
In German Shepherd Dogs the anconeal process develops as a separate centre of ossification, which should be fused to the ulna by twenty weeks. Failure of fusion leads to an ununited anconeal process which is part of the elbow osteochondrosis complex. Degenerative joint disease often occurs, leading to a lameness which is seen from four to five months of age.

Vaccine-associated vasculitis with hypertrophic osteopathy
This vasculitis, which is associated with routine vaccinations, leads to initial gastrointestinal

DISEASE SUMMARIES

signs, which later develop into lameness and hypertrophic osteodystrophy.

Von Willebrand heterotopic osteochondrofibrosis

In this condition a mass of bony, fibrous or cartilaginous tissue develops near the hip muscles. A severe lameness can result, which is mainly mechanical in nature.

NEOPLASTIC CONDITIONS

Actinic keratosis

These lesions are often associated with chronic sun exposure, so are generally seen in pale-skinned areas of animals with outside access. Lesions may be single or multifocal, and plaque-like or papillomatous with hyperkeratosis. They may progress to squamous cell carcinoma which has the potential for local invasion and distant metastasis.

Adrenocortical tumour

Adrenocortical tumours are responsible for 15–20% of hyperadrenocorticism cases in the dog, and 20% in the cat (see under Endocrine conditions). They are usually unilateral (although 10% of cases have bilateral tumours) and may be adenomas or carcinomas. The latter may be invasive and metastasise.

Anal sac adenocarcinoma

Anal sac adenocarcinoma is a malignant tumour which is palpable as a discrete or infiltrative mass in the anal sac. These tumours are often associated with hypercalcaemia and metastasise early to the sublumbar lymph nodes, spleen and lung. They are rare in the cat.

Anaplastic sarcoma

A poorly-differentiated malignant soft-tissue tumour derived from the mesenchymal connective tissues of the body.

Basal cell tumour

These common skin tumours arise from the basal epithelial cells which give rise to the epidermis. They are usually well-circumscribed, firm, freely-mobile masses found in the dermis

and subcutis around the head and neck. They are generally slow-growing and benign in behaviour, rarely metastasising.

Benign fibrous histiocytoma
(see plate 19)

These rare skin tumours may be reactive proliferations rather than true neoplasias. Lesions can be solitary or multiple and predilection sites include the face, legs and scrotum.

Canine anterior uveal melanoma

See under Ocular conditions.

Canine cutaneous histiocytoma
(see plate 20)

These skin tumours are commonly seen in young dogs, and appear as solitary, firm, well-circumscribed intradermal nodules on the head, limbs or trunk. Occasionally the surface will ulcerate. They are benign and most will regress spontaneously over a period of months.

Chemodectoma

Chemodectomas are derived from the chemoreceptor cells of the aortic and carotid bodies which detect changes in the blood pH, oxygen and carbon dioxide levels. Chemodectoma of the aortic body arises at the heart base and is reported more frequently than carotid body tumours which arise at the bifurcation of the carotid artery and present as a cervical mass. Both are relatively uncommon in the dog and cat, but brachycephalic dogs appear predisposed. Chemodectomas may be locally invasive and have the potential to metastasise.

Chondrosarcoma

This is the second most common primary bone tumour of dogs accounting for 5–10% of cases. It is generally slower growing and metastasises less frequently than the osteosarcoma.

Colorectal cancer

Intestinal canacer is not common in the dog or cat. In the dog, cancer of the large intestine is more common than that of the small intestine, adenocarcinoma / carcinoma being the most common malignant tumour. In cats most tumours arise in the small intestine.

Cutaneous papillomas

These are pedunculated or vegetative skin growths found in older dogs and are distinct from the virally-induced papillomas found on the mucous membranes of young dogs. They are considered benign.

Cutaneous plasmacytoma

These neoplasms are derived from plasma cells. They occur commonly on the digits, the lips, the chin and the ear canal.

Fibromatous epulis

A common oral tumour of the dog presenting as a firm gingival mass. These tumours are benign, neither invading locally nor metastasising.

Fibroma

These are uncommon benign neoplasms. They are usually solitary, well-circumscribed lesions.

Fibrosarcoma

A fibrosarcoma is a malignant tumour derived from fibrous tissues and may be found in many sites including the bone, skin, spleen and oral cavity. Tumour behaviour varies with the site and histological grade. In general, fibrosarcomas are locally invasive but have a relatively low rate of metastasis (25% has been suggested for oral fibrosarcoma).

Haemangioma

Haemangiomas are benign tumours arising from the vascular endothelial cells of the dermis and subcutis. They are common in dogs but rare in cats. They appear as well-circumscribed blue/purple masses.

Haemangiosarcoma

This is a highly malignant tumour arising from vascular endothelial cells. Primary sites include the right atrium of the heart, spleen, liver, skin, bone, nervous system, kidney, bladder and oral cavity. Metastasis to a wide variety of sites is common, in many cases micrometastasis having occurred by the time of diagnosis.

Haemangiopericytoma

These common tumours are derived from vascular pericytes. They are usually well-circumscribed and are often found on the limbs. Metastasis is rare, but they frequently recur locally, so treatment of choice is wide surgical excision or amputation.

Histiocytosis

A disorder of histiocytes which takes two forms, both relatively rare. In *Malignant histiocytosis*, proliferation of histiocytes results in solid tumour masses in a variety of organs including the spleen, liver, lymph nodes and lung. The disease is rapidly progressive and fatal. It has been most commonly reported in the Bernese Mountain Dog, but occasionally in other breeds. *Systemic histiocytosis* follows a more chronic, fluctuating course and involves the skin, eyes and peripheral lymph nodes. Systemic histiocytosis has only been reported in the Bernese Mountain Dog and is more often seen in younger dogs than the malignant form.

Insulinoma

See under Endocrine conditions.

Intestinal adenocarcinoma

See under Gastrointestinal conditions.

Keratoacanthoma

Also known as intracutaneous cornifying epithelioma. These benign cutaneous neoplasms can be solitary or multiple.

Limbal melanoma

See under Ocular conditions.

Lipoma (see plate 21)

Benign tumours of fat cells which are generally found in the subcutaneous tissues. They are common, affecting up to 16% of dogs. Infiltrative lipomas are locally invasive making surgical excision more difficult, but they do not metastasise.

Liposarcoma

These rare malignant tumours arise from the subcutaneous lipoblasts. These tumours are infiltrative but rarely metastasise.

Lymphosarcoma

Lymphosarcoma is a malignant lymphoproliferative disease also commonly termed malignant lymphoma. Lymphosarcoma is the most common haematopoietic tumour in the dog and cat. Lymphosarcoma may be classified anatomically by the location of the disease (multicentric, mediastinal, alimentary, cutaneous or extranodal), histologically or immunophenotypically as B-cell or T-cell.

Malignant histiocytosis
See *Histiocytosis*.

Mammary tumours
These are common in both the dog and the cat. Mammary tumours are derived from the epithelial and sometimes myoepithelial tissues of the mammary glands. In dogs approximately 50% are benign, in cats over 80% are malignant. Entire animals or those spayed after several seasons are predisposed. Behaviour varies depending on the histological grade, but malignant mammary tumours may be very aggressive, metastasising to the local lymph nodes, lungs and occasionally the abdominal organs and bone.

Mast cell tumours (see plates 22 and 23)
Mast cell tumours are relatively common in dogs, representing up to 20% of skin tumours. They may present in a wide variety of forms so need to be included in the differential of all skin masses. Behaviour varies from benign to highly-aggressive malignant tumours which have the potential to metastasise (usually to the liver, spleen or kidney). Cutaneous mast cell tumours are less common in the cat, but systemic and intestinal forms of mast cell tumour may also be seen in this species.

Melanoma
Melanomas represent 4–6% of canine skin tumours and 1–2% of all feline skin tumours. They present as firm, pigmented dermal masses and are more common in dark-skinned dogs. Those found on the digits and close to mucocutaneous junctions tend to be more malignant and may metastasise to local lymph nodes, lungs and other more distant sites.

Myxoma/myxosarcoma
These rare neoplasms arise from fibroblasts and occur more frequently on the limbs, dorsum or inguinal regions. Myxomas are benign and myxosarcomas are malignant.

Nasal cavity tumours
The most common nasal cavity tumours diagnosed in the dog are carcinomas (in particular adenocarcinomas). Other types include sarcomas (fibrosarcoma, chondrosarcoma or osteosarcoma), lymphoma and melanoma. Most are malignant, causing local invasion and progressive destruction, but are slow to metastasise. Dolichocephalic dogs, particularly of large and medium size, are reported to be at increased risk. In the cat, adenocarcinoma is the most common tumour followed by lymphoma.

Non-epitheliotropic lymphoma
This uncommon neoplasia is a form of cutaneous lymphosarcoma. It is usually generalised or multifocal. Nodules are seen in the dermis, and spread to the lymph nodes and internal organs may occur.

Osteosarcoma
Osteosarcoma is the most common of the malignant primary bone tumours in the dog. It is rapid in growth and highly invasive and destructive. Osteosarcoma of the appendicular skeleton of dogs is highly malignant and metastasises early (commonly to the lungs). In common with other primary bone tumours, appendicular osteosarcoma is more common in large- and giant-breed dogs. Osteosarcoma of the axial skeleton (including the skull) is generally considered less malignant. Osteosarcoma in the cat is also less aggressive. See also under Musculoskeletal conditions.

Pancreatic carcinoma
A tumour of the duct cells of the pancreas. Uncommon, but usually highly malignant.

Parathyroid tumours
Parathyroid tumours are uncommon in the dog and cat. Functional adenomas are the most common type of parathyroid tumour resulting in primary hyperparathyroidism and hypercalcaemia (see *Primary hyperparathyoidism* under Endocrine conditions). Adenomas are benign and well-encapsulated. Adenocarcinomas may invade locally and metastasise.

Perianal (hepatoid) gland adenoma

These are benign tumours that arise from the modified sebaceous glands of the perianal area. They appear as well-circumscribed raised lesions which may ulcerate. Perianal gland adenocarcinomas may occur, but are less common.

Phaeochromocytoma

See under Endocrine conditions.

Pilomatricoma

A rare benign tumour of the hair follicle. Pilomatricoma presents as a solitary, firm mass in the dermis or subcutis, without ulceration of the overlying epidermis. They usually occur over the back and limbs of dogs. They are rare in cats.

Pituitary tumours

The most common pituitary tumour in the dog is the adenoma of the corticotrophic cells of the anterior lobe. These tumours are generally functional, resulting in an overproduction of adrenocorticotrophic hormone (ACTH) and hyperadrenocorticism (see under Endocrine conditions). Carcinomas do occur and are generally non-functional but are more invasive and likely to metastasise. In the cat, pituitary tumours may be associated with hyperadrenocorticism as above, but tumours of the somatotrophic cells of the anterior pituitary also occur resulting in an overproduction of growth hormone and acromegaly.

Primary bone tumours

Primary bone tumours are relatively uncommon in the dog and represent <5% of all tumours. The most common tumours are osteosarcomas and chondrosarcomas, others, including fibrosarcomas and haemangiosarcomas, occur less frequently. In dogs, the risk of primary bone tumours of the appendicular skeleton increases with body size/weight. They generally occur in older dogs, but in giant breeds they may be seen at an earlier age. Primary bone tumours are uncommon in the cat. See also *Osteosarcoma* and *Fibrosarcoma*.

Primary brain tumours

See under Neurological conditions.

Renal cystadenocarcinoma

See under Renal and Urinary conditions.

Schwannoma

This rare neoplasm arises from the Schwann cells of the nerve sheath and can be dermal or subcutaneous. In dogs they occur most commonly on the limbs, head and tail. They are often alopecic and occasionally pruritic or painful.

Sebaceous gland tumours

One of the most common skin tumours of the dog, but less common in the cat. They may be single or multiple. There are various histologic types: *sebaceous hyperplasia* presents as small, lobulated wart-like lesions; *sebaceous epitheliomas* present as firm dermal masses with hairless overlying skin. Other types include sebaceous gland adenomas and adenocarcinomas. With the exception of adenocarcinomas, sebaceous gland tumours are generally benign in behaviour.

Squamous cell carcinoma of the skin

These are relatively common malignant tumours which arise from keratinocytes. Various predisposing factors have been identified, such as exposure to ultraviolet light, pollutants and pre-existing chronic dermatitis.

Squamous cell carcinoma of the digit

Squamous cell carcinoma is the most common cutaneous tumour of the digit in dogs. It is locally invasive, resulting in bone lysis, and metastasises more frequently than squamous cell carcinomas found in other cutaneous sites.

Sweat gland tumours

These may be adenomas or adenocarcinomas. They are uncommon in the dog and rare in the cat. They may present as small solitary nodules in the dermis and subcutis with or without ulceration. An inflammatory form of adenocarcinoma is poorly circumscribed and more infiltrative. Adenocarcinomas are highly invasive and may metastasise to local and regional lymph nodes, and occasionally to more distant sites, e.g. the lungs.

Systemic histiocytosis

See *Histiocytosis.*

Testicular neoplasia

Testicular neoplasia is common in the dog. There are three main tumour types: Sertoli cell tumours, seminomas and interstitial cell tumours. Certain breeds seem at increased risk. The incidence of Sertoli cell tumour and seminoma is higher in undescended testes than normally descended testes.

Thymoma

Thymoma is a tumour of the epithelial cells of the thymus gland which is situated in the cranial mediastinum. It is uncommon in both dogs and cats. Thymomas are generally benign and slow growing. Symptoms relate to the presence of a cranial mediastinal mass and may vary: cough, dyspnoea, regurgitation and occasionally obstruction of the cranial vena cava leading to facial and forelimb oedema ('precaval syndrome'). Autoimmune conditions such as *Myasthenia gravis* may be associated with thymoma.

Thyroid Carcinoma

See *Thyroid neoplasia in dogs* under Endocrine conditions.

Trichoblastoma

These are common benign skin tumours, appearing as solitary, domed masses. They may become dark in colour and ulcerate.

Trichoepithelioma

A benign tumour of the hair follicle. They present as solitary, firm masses in the dermis or subcutis, often with ulceration of the overlying epidermis. They usually occur over the back and limbs of dogs, but are rare in cats.

Tricholemmoma

This rare, benign tumour occurs most commonly on the head and neck.

NEUROLOGICAL CONDITIONS

Afghan myelopathy

A progressive disease of the white matter of the spinal cord. Symptoms include pelvic limb ataxia and paresis progressing to thoracic limb involvement, tetraplegia and eventually death from respiratory paralysis.

Ambylopia and quadriplegia

This is a lethal inherited condition of Irish Setters. Puppies are unable to walk and progression to visual impairment, nystagmus and seizures occurs.

Arachnoid cysts

Arachnoid cysts are a rare cause of focal spinal cord compression in young dogs. Neurological deficits depend on the site of the lesion.

Atlantoaxial subluxation

This is seen primarily in young dogs of Toy breeds which present with neck pain and neurological deficits in all four limbs due to cervical spinal cord compression. A variety of congenital defects including a lack of or hypoplasia of the dens and shortening of the axis lead to instability of the atlantoaxial articulation. The condition may also be acquired in any breed as a result of fracture of the dens or damage to the ligamentous support. (See also *Odontoid process dysplasia* under Musculoskeletal conditions.)

Birman cat distal polyneuropathy

A degenerative polyneuropathy which results in hypermetria in all limbs, progressive pelvic limb ataxia and a tendency to fall. The condition is believed to be hereditary.

Cerebellar degeneration

Cerebellar cells can undergo premature aging, degeneration and death (termed abiotrophy) leading to signs of cerebellar dysfunction (intention tremor, ataxia, hypermetria and menace deficits). In most cases the condition is believed to be hereditary.

Cerebellar malformation

Congenital malformations of the cerebellum include hypoplasia and aplasia of the whole or part of the cerebellum. Some may have a genetic basis, others result from a teratogen. Clinical signs are seen as soon as the animal becomes mobile and are non-progressive. They include hypermetria, head tremor and a wide-based

DISEASE SUMMARIES

stance. There is no treatment, but animals may make suitable pets if not severely affected.

Cervical vertebral malformation (wobbler syndrome)

This is a developmental malformation and malarticulation of the caudal cervical vertebrae seen in large- and giant-breed dogs, particularly the Dobermann and Great Dane. Clinical signs result from spinal cord compression and include neck pain and gait abnormalities (e.g. ataxia and paresis) which are worse in the pelvic limbs.

Congenital deafness

This has been observed in numerous breeds (especially Dalmatians and blue-eyed white cats) and usually results from a partial or complete failure of development of the organ of Corti.

Congenital vestibular disease

Young animals may present with signs of peripheral vestibular dysfunction including head tilt, circling, and falling. Nystagmus is not a common feature of the congenital condition. There is no treatment, symptoms may improve with time as the animal compensates.

Vestibular disease may also be acquired secondarily to a variety of causes including middle-ear infections in breeds predisposed to ear disease. An idiopathic form may be seen in older dogs.

Dalmatian leukodystrophy

This rarely reported progressive neurological condition results in visual deficits and progressive weakness. On gross pathology there is atrophy of the brain, lateral ventricle dilation and cavitation of the white matter of the cerebral hemispheres.

Dancing Dobermann disease

This is believed to be a neuromuscular disease of the gastrocnemius muscle, the underlying cause is not known. It has only been reported in Dobermann Pinschers and affected dogs initially flex one pelvic limb whilst standing. As progression occurs to involve the other pelvic limb the dog is seen to alternately flex and extend each pelvic limb in a dancing motion.

Degenerative myelopathy

A degenerative disease primarily seen in German Shepherd Dogs over five years of age. Diffuse degeneration of the white matter of the thoracolumbar spinal cord results in progressive pelvic limb ataxia, paresis and loss of conscious proprioception. The cause in unknown.

Demyelinating myelopathy of Miniature Poodles

A rare, possibly inherited condition characterised by diffuse spinal cord demyelination. Pelvic limb paresis progresses to paraplegia and tetraplegia. Spinal reflexes are hyperactive.

Dermoid sinus

A dermoid sinus is a developmental defect arising from the incomplete separation of the skin and neural tube. It may be found midline in the cervical, cranial thoracic or sacrococcygeal regions. In cases where the sinus communicates with the dura mater, neurological signs may be seen. The condition is most commonly found in the Rhodesian Ridgeback and is believed to be hereditary in this breed.

Discospondylitis (see figure 25)

Infection of the intervertebral disc with osteomyelitis of adjoining vertebral bodies. Infection occurs secondarily to spinal surgery, foreign body migration or septic emboli from the skin, urinary/genital tract, or from a concurrent endocarditis. Clinical signs may include pyrexia, anorexia, spinal pain and paresis.

Distal symmetrical polyneuropathy

This distal polyneuropathy has been reported in young adult Great Danes and other large breeds of dog. Symptoms include pelvic limb paresis that progresses to tetraparesis, and atrophy of limb and head muscles. There is no treatment.

Eosinophilic meningoencephalitis

This condition has been reported in six male dogs, three of which were Golden Retrievers. Cerebrospinal fluid analysis demonstrated pleocytosis with an eosinophil percentage of 21–98%. There was a concurrent peripheral blood eosinophilia in four of the cases. Symptoms included behavioural abnormalities and seizures.

DISEASE SUMMARIES

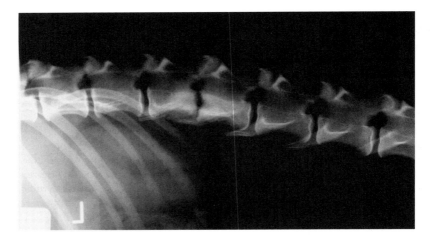

Figure 25
Lateral radiograph of the thoracolumbar spine of a dog demonstrating discospondylitis.
Courtesy of Andy Moores.

Episodic falling

Seen in Cavalier King Charles Spaniels in the UK. During exercise, a bounding hind-limb gait develops. This progresses to a bunny-hop with arched spine, and eventually collapse often with the thoracic limbs crossed over the back of the head. There is no loss of consciousness and recovery is rapid. Some improvement may be seen with diazepam. The cause is unknown.

Giant axonal neuropathy

This is a rare inherited neuropathy of German Shepherd Dogs. The cause is unknown. Distal nerves in the pelvic limbs and long tracts of the central nervous system are affected first, giving rise to paresis, loss of spinal reflexes and pain perception in the pelvic limbs. Megaoesophagus and loss of bark occur later. There is no treatment.

Glycogenosis (glycogen storage disease)

A group of rare diseases resulting from a deficiency of one or more enzymes involved in glycogen degradation or synthesis. Glycogen accumulates in a variety of tissues including the central nervous system, muscle and liver resulting in clinical signs including seizures and muscular weakness.

Granulomatous meningoencephalitis

This is an inflammatory condition of unknown cause. The disease may be focal or diffuse and may affect any part of the central nervous system, leading to a wide range of clinical signs including seizures, ataxia, nystagmus and visual deficits. The disease is usually chronic and progressive. Small-breed dogs are most commonly affected with Poodles representing about 30% of diagnosed cases.

Hemivertebrae

Hemivertebrae are congenitally malformed vertebrae most commonly seen at the level of thoracic vertebrae 7–9. Neurological signs, e.g. pelvic limb ataxia, paresis, faecal and urinary incontinence, may result from spinal cord compression.

Hereditary ataxia

Progressive ataxia results from degeneration of the white matter of the cervical and thoracic spinal cord in young Smooth-haired Fox Terriers and Jack Russell Terriers.

Hound ataxia

A degenerative myelopathy seen in Foxhounds and Beagles in the UK. Degenerative changes are most severe in the mid-thoracic spinal cord

DISEASE SUMMARIES

but may extend to involve the brainstem, caudal cerebellar peduncles or sciatic nerve. Signs include pelvic limb weakness and ataxia. Muscle atrophy and loss of spinal reflexes is not seen. The cause is unknown but a link has been suggested to an all-tripe diet.

Hydrocephalus

Hydrocephalus occurs where there is dilation of all or part of the ventricular system of the brain, and may be congenital or acquired (usually secondary to neoplasia or inflammatory disease). Symptoms include a domed cranium, seizures and altered mental status.

Hyperaesthesia syndromes

Increased sensitivity to tactile and painful stimulation may result in self-mutilation which varies in severity from rippling of the skin when touched or excessive licking to auto-amputation. Some cases are due to underlying neuropathies or are forms of seizure; however, in others no underlying cause is identified. Treatments tried include phenobarbitone, megoestrol acetate and prednisolone. Success has been variable.

Hyperlipidaemia

Hyperlipidaemia (high blood lipid levels) is a familial condition of Miniature Schnauzers and cats which is believed to be associated with a reduced activity of lipoprotein lipase resulting in defective lipid metabolism. Affected animals may experience seizures as well as abdominal distress and pancreatitis.

Hyperoxaluria

A condition seen in Domestic Short Hair cats in which young cats develop acute renal failure and neurological disease. Signs include anorexia, depression, enlarged painful kidneys, weakness, reduced spinal reflexes and poor response to pain. Oxalate crystals are found deposited in the kidney tubules, and swellings of the proximal axons of the ventral horn cells are found in the spinal cord on post-mortem. There is no treatment and the condition carries a grave prognosis.

Hypertrophic neuropathy

An inherited neuropathy reported in the Tibetan Mastiff which results in generalised

weakness, hyporeflexia and dysphonia from seven to ten weeks of age. There is no treatment and the prognosis is guarded.

Hypoglycaemia

Hypoglycaemia is a common metabolic cause of seizures. It may result from a variety of causes including insulinoma, hypoadrenocorticism, severe liver disease and sepsis. Young dogs of Toy breeds may develop hypoglycaemia easily when stressed, fed an inadequate diet or affected by gastrointestinal disease. Hunting dogs which are not fed on the morning of a hunt may also be predisposed to hypoglycaemia as a result of physical exertion.

Hypomyelination

Hypomyelination of the central nervous system has been seen in several breeds of dog and is known to be hereditary in some cases. Signs usually start at a few weeks of age with generalized body tremors which worsen with excitement. *Hypomyelination of the peripheral nervous system* has been seen in two Golden Retriever littermates with pelvic limb weakness and depressed spinal reflexes.

Idiopathic facial paralysis

Paralysis of the facial nerve results in drooping of the lip, paralysis of the eyelids and impaired ear movement on the affected side. Acute onset facial paralysis may occur in adult dogs without evidence of an underlying cause.

Intervertebral disc disease (see figures 26a and 26b)

Degeneration of the intervertebral discs resulting in extrusion or protrusion of the nucleus pulposus may result in spinal cord compression and pain/paresis. Nuclear extrusion occurs early in chondrodystrophoid breeds, e.g. Pekingese, Dachschunds, Beagles, Welsh Corgis, French Bulldogs, some Spaniels and Basset Hounds giving rise to signs in younger dogs.

Leukoencephalomyelopathy of Rottweilers

This is believed to be an inherited condition. Degeneration of the myelin of the spinal cord, brainstem, cerebellum and sometimes optic

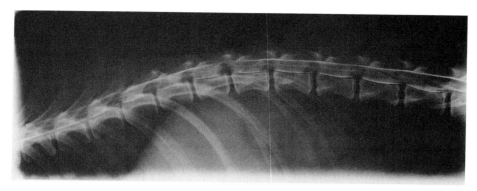

Figure 26a (above)
Myelogram of an eleven-year-old neutered
male Bichon Frise showing loss of the dorsal
column of contrast at T12–T13 consistent
with disc herniation at this site (lateral view).

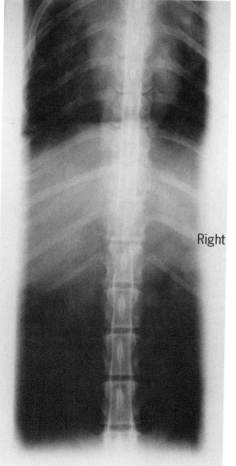

Right

Figure 26b (left)
Dorsoventral view showing extradural
compression on the right side at the level of
T12–T13.

DISEASE SUMMARIES

tracts results in ataxia, tetraparesis and loss of conscious proprioception, with increased spinal reflexes and muscle tone. Vision is usually unaffected. The condition progresses over 6–12 months.

Lissencephaly

A developmental anomaly where the cerebral cortex has reduced or absent gyri or sulci resulting in a smooth appearance. Clinical signs are usually seen from a few months of age and may include behavioural abnormalities, lack of training, aggressive behaviour, visual deficits and seizures.

Lumbosacral stenosis

Stenosis (narrowing) of the lumbosacral vertebral canal and/or intervertebral foramina causes compression of the lumbosacral nerve roots. Clinical signs may include pain on palpation of the area, pelvic limb paresis or lameness, tail paralysis, hypotonia of the anal sphincter and bladder atonicity ('lumbosacral syndrome'). It is most commonly seen in adult German Shepherd Dogs.

Lysosomal storage diseases

These rare diseases result from a failure of normal metabolic processes due to a deficiency of an enzyme within the lysosomes of neuronal tissues. As a result, substrate accumulates, causing cellular dysfunction and eventually death. One of a variety of lysosomal enzymes may be affected. Symptoms usually occur before one year of age and may include ataxia, tremors, seizures, dementia and blindness. Most lysosomal storage diseases are believed to be inherited as an autosomal recessive trait.

Meningitis and polyarteritis

This is a vasculitis of meningeal arteries which results in clinical signs of recurrent fever, anorexia and cervical rigidity. In some cases paresis or tetraparesis may be seen. An immune-mediated aetiology has been suggested and some cases may respond to high-dose, long-term prednisolone treatment.

Meningoencephalocoele

A lethal malformation where part of the brain and meninges is herniated through a defect in the skull.

Multisystem neuronal degeneration

A slowly progressive degenerative disease of young Cocker Spaniels. Diffuse neuronal loss throughout the subcortical, brainstem and cerebellar nuclei results in symptoms including loss of recognition of the owner, apathy, hyperactivity, hypersexuality and aggression.

Muscle cramping

An inherited disorder of Scottish Terriers. Affected dogs are normal at rest but exercise may provoke muscle spasms which in its mildest form appear as pelvic limb stiffness. Severe attacks cause rigidity of all muscles including facial muscles causing the dog to fall over into a tightly curled ball. Consciousness is maintained and the animal makes a spontaneous recovery. The cause is unknown but it is believed to be a disorder of central nervous system neurotransmitters. A similar condition has been reported in Dalmatians and Norwich Terriers.

Myasthenia gravis

Decreased numbers of acetylcholine receptors on the post-synaptic muscle membrane leads to defective neuromuscular transmission. The disease can be congenital or acquired. Clinical signs in dogs include muscle weakness on exercise which improves with rest, and megaoesophagus. The onset may be chronic or acute and the condition can be generalised or focal. Signs in cats include drooling, ventroflexion of the neck, regurgitation, weakness and lameness.

Narcolepsy/cataplexy

Narcolepsy is characterised by excessive sleepiness at inappropriate times, whilst cataplexy is acute flaccid paralysis from which the animal makes a complete recovery after a few seconds to several minutes. In dogs, cataplexy seems to be the more prominent and is often associated with excitement, e.g. eating or playing.

Neuroaxonal dystrophy

A degenerative central nervous system disorder of unknown cause, seen primarily in Rottweilers. Pathological findings include swellings of the distal axons within the central nervous system and cerebellar atrophy. Symptoms include ataxia, hypermetria and intention tremors which may be slowly progressive over several years.

DISEASE SUMMARIES

Partial seizures

Partial seizures result from a focal discharge from the brain. The appearance of the seizure varies with the location of the discharge but may include fly-biting, star-gazing, tail-chasing or self-mutilating behaviour.

Polyradiculoneuritis

This is an inflammatory condition affecting multiple nerve roots resulting in pelvic limb weakness which rapidly progresses to quadriplegia. An idiopathic form may be seen in any breed, however the condition has been seen following raccoon bites in hunting breeds such as the Coonhound. An immunological reaction to raccoon saliva may be the underlying cause in these cases.

Primary brain tumours

Primary brain tumours are derived from tissues of the nervous system including nerve cells, glial cells, meninges and neuroepithelial cells. They are generally solitary and most cases will present with signs of a space-occupying lesion in the brain, the specific signs varying with the location. Meningiomas and gliomas are the most common primary brain tumours in dogs. Meningiomas are the most common primary brain tumours in the cat and may be single or multiple in this species.

Progressive axonopathy

See *Sensory neuropathy*.

Pug encephalitis

A rare, necrotising meningoencephalitis of unknown aetiology seen in Pugs. Symptoms are often acute in onset and include seizures, depression, head-pressing, circling, blindness with normal pupillary reflexes and opisthotonus. The condition is progressive and there is no treatment. Most cases are euthanased.

Pyogranulomatous meningoencephalomyelitis

An acute, rapidly progressive disease of unknown cause seen in mature Pointers. Mononuclear and polymorphonuclear inflammatory infiltrates are found throughout the central nervous system but especially in the cervical spinal cord and lower brainstem. Dogs suffer from cervical rigidity, ataxia and sometimes seizures. The prognosis is poor. A temporary remission in response to antibiotics may be seen.

Rottweiler distal sensorimotor polyneuropathy

A polyneuropathy of Rottweilers resulting in paraparesis progressing to tetraparesis, reduced spinal reflexes, hypotonia and neurogenic atrophy of limb muscles. The condition progresses over twelve months.

Sacrocaudal dysgenesis

Congenital malformation of the sacrococcygeal spinal cord and vertebral column which results in locomotor problems in the hind legs and faecal and urinary incontinence.

Sensory neuropathy

Sensory neuropathies have been seen in a number of breeds. In Pointers signs of self-mutilation associated with loss of pain sensation predominate, whereas in Dachshunds loss of proprioception and ataxia may be seen. In Boxers the condition is termed *progressive axonopathy* and is characterised by pelvic limb hyporeflexia, hypotonia and proprioceptive loss.

Shaker dog disease

This condition has been most commonly observed in dogs with white hair coats, particularly Maltese and West Highland White Terriers. Dogs develop a fine whole-body tremor which may worsen with excitement and stress. Other signs may include nystagmus, menace deficits, proprioceptive deficits and seizures. There may be an underlying mild lymphocytic encephalitis and affected animals are usually responsive to immunosupressive doses of corticosteroids with benzodiazepines.

Spina bifida

This is a developmental defect resulting from the failure of the two halves of the dorsal spinous processes to fuse, most commonly in the lumbar spine. Protrusion of the spinal cord or meninges may result in symptoms including pelvic limb ataxia, paresis and urinary or faecal incontinence. If no protrusion occurs the condition is termed 'spina bifida occulta'.

Spinal dysraphism

This is a congenital malformation of the spinal cord resulting in a wide-based stance and bunny-hopping gait of the hind-limbs. It may be associated with hemivertebrae or spina bifida. The condition is non-progressive.

Spinal muscular atrophy

This is a condition where premature degeneration of various neuronal cell populations of the brainstem and ventral horn of the spinal cord result in generalised weakness which may progress to muscular atrophy and tetraparesis/plegia.

Spongiform degeneration

Spongiform degenerations are rare disorders resulting in vacuolation of the brain and spinal cord which may result in a wide variety of neurological signs.

Springer Spaniel rage syndrome

Seen in young adult Springer Spaniels which become aggressive to people including their owners. No intracranial lesion has been found to explain this behaviour.

True epilepsy

Recurrent seizures caused by functional disorders of the brain. The high incidence in certain breeds of dog suggests an inherited basis.

OCULAR CONDITIONS

BVA/KC/ISDS Eye Scheme

The British Veterinary Association/Kennel Club/International Sheep Dog Society Eye Scheme has been set up to enable breeders to reduce the frequency of inherited eye disease by screening dogs for these conditions prior to breeding. Screening is carried out by appointed eye panelists. A list of panelists can be obtained from the Kennel Club or British Veterinary Association.

Schedule 1 is a list of eye diseases of which it is considered that enough evidence exists to show that the condition is inherited in the breeds shown. Schedule 3 is a list of conditions under investigation for the possibility of inheritance in the breeds shown.

Conditions included in the scheme are those of the eye itself only, eyelid and lacrimal conditions are not included.

Canine anterior uveal melanoma

Melanocytic tumours of the iris or ciliary body. Most are unilateral and benign, however they may cause secondary glaucoma.

Caruncular trichiasis

Hairs growing from the conjunctiva at the medial canthus which may cause ocular irritation.

Cataract

An opacity which may affect all or part of the lens or lens capsule, unilaterally or bilaterally. Cataracts may be primary (where a hereditary basis is suspected) or secondary, e.g. to ocular inflammation, metabolic disease or congenital anomalies such as persistent pupillary membranes or persistent hyaloid artery.

Cataracts may be detected first in a variety of different areas of the lens and may progress at different rates. A complete cataract involves the whole lens and obscures the fundus, resulting in blindness in the affected eye.

Central progressive retinal atrophy (CPRA) or retinal pigment epithelial dystrophy (RPED)

Abnormal accumulation of pigment within the retina resulting in a progressive retinal degeneration and visual deficiencies. The condition was previously seen most commonly in England, but is now infrequently seen.

Chédiak-Higashi syndrome

A condition seen in the Persian cat. Symptoms may include ocular and cutaneous albinism, cataracts, susceptibility to infection and bleeding tendencies. See also under Haematological/Immunological conditions.

Chronic superficial keratitis (pannus)

A bilateral progressive inflammatory disease of the cornea. A fleshy, vascular lesion spreads towards the central cornea from the temporal limbus. Corneal pigmentation follows and, if severe, vision loss occurs. It is suspected to have an immune-mediated basis and is influenced by ultraviolet radiation. The condition is more severe in dogs living at high altitude. May be seen with *Plasma cell infiltration of the nictitating membrane (plasmoma)*.

Coloboma
A congenital absence of part of an ocular structure which may affect the eyelid, iris, choroid, lens or optic disc.

Collie eye anomaly (see plate 24)
A congenital condition characterised by abnormal development of the eye. The severity and effect on vision is variable. Mild cases may have only choroidal hypoplasia. More severe cases may also have optic nerve colobomas, retinal detachment and intraocular haemorrhage.

Congenital, subepithelial, geographic corneal dystrophy
A transient, non-inflammatory corneal opacity seen in puppies younger than ten weeks and absent by 12–14 weeks.

Convergent strabismus (esotropia)
Abnormal deviation of the eyeballs medially.

Corneal dystrophy
A primary, non-inflammatory bilateral opacity of the cornea. The term 'dystrophy' implies an hereditary nature of the condition. However, in many cases of corneal dystrophy firm evidence of inheritance is lacking, although no underlying disease can be found.

Different layers of the cornea may be affected giving *epithelial, endothelial* and *stromal* dystrophies. The appearance, age of onset and rate of progression vary with the breed. Visual disturbance may occur if the lesion becomes extensive.

Corneal sequestrate (see plate 25)
A disease of the cornea seen in the cat. The disease is characterised by the development of a pigmented lesion in the centre of the cornea.

Dermoid
A congenital defect in which palpebral skin

is abnormally located on the conjunctiva or cornea, often at the limbus, and may cause irritation due to the hairs growing from its surface.

Diamond eye
See *Macropalpebral fissure*.

Distichiasis
Abnormally positioned cilia (eyelashes) which emerge through or close to Meibomian gland orifices. They are often of no clinical significance but in some cases may cause ocular irritation.

Ectopic cilia
Cilia (eyelashes) which emerge directly through the palpebral conjunctiva to cause corneal irritation, ulceration and pain.

Ectropion
Eversion of all or part of the eyelid margin leading to exposure of the conjunctival tissues. In some cases this predisposes to conjunctivitis, epiphora and precorneal tear film deficiencies.

Entropion
An inward rolling of all or part of the eyelid margin resulting in irritation of the conjunctival and corneal surfaces.

Eversion of the cartilage of the nictitating membrane
Scrolling of the cartilage of the third eyelid which may result in chronic conjunctivitis. Seen most commonly in young large-breed dogs.

Fibrosing esotropia
Fibrosis of the extraocular muscles, particularly the medial rectus, leads to medial deviation of the eyeball. It is generally bilateral, but may be unilateral. It is most commonly seen in the Shar Pei.

Glaucoma (canine)
A group of diseases characterised by degeneration of the retinal ganglion cells and optic nerve resulting in progressive loss of vision. The condition is associated with an increase in intraocular pressure. Primary glaucoma develops without the presence of other intraocular disease and may be hereditary, with potential for bilateral

involvement. Primary glaucomas may be divided by the appearance of the iridocorneal filtration angle into 'open-angle' and 'closed-angle' glaucomas. Causes of secondary glaucomas include lens luxation, uveitis, neoplasia and cataracts.

Generalised progressive retinal atrophy (GPRA)

Degeneration of the retinal cells. An autosomal recessive inheritance is suspected in most breeds. Different breeds are affected at different ages by different types of GPRA. However, all cases are bilateral and progress to blindness. The earliest clinical sign is night blindness with day vision being lost a variable time later.

Ophthalmoscopically there is attenuation of retinal vessels and tapetal hyper-reflectivity. In the later stages, the condition is often accompanied by cataracts. More than 100 breeds of dog have been identified as suffering from GPRA; however, only those where the condition is seen relatively frequently, or is well-described, have been included in Part I.

Goniodysgenesis (pectinate ligament dysplasia)

Abnormal development of the iridocorneal filtration angle which may predispose to closed-angle glaucoma later in life.

Hereditary retinal dystrophy of Briards (congenital stationary night blindness)

A retinal dystrophy causing congenital night blindness with a variable effect on day vision. In most cases there is no progression of visual impairment. Nystagmus may be present.

Hemeralopia

Day blindness with no ophthalmoscopically visible abnormality. The condition results from selective degeneration of the cone photoreceptors of the retina. Dogs are able to see in dim light.

Idiopathic epiphora

The failure of normal tear drainage leading to overflow of tears over the lower lid, without evidence of increased tear production or obstruction of the drainage system.

Iris cyst

Cysts of the iris and ciliary body are usually benign and may be single or multiple, unilateral or bilateral. They may be congenital, or acquired secondarily to ocular inflammation or trauma.

Keratoconjunctivitis sicca (dry eye)
(see plates 26 and 27)

A common disease, characterised by reduced aqueous tear production resulting in drying and inflammation of the conjunctiva and cornea. The condition may be congenital (rarely), or result from infectious, drug-induced, neurological or immune-mediated causes. A genetic influence is suggested by the high incidence in a number of breeds.

Lacrimal punctal aplasia (imperforate lacrimal punctum)

A congenital anomaly where there is a failure of the lacrimal punctum (tear duct) to open. It may affect upper, lower or both punctae and may be unilateral or bilateral. The lower punctum is most commonly affected, resulting in epiphora (overflow of tears).

Lens luxation

Displacement of the lens from its normal position, which may be primary (and in some breeds inherited) or secondary to trauma, cataract formation, glaucoma, neoplasia or uveitis. Lens luxation is a potentially serious condition and may result in raised intraocular pressure and glaucoma. Where both lens luxation and glaucoma occur, it is not always clear which condition is primary. Primary lens luxation is usually bilateral though both lenses do not usually luxate simultaneously.

Limbal melanoma

These tumours are usually pigmented and found in the limbal region. They may invade the cornea. In older dogs they tend to remain static or grow slowly, in younger dogs growth is more rapid.

Lysosomal storage disease

An inherited deficiency of a specific degradative enzyme leads to the accumulation of its

DISEASE SUMMARIES

substrate in cells, causing progressive cellular malfunction from an early age. Various enzymes may be involved and in some cases the eyes may be affected.

Macropalpebral fissure (euryblepharon)

An abnormally large palpebral fissure. In some cases (e.g. brachycephalic breeds), this occurs as a result of exophthalmos (protrusion of the globe), in others it results from overlong eyelid margins and may allow both entropion and ectropion to develop, resulting in 'diamond eye' in severe cases. The precorneal tear film is often disturbed, and corneal and conjunctival disease may occur secondarily.

Medial canthal pocket syndrome

The combination of a narrow skull with deep set eyes leads to the formation of a conjunctival pocket at the medial canthus, allowing the collection of debris which may cause recurrent conjunctivitis.

Microcornea

A congenital abnormally small cornea which may be associated with other ocular defects.

Micropalpebral fissure (blepharophimosis)

A congenital defect resulting in an abnormally small palpebral fissure.

Micropapilla

A congenitally small optic disc which is not associated with visual impairment. It may be difficult to distinguish from optic nerve hypoplasia ophthalmoscopically.

Microphakia

A congenital defect resulting in an abnormally small lens, which may be associated with other intraocular defects.

Microphthalmia

A congenitally small eye, often seen with other ocular defects, e.g. microcornea, anterior chamber defects, cataract, persistent pupillary membranes and retinal defects (*Multiple ocular defects*).

Multiple ocular defects

Several congenital defects present in the same eye.

Nasal fold trichiasis

Prominent nasal folds in some breeds (notably the Pekingese) which allow the facial hair to come into contact with ocular tissues, causing irritation.

Neuronal ceroid lipofuscinosis

An inherited lipid-storage disease resulting in retinal degeneration and encephalopathy.

Nodular episclerokeratitis (fibrous histiocytoma, nodular granulomatous episclerokeratitis, proliferative keratoconjunctivitis)

Single or multiple, raised fleshy masses originating at the limbus and invading the cornea. Involvement of the nictitating membrane may occur. Usually a bilateral condition.

Nystagmus

Involuntary repetitive ocular movements.

Ocular melanosis

Large numbers of melanocytes infiltrate the iridocorneal angle, episclera, choroid and iris, predisposing to glaucoma (pigmentary glaucoma). Primarily seen in middle-aged Cairn Terriers.

Optic nerve coloboma

A congenital defect of the optic nerve head. The optic disc may appear irregular with a deep cavity. This defect may affect vision if large.

Optic nerve hypoplasia

A congenitally small optic disc with reduced numbers of optic nerve axons and visual impairment.

Pannus

See *Chronic superficial keratitis.*

Persistent hyaloid artery (PHA)

A congenital defect resulting from the failure of the hyaloid artery to regress. The remnant is seen as a segment (which may or may not contain blood) within the vitreal cavity between the optic disc and the lens. A cataract may form at the point of attachment to the lens capsule.

Persistent hyperplastic primary vitreous (PHPV)

A congenital condition in which there is abnormal development and regression of the hyaloid system and primary vitreous. It is often associated with *persistent hyperplastic tunica vasculosa lentis (PHTVL)* in which there is persistence of an embryonic vascular system attached to the posterior lens capsule. The condition is rare, but is seen more frequently in Dobermanns and Staffordshire Bull Terriers. The condition varies in severity. In its most severe form it is associated with microphthalmia and other ocular defects.

Persistent pupillary membranes (PPM)

Persistent pupillary membranes are uveal remnants which fail to regress normally in the first six weeks of life and persist in the anterior chamber (either unilaterally or bilaterally). Strands which bridge from iris-to-iris are generally of no clinical significance, however iris-to-cornea or iris-to-lens strands may cause focal corneal and lenticular opacities respectively. PPMs are a relatively common finding but severe visual impairment is rare.

Pigmentary keratitis

Corneal pigmentation is usually seen with chronic keratitis. Pigmentary keratitis is particularly common in brachycephalic breeds and may represent a pigmentary or epithelial dystrophy in these breeds.

Pigmentary uveitis

Inflammation of the iris and ciliary body associated with abnormal pigment deposition. Seen most commonly in the Golden Retriever and often seen in conjunction with iris cysts. Cataract and glaucoma are common sequelae.

Plasma cell infiltration of the nictitating membrane (plasmoma)

Bilateral plasma cell infiltration of the nictitating membrane resulting in follicle formation and depigmentation. Often associated with *Chronic superficial keratitis (pannus)*.

Posterior lenticonus

A congenital abnormality where there is a conical protrusion of the posterior lens capsule and cortex into the vitreous. It may be associated with other ocular abnormalities and may be unilateral or bilateral.

Prolapse of the gland of the nictitating membrane ('cherry eye')

Prolapse of the tear gland normally located behind the nictitating membrane results in exposure and irritation of the gland. It is usually seen in young dogs, less than two years of age.

Proptosis

Anterior displacement of the globe with entrapment of the eyelids behind it. It usually results from trauma and occurs more easily in brachycephalic breeds.

Pseudopapilloedema

An enlarged optic nerve head due to excessive myelination of the optic nerve axons. No effect on vision.

Refractory corneal ulceration (indolent ulcer, Boxer ulcer, recurrent corneal erosion syndrome)

Slow-healing, superficial corneal ulcers which may represent a form of corneal epithelial dystrophy. Originally described in the Boxer, but also occurs in other breeds. Usually seen in middle-aged dogs.

Retinal detachment

Separation of the retina from the underlying tissues resulting in loss of function of the detached portion. May be partial or complete.

Retinal dysplasia

Abnormal differentiation of the retina present at birth. Retinal dysplasia may be inherited in some breeds. It may occur alone, or with other ocular defects or, in some cases, with skeletal defects. Three main forms exist:

- Multifocal retinal dysplasia: retinal folds exist as focal or multifocal lesions and appear as dots or linear streaks. Usually not associated with vision loss.

DISEASE SUMMARIES

- Geographic retinal dysplasia: involvement of a larger irregular area of retina with some retinal elevation. May be associated with visual deficiencies.
- Total retinal dysplasia with detachment: the whole retina is involved and results in complete retinal detachment and vision loss.

Systemic histiocytosis (see also *Histiocytosis* under Neoplastic conditions)

A multisystemic disease characterised by infiltration of affected tissues with histiocytes. Ocular tissues may be affected, leading to uveitis, chemosis, episcleritis and conjunctivitis. The disease is primarily seen as a familial disease in the Bernese Mountain Dog.

Tapetal degeneration

An inherited condition seen in Beagles, wherein there is progressive degeneration of tapetal cells without any affect on vision.

Trichiasis

A condition in which normal hairs arising from the periocular or facial areas deviate to contact and irritate the cornea and conjunctiva.

Uveodermatological syndrome

This is believed to be an immune-mediated disorder similar to Vogt-Koyanagi-Harada syndrome seen in humans. Melanocytes are targeted by the immune system. Ocular signs include anterior uveitis, uveal depigmentation and retinal damage. Dermatological signs may include vitiligo (depigmentation) of the eyelids, nasal planum and lips. See also under Dermatological conditions.

Vitreal syneresis

Degeneration of the vitreous results in liquefaction. This is a common age-related finding and usually of no clinical significance. However, in some cases, extension of the abnormal vitreous into the anterior chamber may predispose to glaucoma. Rarely, it may predispose to retinal detachment.

RENAL AND URINARY CONDITIONS

Calcium oxalate urolithiasis
(see figure 27)

Calcium oxalate uroliths are commonly found in both dogs and cats. In dogs, hypercalciuria predisposes to calcium oxalate urolith formation and may occur due to excessive intestinal absorption of calcium (absorptive calciuria), impaired renal reabsorption of calcium (renal leak calciuria), or hypercalcaemia (resorptive calciuria). Calcium oxalate uroliths tend to be radiodense, often rough and round or oval in shape and are not pH sensitive.

Calcium phosphate urolithiasis

Calcium phosphate uroliths are uncommon in both dogs and cats but where they occur the most common forms are hydroxyapatite and brushite. These uroliths are very radiodense, smooth and round or faceted. With the exception of brushite, they are less soluble in alkaline urine. Conditions resulting in hypercalciuria will predispose to their formation. Calcium phosphate is more commonly found as a minor component of struvite or calcium oxalate uroliths.

Cystine urolithiasis

Cystinuria occurs as a result of an inherited defect in cystine transport in the renal tubules. Cystinuria predisposes to cystine urolithiasis. Most cystine uroliths are relatively radiolucent, smooth and oval and are more likely to form in acid urine. They represent 1–3% of canine uroliths in the USA, but the incidence varies geographically, being higher in other parts of the world. They are relatively uncommon in cats.

Ectopic ureters

A congenital anomaly involving one or both ureters. There is failure of the affected ureter to terminate in the trigone region of the bladder, opening instead into the urethra, vagina or uterus. Continuous or intermittent urinary incontinence may be seen as a result, usually in the juvenile bitch. Urinary incontinence is less commonly associated with ectopic ureters in the

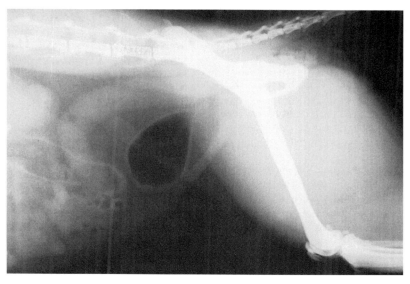

Figure 27
Pneumocystogram of a four-year-old neutered male Domestic Short Hair cat showing the presence of radiodense calcium oxalate calculi.

male because of the longer length of the urethra and stronger urethral sphincter.

Familial renal disease

Familial diseases include those that occur in related individuals with a greater frequency than chance alone would allow. Familial renal disease should be suspected whenever chronic renal failure occurs in an immature or young animal. If chronic renal failure develops before physical maturity, stunting will develop. Familial renal diseases vary in clinical signs and pathology depending on the breed:

- Glomerular basement membrane disorder: the main lesion in this condition is a thickening and splitting of the glomerular basement membrane, usually resulting in early-onset proteinuria and leading to renal failure.
- Periglomerular fibrosis: periglomerular fibrosis progresses to generalised interstitial fibrosis and results in renal failure.
- Membranoproliferative glomerulonephritis: glomerulonephritis results from the presence of immune complexes in the glomerular

capillary walls, leading to glomerular damage. Glomerulonephritis may be classified histologically as membranous, proliferative or membranoproliferative. In most cases there is significant proteinuria leading to hypoalbuminaemia which, if severe, is manifest as peripheral oedema or ascites (nephrotic syndrome). The condition may progress to renal failure.

- Renal amyloidosis: see page 226.
- Renal dysplasia: the term renal dysplasia refers to conditions where there is disorganised development of the renal parenchyma resulting in the persistence of structures inappropriate to the stage of development, e.g. immature glomeruli.

Fanconi's syndrome

Fanconi's syndrome results from renal tubular dysfunction resulting in abnormal reabsorption of many solutes including glucose, amino acids and phosphate. Low blood levels of the solutes involved may result. All cases are polyuric and polydipsic. The condition may progress to acute renal failure or pyelonephritis.

DISEASE SUMMARIES

Hyperoxaluria
See under Neurological conditions.

Hypospadias
See under Reproductive conditions.

Polycystic kidney disease (see plate 28)
In this disorder, large portions of the renal parenchyma are replaced by multiple cysts. Both kidneys are generally involved and in some cases cysts are found in the liver as well. Kidneys may be palpably enlarged and irregular, and the diagnosis can be confirmed by ultrasound. The condition progresses to renal failure. Renal cysts may also be seen in cases of renal dysplasia or neoplasia.

Primary renal glucosuria
See *Renal glucosuria*.

Reactive systemic amyloidosis
See *Renal amyloidosis*.

Renal amyloidosis
Amyloidosis results from the deposition of an insoluble fibrillar protein (amyloid) in a variety of organs, resulting in their dysfunction. *Reactive systemic amyloidosis* is a systemic syndrome which is familial in the Abyssinian cat and Shar Pei dog, in which amyloid deposition can be found in many organs. Amyloid deposits in the kidney lead to progressive renal dysfunction. In most cases there is glomerular involvement, resulting in moderate to severe proteinuria and sometimes nephrotic syndrome. In most breeds, renal amyloidosis is seen in older dogs; however, in the Shar Pei dog and Abyssinian cat it is seen at an earlier age.

Renal cystadenocarcinoma
This is a condition of bilateral and multifocal primary renal neoplasia which is seen primarily in the German Shepherd Dog. Cases present at 5–11 years of age with anorexia, weight loss and polydipsia. The renal condition is associated with generalised cutaneous nodules (nodular dermatofibrosis) and, in females, with multiple uterine leiomyomas.

Renal glucosuria
Glucosuria with normal blood glucose levels is uncommon in dogs and cats. It indicates tubular dysfunction and may be seen as part of Fanconi's syndrome, familial renal conditions or as an isolated defect with normal renal function (primary renal glucosuria).

Renal telangiectasia
Abnormal development of blood vessels leads to the formation of cavernous spaces filled with blood clots which appear macroscopically as red or black nodules in the kidney and sometimes in other tissues. Affected individuals present with marked haematuria.

Sacrocaudal dysgenesis
See under Neurological conditions.

Silica urolithiasis
Silica uroliths are uncommon. They have a characteristic jackstone appearance, are relatively radiodense and are less soluble in acid urine. There may be a link between dietary ingredients (notably corn gluten feed and soybean hulls) and silica urolith formation. A higher prevalence in large-breed dogs may be explained by the tendency to feed dry diets containing large quantities of plant ingredients such as these.

Struvite (magnesium ammonium phosphate) urolithiasis
Struvite uroliths are relatively common in cats and dogs. They are generally radiodense, smooth, round or faceted stones. Alkaline urine and (in dogs) urinary tract infection with urease-producing bacteria favour their formation.

Unilateral renal agenesis
Congenital absence of one kidney. Often an incidental finding, but individuals are predisposed to renal failure if the remaining kidney becomes compromised.

Urate urolithiasis
Ammonium urate, sodium urate, calcium urate and uric acid uroliths are relatively radiolucent and usually found as multiple, small, smooth, round or oval stones of brown-green colour.

They tend to form more in acid urine and where there is concurrent infection with urease producing bacteria. Dalmatians are predisposed to the development of urate uroliths because of a reduced capacity to convert uric acid to allantoin in the liver, leading to high levels of urinary uric acid excretion. Animals with hepatic portal vascular anomalies are predisposed to ammonium urate uroliths, owing to the reduced hepatic ability to convert ammonia to urea and uric acid to allantoin. This leads to increased urinary excretion of these substances.

Urethral prolapse

Prolapse of the urethral mucosa through the external urethral orifice may occur in young male dogs. Brachycephalic breeds may be predisposed.

Urethral sphincter mechanism incompetence

A weak urinary sphincter allows urine leakage, usually when the animal is relaxed and lying down. The condition is the most common cause of urinary incontinence in the adult dog and is most commonly diagnosed in neutered females of medium to large breeds. In many cases, the condition is responsive to reproductive hormone administration.

Urethrorectal fistula

An uncommon condition in which a fistula connects the lumen of the urethra with the lumen of the large bowel. Most cases are congenital but the condition may be acquired secondary to trauma or neoplasia. Affected animals may pass urine via both the anus and the penis or vulva, and are predisposed to urinary tract infection.

Urolithiasis

The formation of stones (uroliths) anywhere within the urinary tract.

REPRODUCTIVE CONDITIONS

Azoospermia with spermatogenic arrest

In azoospermia, the ejaculate appears normal but contains no spermatozoa. Azoospermia with spermatogenic arrest occurs in dogs that were previously fertile but have become azoospermic. It is believed to be the result of an autoimmune orchitis.

Congenital preputial stenosis

A congenital defect wherein there is an abnormally small preputial opening. This may interfere with normal urination and result in a failure to mate due to an inability to extrude the penis.

Cryptorchidism

Cryptorchidism is defined as a failure of one or both testes to descend into the scrotum. The undescended testis may be found in the inguinal canal or abdomen. Non-genetic factors may play a part, but the high incidence in some breeds of dog, and in families within those breeds, suggests a genetic influence. A sex-limited autosomal mode of inheritance has been suggested.

Dystocia

Dystocia can be defined as a difficulty or an inability in giving birth. It may result from a wide range of maternal or foetal factors. Brachycephalic breeds are predisposed due to a combination of a narrow maternal pelvis and a large foetal head and shoulders. Small nervous breeds may be predisposed due to a tendency to psychological inhibition and primary uterine inertia.

Hypospadias

Hypospadias results from incomplete fusion of the urethral folds during the formation of the male urethra such that the urethra opens abnormally on the underside of the penis, proximal to the glans penis. It may be seen with other congenital defects in intersex states.

Male pseudohermaphrodite syndrome

A pseudohermaphrodite is an individual in whom the chromosomal and gonadal sex agree, but the phenotypic sex is reversed. Therefore a male pseudohermaphrodite has a Y chromosome, testes (usually undescended) and female genitalia.

Penile hypoplasia

This is a rare congenital disorder that has been reported in the Cocker Spaniel, Collie,

DISEASE SUMMARIES

Dobermann and Great Dane. It may be seen as part of some intersex states.

Testicular neoplasia

See under Neoplastic conditions.

Urethral prolapse

See under Renal and Urinary conditions.

Vaginal hyperplasia (see plate 29)

Vaginal hyperplasia is an exaggerated response of the vaginal mucosa to normal circulating oestrogen during proestrus or oestrus. Vaginal oedema and thickening occurs and may result in a degree of vaginal prolapse. Boxers and Mastiff breeds seem to be most commonly affected.

XO syndrome

XO syndrome occurs when there has been nondisjunction during development of the gametes (eggs or sperm) resulting in one gamete containing two sex chromosomes (e.g. an egg with two X chromosomes or a sperm with an X and a Y chromosome) and the other gamete containing no sex chromosomes. When the latter is fertilised with an X-containing gamete (egg or sperm) an XO zygote is the result. This individual is a phenotypic female who may be infertile or demonstrate prolonged proestrus.

XXX syndrome

XXX syndrome occurs when there has been non-disjunction during development of the gametes (eggs or sperm) resulting in one gamete containing two sex chromosomes (e.g. an egg with two X chromosomes or a sperm with an X and a Y chromosome) and the other gamete containing no sex chromosomes. When the XX egg is fertilised by an X-containing sperm, an XXX zygote is the result. This individual is a phenotypic female who may have underdeveloped genitalia and may fail to cycle.

XX sex reversal

Sex reversal refers to the situation where the chromosomal and phenotypic sex do not agree. In XX sex reversal a phenotypic male is chromosomally a female.

RESPIRATORY CONDITIONS

Adult respiratory distress syndrome (ARDS)

This condition has been reported in related Dalmatians. Progressive pulmonary failure occurred, leading to death in three weeks. No known risk factors for ARDS could be identified.

Agenesis of the nares

This congenital condition can predispose to laryngeal collapse. Dyspnoea, mouth breathing and snoring are seen.

Aspergillosis

This fungal infection causes chronic nasal discharge. See also under Infectious conditions.

Brachycephalic upper airway syndrome

This term is used to describe a group of anatomical deformities which lead to respiratory compromise in brachycephalic breeds. These deformities include stenotic nares, laryngeal deformities and hypoplastic trachea. The clinical signs are of upper airway obstruction, and secondary complications; concurrent conditions such as laryngeal oedema and bronchopneumonia can occur in severely affected dogs.

Bronchiectasis

This is a dilatation of the bronchi, occurring as a complication of chronic bronchitis or bronchopenumonia. The changes are irreversible once present.

Bronchial cartilage hypoplasia

This condition presents early in life, usually causing severe respiratory distress.

Chylothorax (see plate 30)

This condition is quite common. Clinical signs are the same as for other pleural effusions, dyspnoea being especially common.

Collapsed trachea

This condition can occur in young dogs with a severe form of the condition, or later in life in those less severely affected. Clinical signs include coughing and inspiratory stridor. A characteristic 'goose-honk' cough may be heard.

DISEASE SUMMARIES

Feline asthma

Also known as feline bronchitis, allergic bronchitis. This condition can present with mild, chronic or acute severe signs. Coughing and dyspnoea are seen.

Hypoplastic trachea

This is part of the brachycephalic upper airway syndrome.

Laryngeal paralysis

This condition is usually idiopathic, but may be related to generalised myopathies or neuropathies. Stridor, aggravated by excitement and exercise, is the main clinical sign, although severe cases may progress to cyanosis and collapse.

Lung lobe torsion

This rare condition is more common in large, deep-chested breeds. Presenting signs include dyspnoea and pleural effusion. There may be an accompanying chylothorax.

Malignant histiocytosis (see also *Histiocytosis* under Neoplastic conditions)

This disease is thought to be a proliferation of histiocytic cells. Respiratory signs, such as cough or respiratory distress, are seen, as well as anaemia, weight loss and neurological problems.

Nasal dermoid sinus cyst

This newly-described condition causes chronic nasal discharge. Complete surgical excision leads to a good prognosis.

Nasopharyngeal polyps

These polyps are uncommon but cause chronic respiratory disease.

Primary ciliary dyskinesia

In this condition, the mechanism for removing mucus from the airways is defective, leading to respiratory infections. Other conditions associated with defective ciliary function include loss of hearing and loss of sperm motility, with consequent infertility.

Pneumonia due to *Pneumocystis carinii*

Pneumocystis carinii is a protozoal organism, infection with which may result in pneumonia in the presence of immunosurpression (see also under Haematological/Immunological conditions).

Pulmonary interstitial fibrosis

This condition may be secondary to chronic respiratory disease, leading to the replacement of alveolar walls and lung interstitium with fibrous tissue. This leads to a reduced inspiratory capacity. Clinical signs of cough and exercise intolerance progress slowly.

Spontaneous thymic haemorrhage

This may occur in young dogs at the time of thymic involution, and may be fatal.

DISEASE SUMMARIES

Sources

Textbooks

American College of Veterinary Ophthalmologists (1992) *Ocular Disorders Proven or Suspected to be Hereditary in Dogs*. Canine Eye Registration Foundation, West Lafayette.

August, J.R. (1994) *Consultations in Feline Internal Medicine 2*. WB Saunders Co., Philadelphia.

August, J.R. (1997) *Consultations in Feline Internal Medicine 3*. WB Saunders Co., Philadelphia.

August, J.R. (2001) *Consultations in Feline Internal Medicine 4*. WB Saunders Co., Philadelphia.

Bainbridge, J. & Elliott, J. (1996) *Manual of Canine and Feline Nephrology and Urology*. BSAVA Publications, Cheltenham.

Barlough, J.E. (1988) *Manual of Small Animal Infectious Diseases*. Churchill Livingstone, London.

Bonagura, J.D. (2000) *Kirk's Current Veterinary Therapy XIII, Small Animal Practice*. WB Saunders Co., Philadelphia.

Braund, K.G. (1994) *Clinical Syndromes in Veterinary Neurology*, 2nd edn. Mosby Publishers, St Louis.

Brinker, W.O., Piermattei, D.L. & Flo, G.L. (1997) *Handbook of Small Animal Orthopaedics and Fracture Repair*, 3rd edn. WB Saunders Co., Philadelphia.

Chrisman, C.L. (1991) *Problems in Small Animal Neurology*, 2nd edn. Lea and Febiger, Philadelphia.

Coughlan, A. & Miller, A. (1998) *Manual of Small Animal Fracture Repair and Management*. BSAVA Publications, Cheltenham.

Davidson, M., Else, R. & Lumsden, J. (1998) *Manual of Small Animal Clinical Pathology*. BSAVA Publications, Cheltenham.

Day, M.J. (1999) *Clinical Immunology of the Dog and Cat*. Manson Publishing, London.

Day, M., Mackin, A. & Littlewood, J. (2000) *Manual of Canine and Feline Haematology and Transfusion Medicine*. BSAVA Publications, Cheltenham.

Dunn, J. (1999) *Textbook of Small Animal Medicine*. WB Saunders Co., Philadelphia.

Ettinger, S.J. & Feldman, E.C. (2000) *Textbook of Veterinary Internal Medicine*, 5th edn. WB Saunders Co., Philadelphia.

Feldman, E.C. & Nelson, R.W. (1986) *Canine and Feline Endocrinology and Reproduction*, 2nd edn. WB Saunders Co., Philadelphia.

Gelatt, K.N. (1998) *Veterinary Ophthalmology*, 3rd edn. Lippincott, Williams & Wilkins, Philadelphia.

Gershwin, L.J., Krakowa, S. & Olsen, R.G. (1995) *Immunology and Immunopathology of Domestic Animals*, 2nd edn. Mosby Publishers, St Louis.

Guilford, W.G., Center, S.A., Strombeck, D.R., Williams, D.A. & Meyer D.J. (1996) *Strombeck's Gastroenterology*, 3rd edn. WB Saunders Co., Philadelphia.

Houlton, J.E. (1994) *Manual of Small Animal Arthrology*. BSAVA Publications, Cheltenham.

Martin, M. & Corcoran, B. (1997) *Cardiorespiratory Diseases of the Dog and Cat*. Blackwell Science, Oxford.

Morris, J. & Dobson, J. (2001) *Small Animal Oncology*. Blackwell Science, Oxford.

Morrison, W.B. (1998) *Cancer in Dogs and Cats*. Williams & Wilkins, Baltimore.

Osborne, C.A. & Finco, D.R. (1995) *Canine and Feline Nephrology and Urology*. Williams & Wilkins, Baltimore.

Osborne, C.A., Lulich, J.P. & Barteges, J.W. (1999) *The Veterinary Clinics of North America – The ROCKet Science of Canine Urolithiasis*. WB Saunders Co., Philadelphia.

Paterson, S. (2000) *Skin Diseases of the Cat*. Blackwell Science, Oxford.

Petersen-Jones, S. & Crispin, S. (1993) *Manual of Small Animal Ophthalmology*. BSAVA Publications, Cheltenham.

Petersen-Jones, S. & Crispin, S. (2002) *Manual of Small Animal Ophthalmology*, 2nd edn. BSAVA Publications, Cheltenham.

Ramsey, I. & Tennant, B. (2001) *Manual of Canine and Feline Infectious Diseases*. BSAVA Publications, Cheltenham.

Rubin, L.F. (1989) *Inherited Eye Diseases in Purebred Dogs*. Williams & Wilkins, Baltimore.

Scott, D.W., Miller, W.H. & Griffin, C.E. (2001) *Muller & Kirk's Small Animal Dermatology*, 6th edn. WB Saunders Co., Philadelphia.

Seymour, C. & Gleed, R. (1999) *Manual of Small Animal Anaesthesia and Analgesia*. BSAVA Publications, Cheltenham.

Thomas, D.A., Simpson, J.W. & Hall, E.J. (1996) *Manual of Canine and Feline Gastroenterology*. BSAVA Publications, Cheltenham.

Torrance, A.G. & Mooney, C.T. (1998) *Manual of Canine and Feline Endocrinology*, 2nd edn. BSAVA Publications, Cheltenham.

Wheeler, S.J. (1995) *Manual of Small Animal Neurology*. BSAVA Publications, Cheltenham.

Papers
Cardiovascular

Moise, N.S., Gilmour, R.F., Riccio, M.L. & Flahive, W.F. Jr. (1997) Diagnosis of inherited ventricular tachycardia in German Shepherd Dogs. *Journal of the American Veterinary Medical Association*, **210**:3, 403–10.

Patterson, D.F. (1989) Hereditary congenital heart defects in dogs. *Journal of Small Animal Practice*, **30**:3, 153–65.

Rozengurt, N. (1994) Endocardial fibroelastosis in common domestic cats in the UK. *Journal of Comparative Pathology*, **110**:3, 295–301.

Sleeper, M.M., Henthorn, P.S., Vijayasarathy, C., *et al.* (2002) Dilated cardiomyopathy in juvenile Portuguese Water Dogs. *Journal of Veterinary Internal Medicine*, **16**:1, 52–62.

Tidholm, A. & Jonsson, L. (1997) A retrospective study of canine dilated cardiomyopathy (189 cases). *Journal of the American Animal Hospital Association*, **33**:6, 544–50.

Dermatological

Brennan, K.E. & Ihrke, P.J. (1983) Grass awn migration in dogs and cats: a retrospective study of 182 cases. *Journal of the American Veterinary Medical Association*, **182**:11, 1201–4.

Lewis, C.J. (1995) Black hair follicular dysplasia in UK bred Salukis. *Veterinary Record*, **137**:12, 294–5.

Miller, D.M. (1995) The occurrence of mast cell tumours in young Shar-Peis. *Journal of Veterinary Diagnostic Investigation*, **7**:3, 360–63.

Miller, W.H. & Scott, D.W. (1995) Follicular dysplasia of the Portuguese Water Dog. *Veterinary Dermatology*, **6**:2, 67–74.

Scarff, D.H. (1994) Sebaceous adenitis in the standard poodle. *Veterinary Record*, **135**:11, 264.

Scott, D.W. & Paradis, M. (1990) A survey of canine and feline skin disorders seen in a university practice: Small Animal Clinic, University of Montreal, Saint-Hyacinthe, Quebec (1987–1988). *Canadian Veterinary Journal*, **31**, 830–35.

Drug reactions

Cribb, A.E. & Spielberg, S.P. (1990) An in vitro investigation of predisposition to sulphonamide idiosyncratic toxicity in dogs. *Veterinary Research Communications*, **14**:3, 241–52.

Genetics

Patterson, D.F., Aguirre, G.A., Fyfe, J.C., *et al.* (1989) Is this a genetic disease? *Journal of Small Animal Practice*, **30**:3, 127–39.

Willis, M.B. (1989) Control of inherited defects in dogs. *Journal of Small Animal Practice*, **30**:3, 188–92.

Haematological/immunological

Bridle, K.H. & Littlewood, J.D. (1998) Tail tip necrosis in two litters of Birman kittens. *Journal of Small Animal Practice*, **39**:2, 88–9.

Day, M.J. (1999) Possible immunodeficiency in Rottweiler dogs. *Journal of Small Animal Practice*, **41**:12, 561–8.

Debenham, S.L., Millington, A., Kijast, J., Andersson, L. & Binns, M. (2002) Canine leucocyte adhesion deficiency in Irish Red and White Setters. *Journal of Small Animal Practice*, **43**:2, 74–5.

Feldman, D.G., Brooks, M.B. & Dodds, W.J. (1995) Haemophilia B (Factor IX deficiency) in a family of German Shepherd Dogs. *Journal of the American Veterinary Medical Association*, **206**:12, 1901–5.

Littlewood, J.D. (1989) Inherited bleeding disorders of dogs and cats. *Journal of Small Animal Practice*, **30**:3, 140–43.

Lobetti, R.G., Leisewitz, A.L. & Spencer, J.A. (1996) *Pneumocystis carinii* in the Miniature Dachshund: case report and literature review. *Journal of Small Animal Practice*, **37**:6, 280–5.

Maggio-Price, L. & Dodds, W.J. (1993) Factor IX deficiency (Haemophilia B) in a family of British shorthair cats. *Journal of the American Veterinary Medical Association*, **203**:12, 1702–4.

Musculoskeletal

Beale, B.S., Goeing, R.L., Herrington, J., Dee, J. & Conrad, K. (1991) A prospective evaluation of four surgical approaches to the talus of the dog in the treatment of osteochondritis dissecans. *Journal of the American Animal Hospital Association*, **26**:2, 221–9.

Bellenger, C.R. (1996) Inguinal and scrotal herniation in 61 dogs. *Australian Veterinary Practitioner*, **26**:2, 58–9.

Brass, W. (1989) Hip dysplasia in dogs. *Journal of Small Animal Practice*, **30**:3, 166–70.

Breit, S. & Kunzel, W. (2001) Breed specific osteological features of the canine lumbosacral junction. *Annals of Anatomy*, **183**:2, 151–7.

Duval, J.M., Budsberg, S.C., Flo, G.L. & Sammarco, J.L. (1999) Breed, sex, and body weight as risk factors for rupture of the cranial cruciate ligament in young dogs. *Journal of the American Veterinary Medical Association*, **215**:6, 811–14.

Franch, J., Cesari, J.R. & Font, J. (1998) Craniomandibular osteopathy in two Pyrenean Mountain Dogs. *Veterinary Record*, **142**:17, 455–9.

Hanson, S.M., Smith, M.O., Walker, T.L. & Shelton, G.D. (1998) Juvenile-onset distal myopathy in Rottweiler dogs. *Journal of Veterinary Internal Medicine*, **12**:2, 103–8.

Hosgood, G., Hedlund, C.S., Pechman, R.D. & Dean, P.W. (1995) Perineal herniorrhaphy: perioperative data from 100 dogs. *Journal of the American Animal Hospital Association*, **31**:4, 331–42.

Jones, B.R. & Alley, M.R. (1988) Hypokalaemic myopathy in Burmese kittens. *New Zealand Veterinary Journal*, **36**:3, 150–51.

Keller, G.G. & Corley, E.A. (1989) Canine hip dysplasia: investigating the sex predilection and the frequency of unilateral CHD. *Veterinary Medicine*, **84**:12, 1164–6.

Malik, R., Allan, G.S., Howlett, C.R., *et al.* (1999) Osteochondrodysplasia in Scottish Fold cats. *Australian Veterinary Journal*, **77**:2, 85–92.

Morgan, J.P. (1999) Transitional lumbosacral vertebral anomaly in the dog: a radiographic study. *Journal of Small Animal Practice*, **40**:4, 167–72.

Morgan, J.P., Wind, A. & Davidson, A.P. (1999) Bone dysplasias in the Labrador Retriever: a radiographic study. *Journal of the American Animal Hospital Association*, **35**:4, 332–40.

Necas, A., Zatloukal, J., Kecova, H. & Dvorak, M. (2000) Predisposition of dog breeds to rupture of the cranial cruciate ligament. *Acta Veterinaria Brno*, **69**:4, 305–10.

Padgett, G.A., Mostosky, U.V., Probst, C.W., Thomas, M.W. & Krecke, C.F. (1995) The inheritance of osteochondritis dissecans and fragmented coronoid process of the elbow joint in
Labdrador Retrievers. *Journal of the American Animal Hospital Association*, **31**:4, 327–30.

Robinson, R. (1977) Genetic aspects of umbilical hernia incidence in dogs and cats. *Veterinary
Record*, **100**:1, 9–10.

Vite, C.H., Melniczek, J., Patterson, D. & Giger, U. (1999) Congenital myotonic myopathy in the
Miniature Schnauzer: an autosomal recessive trait. *Journal of Heredity*, **90**:5, 578–80.

Physiological

Dole, R.S. & Spurgeon, T.L. (1998) Frequency of supernumerary teeth in a dolicocephalic breed: the
grey hounds. *American Journal of Veterinary Research*, **59**:1, 16–17.

Gaughan, K.R. & Bruyette, D.S. (2001) Thyroid function testing in greyhounds. *American Journal of
Veterinary Research*, **62**:7, 1130–33.

Pedersen, H.D., Haggstrom, J., Olsen, L.H., *et al.* (2002) Idiopathic asymptomatic thrombocytopenia
in Cavalier King Charles Spaniels is an autosomal recessive trait. *Journal of Veterinary Internal
Medicine*, **16**:2, 169–73.

Sullivan, P.S., Evans, H.L. & McDonald, T.P. (1994) Platelet concentration and hemoglobin function in greyhounds. *Journal of the American Veterinary Medical Association*, **205**:6, 838–41.

Respiratory

Anderson, D.A. & White, R.A.S. (2002) Nasal dermoid sinus cysts in the dog. *Veterinary Surgery*,
31:4, 303–8.

Braund, K.G., Shores, A., Cochrane, S., Forrester, D., Kwiecien, J.M. & Steiss, J.E. (1994)
Laryngeal paralysis-polyneuropathy complex in young Dalmatians. *American Journal of Veterinary
Research*, **55**:4, 534–42.

Carpenter, J.L., Myers, A.M., Conner, M.W., Schelling, S.H., Kennedy, F.A. & Reimann, K.A.
(1988) Tuberculosis in 5 Basset hounds. *Journal of the American Veterinary Medical Association*,
192:11, 1563–8.

Fossum, T.W., Birchard, S.J. & Jacobs, R.M. (1986) Chylothorax in 34 dogs. *Journal of the American
Veterinary Medical Association*, **188**:11, 1315–18.

Greenfield, C.L., Messick, J.B., Solter, P.F. & Schaeffer, D.J. (1999) Leukopenia in 6 healthy
Belgian Tervuren. *Journal of the American Veterinary Medical Association*, **215**:8, 1121–2.

Harvey, C.E. (1989) Inherited and congenital airway conditions. *Journal of Small Animal Practice*,
30:3, 184–7.

Jarvinen, A.K., Saario, E., Andresen, E., Happonen, I., Saari, S. & Rajamaki, M. (1995) Lung injury
leading to adult respiratory distress syndrome in young Dalmatian dogs. *Journal of Veterinary
Internal Medicine*, **9**:3, 162–8.

Neath, P.J., Brockman, D.J. & King, L.G. (2000) Lung lobe torsion in dogs: 22 cases (1981–1999).
Journal of the American Veterinary Medical Association, **217**:7, 1041–4.

Watson, P.J., Herrtage, M.E., Peacock, M.A. & Sargan, D.R. (1999) Primary ciliary dyskinesia in
Newfoundland dogs. *Veterinary Record*, **144**:26, 718–25.

White, R.A.S. & Williams, J.M. (1994) Tracheal collapse of the dog – is there really a role for
surgery? A survey of 100 cases. *Journal of Small Animal Practice*, **35**:4, 191–6.

Miscellaneous

Egenvall, A., Bonnett, B.N., Shoukri, M., Olson, P., Hedhammar, A. & Dohoo, I. (2000) Age pattern
of mortality in eight breeds of insured dogs in Sweden. *Preventive Veterinary Medicine*, **46**:1, 1–14.

Appendix: Details of some organisations running surveillance schemes for inherited diseases

British Veterinary Association/Kennel Club
Schemes run: Hip dysplasia, elbow dysplasia, eye disease such as PRA and cataracts
Contact details: British Veterinary Association
                    (Canine Health Schemes)
                    7 Mansfield Street
                    London W1M 0AT
                    www.bva.co.uk

Orthopaedic Foundation for Animals
Schemes run: Hip dysplasia, elbow dysplasia, patellar luxation, cardiac disease, autoimmune thyroiditis
Contact details: OFA
                    2300 E. Nifong Boulevard
                    Columbia
                    Missouri 65201–3856
                    USA
                    www.offa.org

Feline Advisory Bureau
Schemes run: Polycystic kidney disease
Contact details: FAB PKD Screening Scheme
                    Taeselbury
                    High St.
                    Tisbury
                    Wilts SP3 6LD
                    UK
                    www.fabcats.org

University of Pennsylvania
Schemes run: Hip dysplasia
Contact details: www.vet.upenn.edu/research/centers/pennhip//

Canine Eye Registration Foundation (CERF)
Schemes run: Canine hereditary eye disease certification in the USA
Contact Details: www.vmdb.org/cerf.html